Musculoskeletal Ultrasound for the Rheumatologist

AF400351

George A. W. Bruyn · Wolfgang A. Schmidt

Musculoskeletal Ultrasound for the Rheumatologist

An Introductory Guide

Third Edition

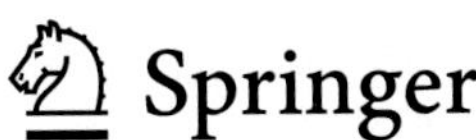 Springer

George A. W. Bruyn
Reumakliniek Lelystad
Lelystad, The Netherlands

Tergooi MC hospital
Hilversum, The Netherlands

Wolfgang A. Schmidt
Medical Center for Rheumatology
in Berlin-Buch
Immanuel Krankenhaus Berlin
Berlin, Germany

ISBN 978-3-031-27739-9   ISBN 978-3-031-27737-5   (eBook)
https://doi.org/10.1007/978-3-031-27737-5

1st and 2nd editions: © Bohn Stafleu van Loghum, Houten, the Netherlands 2007, 2012
3rd edition: © The Editor(s) (if applicable) and The Author(s), under exclusive license to Springer
Nature Switzerland AG 2023
This work is subject to copyright. All rights are solely and exclusively licensed by the Publisher, whether
the whole or part of the material is concerned, specifically the rights of translation, reprinting, reuse
of illustrations, recitation, broadcasting, reproduction on microfilms or in any other physical way, and
transmission or information storage and retrieval, electronic adaptation, computer software, or by similar
or dissimilar methodology now known or hereafter developed.
The use of general descriptive names, registered names, trademarks, service marks, etc. in this publication
does not imply, even in the absence of a specific statement, that such names are exempt from the relevant
protective laws and regulations and therefore free for general use.
The publisher, the authors, and the editors are safe to assume that the advice and information in this book
are believed to be true and accurate at the date of publication. Neither the publisher nor the authors or
the editors give a warranty, expressed or implied, with respect to the material contained herein or for any
errors or omissions that may have been made. The publisher remains neutral with regard to jurisdictional
claims in published maps and institutional affiliations.

This Springer imprint is published by the registered company Springer Nature Switzerland AG
The registered company address is: Gewerbestrasse 11, 6330 Cham, Switzerland

Foreword

Musculoskeletal sonography is making constant progress, and its applications within the field of rheumatology have progressively expanded thanks to the many contributions to research that have recently been published. Research has developed alongside activities focused on education and training, which are no less demanding. The request for training in sonography is in exponential growth. As the learning curve in sonography is virtually endless, there is an urgent need for teaching material that can be of support for those taking their first steps in sonographic training. George Bruyn and Wolfgang Schmidt are the authors of this excellent, very readable and well-organized book that provides a rigorous yet accessible introduction to the rapidly growing field of sonography in rheumatology. Compared with other work in this field, this book stands out for its clear explanations of all the basic steps in performing rheumatological sonography, thus providing a very efficient tool for self-teaching. For anatomical areas of interest, the novice investigator will be able to evaluate the correct positioning of the probe, anatomical landmarks and the representative image that can be obtained.

The quality of the images is very good, bearing witness to the level of excellence reached by the authors, who are renowned pioneers of musculoskeletal sonography. The authors have also succeeded in outlining a panorama that represents the main sonographic expressions within rheumatic disease and this helps the reader to understand the added benefit of sonography in daily practice and its relevant potential in depicting soft tissue involvement in rheumatic diseases.

This book will be extremely useful for all those who are taking their first steps into the fascinating world of rheumatological sonography, but it will also be useful for those who, having already started their experience, would like to compare the quality of their images with that of authoritative experts.

The authors should be congratulated on their excellent work that will surely contribute to the dissemination of sonography in rheumatology.

Professor Walter Grassi
Department of Rheumatology
Università Politecnica delle Marche
Ancona, Italy

Preface to the Third Edition

A decade has passed since the release of the second edition in 2011. In many countries, the clinical significance of ultrasound in the rheumatology office is leaping forward at an impressive rate. At least 94% of adult rheumatology fellowship programs in the United States have now incorporated teaching in musculoskeletal ultrasound. At the same time, however, we are facing the daunting prospects of delivering an accurate state -of -the- art. New publications prompted the authors to re-examine all chapters for up-to-date procedures and learning points. Therefore, the third edition of the Guide has been completely revised. The new edition has kept the same format as the previous ones, dividing the topic into sections, each related to an anatomical area of interest. In addition, two new chapters, i.e., on lung ultrasound and on pelvic injections, have been added.

On a different note, the previous two editions of the «Introductory Guide to Musculoskeletal Ultrasound for the Rheumatologist» were handled by Lydia Nieuwendijk, the publisher at Bohn Stafleu & van Loghum. We aimed to make the Guide accessible for rheumatologists in a global community, and decided to write the Guide in English. However, since Dutch was the language of the Dutch publishing house, changing to English was not a minor nor an accidental challenge. We owe a debt of gratitude to Lydia Nieuwendijk for her guidance over the years. We welcome the new staff of Springer Nature, Elizabeth Pope and Sanjievkumar Mathiyazhagan, who supported us in writing a new edition and guiding us through the drafts of the Guide.

Over the years, translation of the Guide into different languages has been conducted, e.g., in Polish, Korean, Czech, and Turkish. Our immense gratitude goes to Artur Bachta, Taeyoung Kang, Petra Hanova, and Ender Terzioglu. Without their support the translations would have been impossible. Our special thanks go also to Priscilla Wong, Giorgio Tamborrini, Petra Hanova, and Patricia Smith-van der Meijde, who provided us with one or two of their best ultrasound images. We hope that the present book will be viewed as an enhancement of the previous editions.

<table>
<tr><td>Loënga, The Netherlands</td><td>George A. W. Bruyn</td></tr>
<tr><td>Berlin, Germany</td><td>Wolfgang A. Schmidt</td></tr>
<tr><td>December 2022</td><td></td></tr>
</table>

Preface to the Second Edition

The Guide's first edition is left only four years behind us, yet it seems as if light years have passed. We received feedback from many colleagues, ranging from trainees to experienced rheumatologists and others, mostly positive. All comments were taken very seriously. Quickly we realized that as so many initiatives have been initiated and moved on since then, it was about time to think about significantly modifying the first print and adding novel features to a second edition of the Guide. In a field where knowledge and expertise matter, skills have become increasingly important. Therefore, we decided to add a new topic to each of the chapters 5 to 10, i.e, how to carry out ultrasound-guided injections of these various joints. Thus, we take pride in creating a contribution to the dissemination of musculoskeletal sonography. Needless to mention, we welcome the continuing dialogue with the readers of this guide and hope you enjoy this new edition. What else? Well, the authors still have lots of fun while on their collaborative teaching at courses abroad, particularly in the Americas and at the EULAR courses, and they will continue to do so.

<table>
<tr><td>Leeuwarden, The Netherlands</td><td>George A. W. Bruyn</td></tr>
<tr><td>Berlin, Germany</td><td>Wolfgang A. Schmidt</td></tr>
</table>

Preface to the First Edition

This book provides a comprehensive compilation of standard ultrasound scans in rheumatology. In the text, the more important normal and pathological sonography findings of various structures and disorders have been systematically incorporated. During the preparation of this guide, much of the literature relating to sonography imaging of synovitis and erosions of joints was reviewed and abstracted. The bibliography is, of course, not complete; this guide is not meant to be a textbook on musculoskeletal ultrasound.

The format of this book is to present so-called Standard Scans that cover a whole range of anatomical sites: shoulder, elbow, wrist, fingers, hip, knee, ankle, forefoot, and toes. Each Standard Scan is accompanied by a picture of the position of the probe, an anatomical drawing, an ultrasound picture and an explanation of the ultrasound scan. In addition, new indications for ultrasound in rheumatology as vasculitis and connective tissue disease are discussed.

We both contributed an equal amount of experience and work to this book. From 1999, we have been conducting workshops together at the American College of Rheumatology's annual meetings and have been involved in many international courses on musculoskeletal ultrasound. This book summarizes our experience in a short systematic review.

The preparation of the first edition of this book was made possible by the support of Wyeth Pharmaceuticals Netherlands. The collaboration with Cristopher Haydon of the British Medical Society of Ultrasound is gratefully acknowledged. Nathalie Bruyn expertly prepared many photographs and was responsible for the drawings in chapters 5 to 10. We are also grateful to Caroline ter Meulen and Lydia Nieuwendijk, editors at Bohn Stafleu van Loghum.

We would like to express our special gratitude to professor Walter Grassi from the University of Ancona, Italy. His wisdom, enthusiasm and clear vision on the future of musculoskeletal ultrasonography in the area of rheumatology planted the seeds for this work.

Leeuwarden, The Netherlands   George A. W. Bruyn
Berlin, Germany   Wolfgang A. Schmidt

Contents

Chapter 1
Introduction

A patient with a rheumatological inflammatory disorder usually presents with symptoms or signs including pain, stiffness, fatigue, weakness, or joint swelling. In rheumatology, history taking and physical examination are the fundamentals of the diagnostic process in which information from signs and symptoms has to be weighed in terms of positive and negative predictive values. Although exact data are lacking, it is estimated that by means of history and physical examination, a correct tentative diagnosis is made in 80–90% of patients at presentation. In the miscellaneous 10 to 20%, further diagnostic steps, i.e., laboratory tests and imaging techniques, are required for establishing a diagnosis. Ultrasound has proven to be more sensitive than clinical examination to detect synovitis in patients with early rheumatoid arthritis; furthermore, it has been shown to have superior sensitivity compared to conventional radiographs for picking up small erosions in finger joints.

The sensitivity for synovitis and erosions is reported to be comparable with that of MRI in some studies but inferior in others, due to the fact that ultrasound sensitivity is related to the site and the accessibility of the joint. Ultrasound is also able to detect minute fluid collections in joints, entheseal abnormalities like calcifications and enthesophytes, as well as tendon sheath inflammation and thickening of finger pulleys and tendons in psoriatic arthritis. By means of its power Doppler feature, ultrasound can pick up signals of dilated small blood vessels at various anatomical sites including entheses, tendon sheaths and joint synovia. Color Doppler combined with grayscale ultrasound may detect the oedema of arterial walls like that of the temporal artery in temporal arteritis. Grayscale ultrasound may already give a preliminary impression of joint synovitis, but positive power Doppler signals will definitely confirm the active inflammation of the joint. Abnormal structure of the salivary glands related to Sjögren's syndrome can be detected as well as abnormal muscle anatomy encountered in myositis. The proof of the pudding, however, is in the eating. Thus, the legitimate question to reflect on is, does ultrasound make a difference to daily patient care? And if so, can we measure its impact on patient care? For instance, can ultrasound be used to diagnose early (undifferentiated) arthritis and can it help to predict a development into chronic arthritis or self-limiting arthritis?

© The Author(s), under exclusive license to Springer Nature Switzerland AG 2023
G. A. W. Bruyn and W. A. Schmidt, *Musculoskeletal Ultrasound for the Rheumatologist*,
https://doi.org/10.1007/978-3-031-27737-5_1

Data indicate that ultrasound assessment may have a significant impact on clinical decision making, particularly in rheumatologic evaluation for diagnosis.

The evidence for other indications, including disease activity monitoring and aiding in prognosis, is less compelling. Ultrasound monitoring of inflammation did not result in improved outcomes, such as low disease activity/remission or less radiographic progression compared to conventional monitoring with DAS-28 ESR in patients with rheumatoid arthritis.

A very useful feature of ultrasound is guiding the needle pathway for injecting difficult joints and aspirating fluid from specific sites. Furthermore, based on its high resolution, ultrasound is the imaging technique of choice for diagnosing tendon disorders and peripheral nerve lesions. An additional advantage of ultrasound is that the patient does not need extensive preparation, which makes the procedure time-efficient. The only clinical requirements are good equipment and about 15 minutes of time.

Care must be taken to avoid errors in interpreting images. Therefore, knowledge of the pitfalls of the technique is an essential part of the clinician's training. One of the pitfalls are artifacts due to incorrect positioning of the probe. Insight into ultrasound findings in rheumatic disease requires familiarity with the anatomy and pathology of the structures involved. Widely regarded as the expert in rheumatic diseases, it is key that the rheumatologist also masters the cross-sectional anatomy of the musculoskeletal system. Rheumatologist-ultrasonographers have to bear in mind that cross-sectional anatomy is quite different from the classical anatomy lessons back at medical school. Hence, getting used to cross-sectional thinking implies a considerable investment of time for training and practice.

Despite these limitations, including the long and steep learning curve for the operator and the small field of view, musculoskeletal ultrasound obviously bears the potential to significantly improve daily patient care in rheumatology practice.

1.1 Historical Perspective

A number of pioneers, including scientists, engineers and clinicians, have contributed to the development of diagnostic ultrasonography.

During the early 1940s, the Austrian neurologist-psychiatrist Karl Theodore Dussik was probably the first physician to use ultrasound for diagnostic purposes. Although John Wild published a landmark study of breast nodules reporting a diagnostic accuracy of 90%, the Glasgow obstetrician Ian Donald was responsible for the ultrasound boom in medical diagnosis (Fig. 1.1). In 1956, in partnership with a young engineer, Tom Brown, Donald developed the first two-dimensional, direct contact scanner in 1956, which he first demonstrated at a clinico-pathological conference at the University department of Midwifery in Glasgow. Many physicians in the audience were totally opposed to the idea of relying on a machine instead of their hands when examining an unborn baby, until there and then, a Glasgow professor of Internal Medicine happened to make a diagnosis of malignant ascites in a female patient.

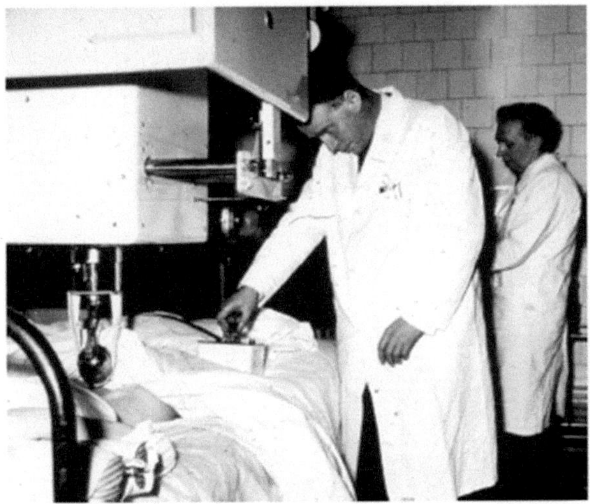

Fig. 1.1 The Glasgow obstetrician Ian Donald with the first automatic ultrasound scanner designed by Tom Brown (1960)

On examining the patient himself with the ultrasound machine, professor Donald informed the audience that the finding looked more like an ovarian cyst. Definite clinical interest was aroused when this diagnosis was confirmed in the operating theatre.

At the same time, another milestone was set at the University of Lund in Sweden, when Inge Edler, one of the most prominent cardiologists of his time, together with the scientist Carl Hertz, introduced M-mode (M for motion) registration. M-mode is a method that uses a single ultrasound beam aimed in a fixed direction through the heart. It marked a breakthrough into the understanding of cardiac disease.

Edler and Hertz applied a transducer to the human chest in the 3rd and 4th intercostal space at the left sternal edge and reported echo motion synchronous with the heartbeat. Many years later in 1969, the Dutch engineer Nicolaas Klaas Bom (Fig. 1.2) improved the early reflectoscope of Edler and Hertz with the introduction of the first linear array transducer at the department of Cardiology of Erasmus University in Rotterdam. Realizing that a moving object is easier to observe than a still object, Bom mounted twenty crystal elements on his prototype, which were switched on sequentially, so producing twenty echo lines. Featuring real-time images of a moving heart for the first time in history, the device produced a spontaneous applause at the European cardiology congress of 1972. By the 1970s, following its successful use in imaging horse tendons in veterinary practice, ultrasound imaging of the musculoskeletal system began to interest radiologists and orthopedic surgeons. Seltzer published the first study on the rotator cuff of rhesus monkeys before and after fluid instillation and Graf reported on the acetabular rim of infants in order to detect congenital hips dysplasia.

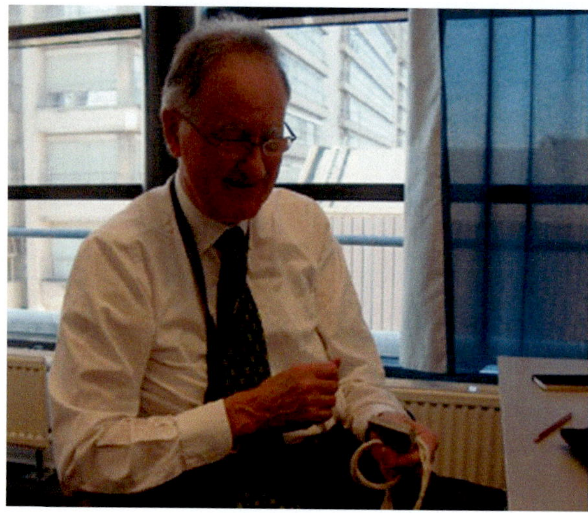

Fig. 1.2 Dutch engineer Nicolaas Bom and the prototype of the first linear array ultrasound probe

However, visualization of smaller joints was still a hazardous endeavour as resolution of images remained poor. Hence, three important technological advances have made inroads regarding the use of ultrasound in rheumatology. Firstly, the advent of high-resolution probes permitted the evaluation of smaller and superficial structures, such as finger tendons, small joints, nerves and pulleys. These "footprint probes" emitted waves with frequencies of 10–20 MHz and more, and came with an axial resolution of 0.1 mm. With these frequencies, reliably assessing the articular capsule or the hyaline cartilage of small joints like the MCP, PIP or MTP joints became feasible. Broadband probes which include a range of frequencies (e.g., 5–10 MHz, 8–14 MHz, 6–24 MHz) were becoming increasingly popular because of the ease in examining superficial and deep structures at the same time.

Secondly, progress in data processing by the computer enormously advanced the technologic scope of ultrasound. An example is the spatial compounding techniques in which the transducer beam is electronically steered to acquire overlapping scans from different angles and produce images with superior spatial resolution. A relatively novel development is the acquisition of volume data sets and the rendering technology for reconstructing 3-dimensional images from 3 planes. Three-dimensional ultrasound is potentially able to reduce the operator dependency of the technique.

Thirdly, the development of the color and power Doppler technique has enabled assessment of soft tissue hyperemia. Power Doppler mode detects low-velocity blood flow at the microvascular level, for instance of synovium or malignant masses. Since inflammation coincides with increased perfusion, power Doppler ultrasound helps to differentiate inflammatory synovitis from degenerative lesions, active from inactive synovitis, and assists in monitoring the response to therapy. Color Doppler ultrasound is used to examine larger vessels for the detection of stenoses and vessel wall abnormalities. In rheumatology, the technique is particularly applied for the study of vasculitis, including temporal arteritis.

Development of ultrasound in rheumatology will not halt at this point. The research agenda prompts grayscale ultrasound and power Doppler to be validated, not only in inflammatory joint disease, but also in other rheumatological disorders including osteoarthritis, vasculitis, myopathies and salivary gland disease. Comparisons with golden standards, including MRI, synovial biopsy, and arthroscopy, as well as reliability studies testing the intra- and interobserver reliability on inflammation in various joints, continue to be carried out in order to validate the technique and thus strengthening and corroborating the role of ultrasound in rheumatology.

Chapter 2
Fundamentals of Musculoskeletal Ultrasound

2.1 Frequency and Wavelength

Ultrasound refers to any sound that is above audible sound in the acoustic spectrum. The human ear is capable of hearing sounds in a frequency range between 20 to 20,000 Hz (Hz), so 20 to 20,000 cycles per second (1000 cycles per second equals 1 kilohertz or 1 kHz). Only young children hear the high range while, with aging, the upper limit drops to about 12,000 cycles per second. Some animals are able to hear frequencies as high as 100,000 cycles per second. Thus, the ultrasonic range of frequencies run from 20 kHz to 1 GHz. Medical applied ultrasound frequencies range from 2,000,000 Hz (2 MHz) to 50,000,000 Hz (50 MHz). These sound waves travel through the human body at a velocity (v) of 1540 m per second, so after 0,0000649 seconds, a distance of 10 cm has been travelled. Most anatomic structures relevant to rheumatology are much closer, often situated in the skin no deeper than 5 cm from the surface.

Frequency (f) and wavelength (λ) are inversely proportional, i.e., f ~ $1/\lambda$, so the higher the frequency of the wave, the shorter its wavelength. There is also a relationship between frequency, beam penetration and resolution. Sound wave beams with a higher frequency penetrate tissues less than lower frequency waves, but a sharper ultrasound image is outlined. Conversely a transducer producing a lower frequency (longer wavelengths) will produce greater depth of penetration but less well-defined images. As already mentioned, in rheumatology most structures of interest are located relatively superficially, so high-frequency ultrasound should be used. To be able to distinguish between two interfaces lying closely together, a distance of at least half a wavelength is needed between the two interfaces.

© The Author(s), under exclusive license to Springer Nature Switzerland AG 2023

G. A. W. Bruyn and W. A. Schmidt, *Musculoskeletal Ultrasound for the Rheumatologist*,
https://doi.org/10.1007/978-3-031-27737-5_2

2.2 Generating Ultrasound Waves

Ultrasound waves are generated by a transducer consisting of a disc with crystals of lead zirconate titanate. These crystals are *piezoelectric*, in other words, they transform electrical potentials into mechanical vibrations and vice versa. Every time an electrical current is passed through the crystals, the disc generates an ultrasound pulse; conversely, when the disc receives a wave of ultrasound, it will deform and a voltage is generated on the transducer surface. To produce a well-directed beam, the disc is mounted at the end of a cylindrical tube, also called a probe. At the other end of the tube, damping material is mounted to damp down the ultrasonic waves generated at the back of the disc.

2.3 Reflection and Transmission

The emitted waves are reflected at the interface of two different tissues. The greater the difference in tissue density, the more reflective the boundary will be, while with similar densities waves pass easily from one tissue to the other.

The mathematical equation determining the amount of reflection and transmission is given by the speed of sound c and the specific acoustic impedance Z of the tissue. The impedance of sound in air is low; in muscle is it 10,000 times higher than in air and in bone Z is so high – about 50,000 times higher to that of air – that the sound beam does not penetrate bone at all.

The boundary between two different tissues is called an acoustic interface. As there is an interface between air and skin, we must apply a coupling medium on the transducer, such as a gel with an impedance similar to human tissue, otherwise only 0.1% of the incident beam energy would be transmitted into the skin tissue and 99.9% would be reflected off the skin surface. Similarly, almost 99% of the sound beam is reflected at the interface of air and muscle, while liquids – such as blood or synovial fluid – do not reflect sound waves.

When the surface of an object is flat - not round - and no air is present between the source and the object, almost all the ultrasound waves will be reflected from reflectors inside the object at right angles; these returning echoes are then detected by the transducer. The crystal reconverts the returning ultrasonic wave which has the same wavelength as the emitted wave, into an electronic potential. Subsequently, the electronic potential is converted by a computer into an ultrasound image. The transducer acts as the receiver of ultrasound echoes about 99.9% of the time, and it emits sound waves in the very small amount of time remaining.

Fig. 2.1   This picture shows the line-up of 8 time gain control slides on the ultrasound machine. The topical hierarchy of the slides corresponds to the gain position on the ultrasound image, i.e., the upper slides control the gain for the upper part of the image, the lower slides for the lower (deeper) tissues on the ultrasound image

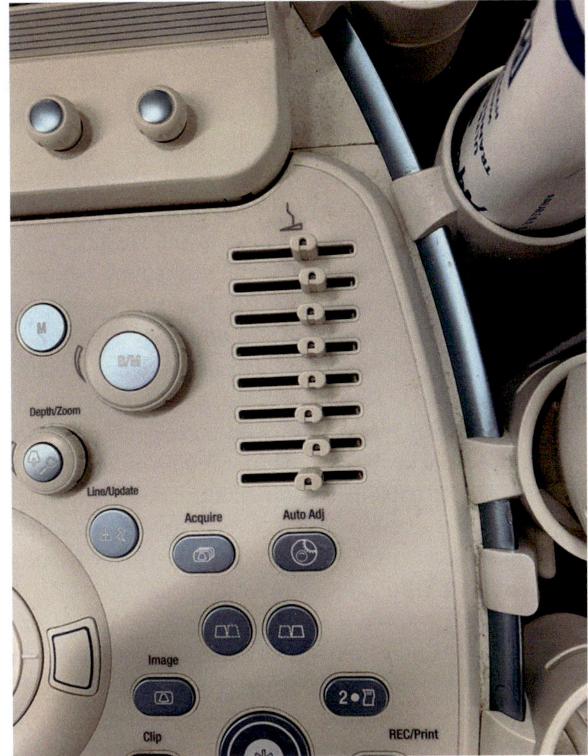

2.4   Attenuation

Ultrasound loses its energy as it propagates through a tissue. This loss of energy is called attenuation. There are three causes of attenuation: diffraction, scattering, and absorption. Attenuation results in echoes from deep body tissues being displayed less intensely then those returning from superficial structures. A function of the ultrasound system called time-gain compensation (Fig. 2.1) will correct the attenuation, and intensifies the echoes returning from deeper structures.

2.5   A Glossary of Ultrasound

It is useful to become familiar with a number of common ultrasound concepts or nomenclatures.

1.   **B-mode or grayscale ultrasound**. B (for brightness)-mode is the precursor of grayscale ultrasound and is limited to defining boundaries of structures and differentiating fluid from solid. Grayscale ultrasound includes the whole range

of possible intensities of the grey, black and white images. However, it cannot differentiate between quiescent and active synovitis.

2. **Doppler ultrasound**. Doppler ultrasound relies on the Doppler principle, which states that sound waves increase in frequency when they reflect from objects (e.g., moving red blood cells) moving towards the transducer and decrease in frequency when they reflect from objects moving away. Using the standard Doppler formula, Δf equals $2vf \cos \theta /c$, the velocity of the flow can be calculated. Because of the cosine in the formula, Doppler will not determine flow which is perpendicular to the ultrasound beam.

3. **Color Doppler ultrasound**. In color Doppler ultrasound, the Doppler effect is combined with real-time imaging. The real-time image is created by rapid movement of the ultrasound beam. The information from Doppler ultrasound is integrated in the grayscale image as a color signal. This signal indicates the direction of blood flow. Red signals indicate flow that is directed towards the ultrasound probe, while blue signals indicate flow directed away from the probe.

4. **Duplex ultrasound**. Duplex ultrasound combines the color Doppler image with spectral Doppler. The flow is displayed as a spectral waveform of changes in velocity during the cardicac cycle. The flow velocity is depicted on the vertical axis with time on the horizontal axis.

5. **Power Doppler**. Power Doppler is a variant of Doppler ultrasound. It differs from the latter in that it will demonstrate flow in any direction, so it is independent of the angle θ between the flow and the probe. Power Doppler ultrasound is very sensitive and may show hyperemia of inflamed tissues. It also differentiates between cysts/ganglions and blood vessels, and in this way can help in ultrasound-guided aspirations, by avoiding blood vessels and correctly picking the site of biopsy. When applying power Doppler ultrasound, care should be taken to avoid unnecessary probe pressure, and ensure complete relaxation of the structure of interest, otherwise an artificial reduced Doppler signal will be the result.

6. **Transducer or probe**. The transducer is the eye of the ultrasound machine. It generates the sound waves in terms of millions per second and receives the echoes. The frequency of the sound wave determines how deep it will penetrate the tissue. The frequency also determines the resolution, so the higher the frequency, the greater the resolution, and the lesser the penetration.

7. **Resolution**. Resolution is the optical ability to distinguish detail, such as the separation of two closely adjacent objects. Axial or vertical resolution distinguishes two objects lying in the same line of the beam at different depths. Axial resolution is dependent of the wavelength of the sound wave, smaller wavelengths result in higher resolution images. Lateral or horizontal resolution refers to the ability to distinguish two objects when they lie side to side. Lateral resolution can be improved by focusing the ultrasound beam. The modern transducers used for musculoskeletal ultrasound reach an axial resolution of 0.1 mm and a lateral resolution of 0.2 mm. 20 MHz transducers reach an axial resolution power of 0.04 mm.

8. **Focus, frequency and depth**. The ultrasound beam is emitted as a cylindrical beam by the transducer. The shape of the cylindrical ultrasound beam may be focused by a concave lens, similar to a camera. The lateral resolution is optimal at this focus point where the beam is at its smallest. Adjusting the focus is done by turning a knob on the ultrasound machine and should be placed at the region of interest. Depth of the image can be adjusted by a special knob so that structures of interest within the field of view may be moved far or closer for optimal visualisation (Fig. 2.2). The frequency although automatically selected by the preset of the structure of interest can also be adjusted with a knob.

9. **Gain**. Overall or **B-mode gain** corrects the attenuation of the ultrasound beam due to scattering and tissue absorption. **Time gain compensation** amplifies the echoes returning to the transducer at a specific depth. The examiner can modify the time gain by adjusting the controls of the ultrasound machine (Fig. 2.2).

10. **Anisotropy**. Anisotropy is a typical ultrasound artifact, usually occurring in sonograms of tendons, and to a lesser degree in nerves and muscles. The tendon may appear hyporeflective, thus simulating disease. However, this is not due to pathology but due to scattering of the beam which is not perpendicular to the surface. Scattered sound waves are not captured by the probe and so the tendon appears dark.

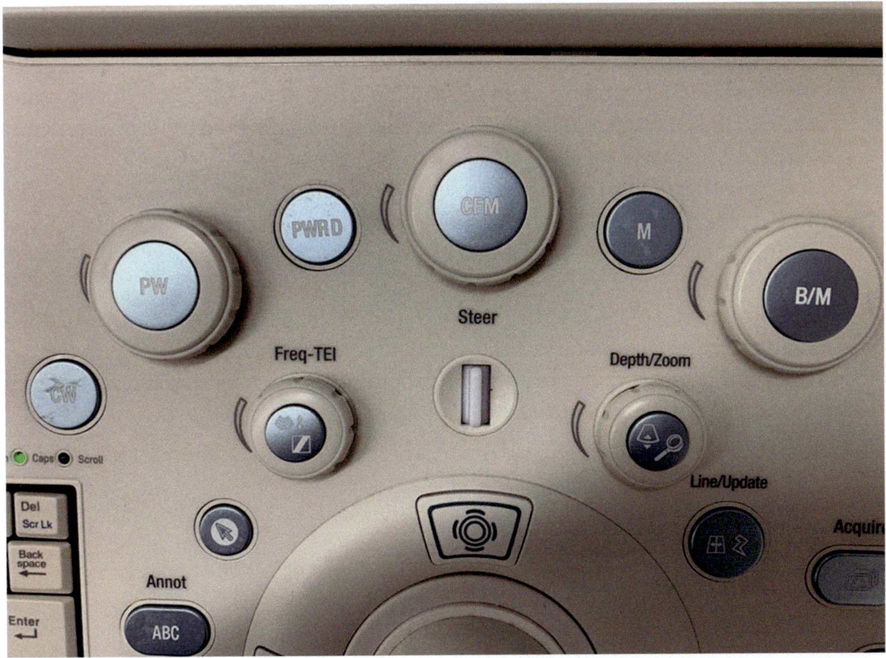

Fig. 2.2 The figure indicates three special knobs, the left one for changing the frequency, the right lower one for selecting the depth, and the right upper one (B/M) knob for adjusting the overall gain

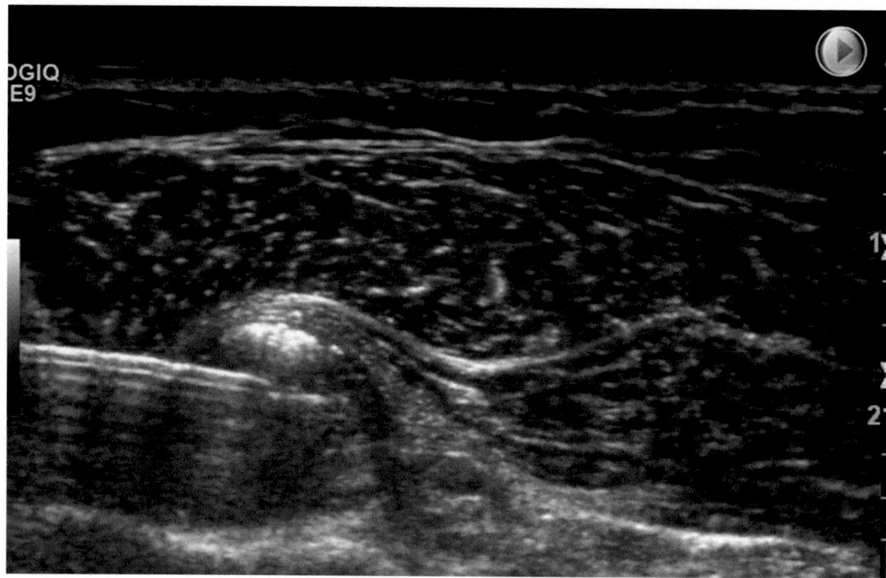

Fig. 2.3 Multiple reverberation artifacts beneath the needle which is introduced from the left side of the image

11. **Refraction**. Refraction is an artifact depicting real structures in the wrong position caused by the bending of an ultrasound wave at the interface of two materials, e.g., the position of the tip of the needle; we can minimize this phenomenon by keeping the incident beam as close to 90° as possible.
12. **Reverberation (Fig. 2.3)**. Reverberation is the phenomenon of the beam bouncing back and forth between the transducer and the object, giving rise to multiple echoes. This can be seen for example when a needle is introduced in the tissue.
13. **Edge shadowing (Fig. 2.4)**. In ultrasound, edge shadowing refers to the shadows behind the edge of spherical, fluid-filled structures.
14. **Comet tail** is an artifact caused by reverberation. It creates characteristic bands of increased echogenicity distal to the object.

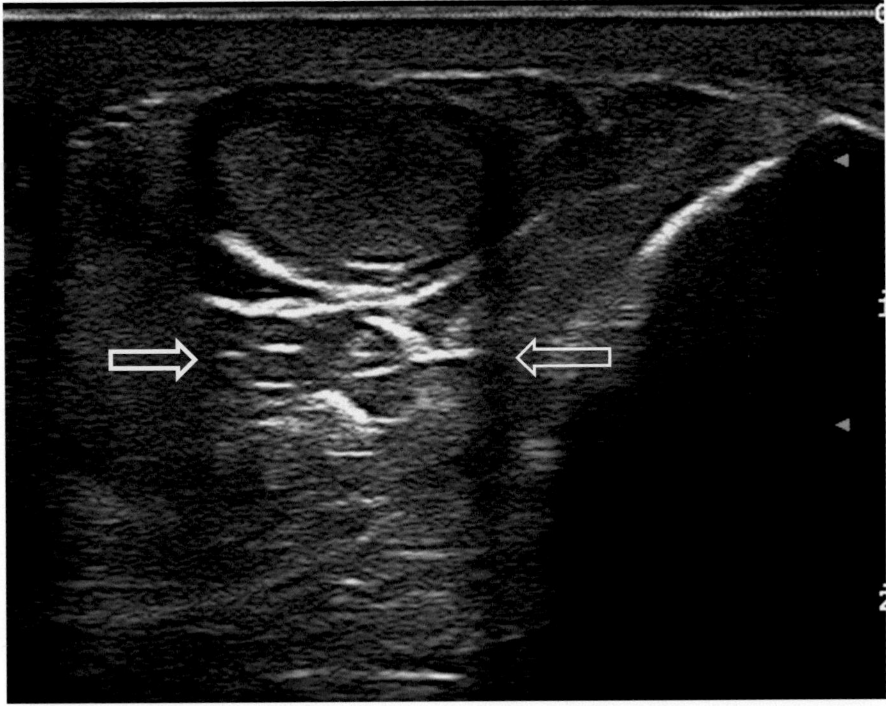

Fig. 2.4 This transverse scan of a peroneus tendinopathy shows an example of edge shadowing, i.e., a hypoechoic shadowing along the sides of the elliptical tendon (arrows). Differential diagnosis is with a tenosynovial sheath widening

15. **Acoustic shadowing (Fig. 2.5)** means that almost all of the beam is reflected when it hits a highly reflective surface, like bone, air, calcifications and calculi. It produces a dark shadow below the highly reflective surface.
16. **Echogenicity (Fig. 2.6)**. A structure may appear anechoic (black), hypoechoic (dark-gray), iso-echoic (gray, akin to liver tissue), a mixture of hyper- and hypoechoic, and hyperechoic or echogenic (white). Bone sharply reflects ultrasound waves and the bony edge appears white. Cartilage appears as a anechoic

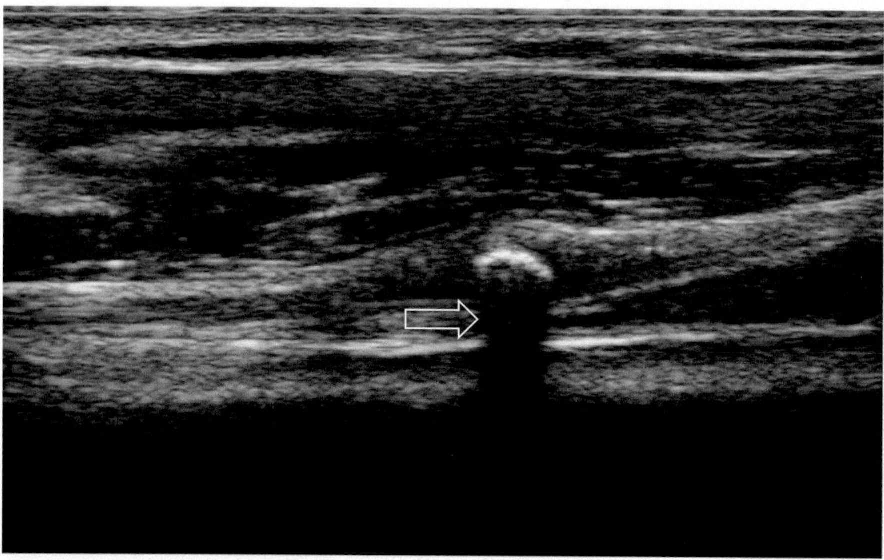

Fig. 2.5 This longitudinal scan shows a hyperechoic structure ($\Rightarrow$) with posterior shadowing. The structure is located anteriorly to the biceps tendon close to its junction with the muscle. It represents a calcification in the pectoralis major tendon

band overlying the bone. Fluid collections are hypo- or anechoic structures that may result in posterior acoustic enhancement, demonstrated by brighter echoes underneath the structure.

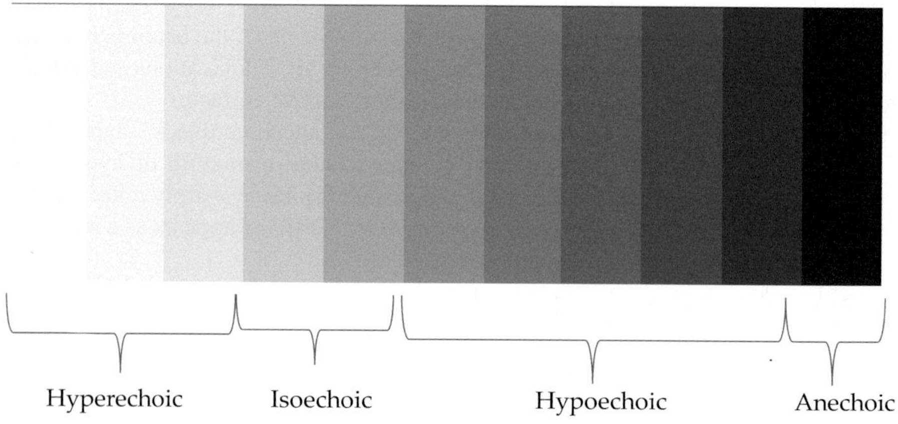

Fig. 2.6 This picture shows the spectrum of greyscale grades that together make up the echogenicity, ranging from hyperechoic to the left to anechoic to the far right

17. **Enhancement** is an artifact resulting from the lack of impedance when sound waves pass through fluid causing increased echoes from underlying structures (Fig. 2.7).
18. **Blooming** is a Doppler artifact when Doppler signals extend beyond the anatomical limit of the vessel. Blooming is gain dependent, so it can be corrected by decreasing the gain.
19. **Aliasing**. Aliasing is a Doppler artifact occurring when velocities of red blood cells are higher than the pulse repetition frequency (PRF). This occurs for example in areas of stenosis, where the reduced lumen of the vessel is seen with a red to blue shift. Red represents flow towards the transducer, within the range of the PRF, and blue velocities beyond the range of the PRF, not reversed flow.
20. **Harmonic imaging**. Harmonic imaging transmits signals at a low frequency and uses the second harmonic signal at a higher frequency, by filtering out the first returning echoes from the received signal to produce an image.

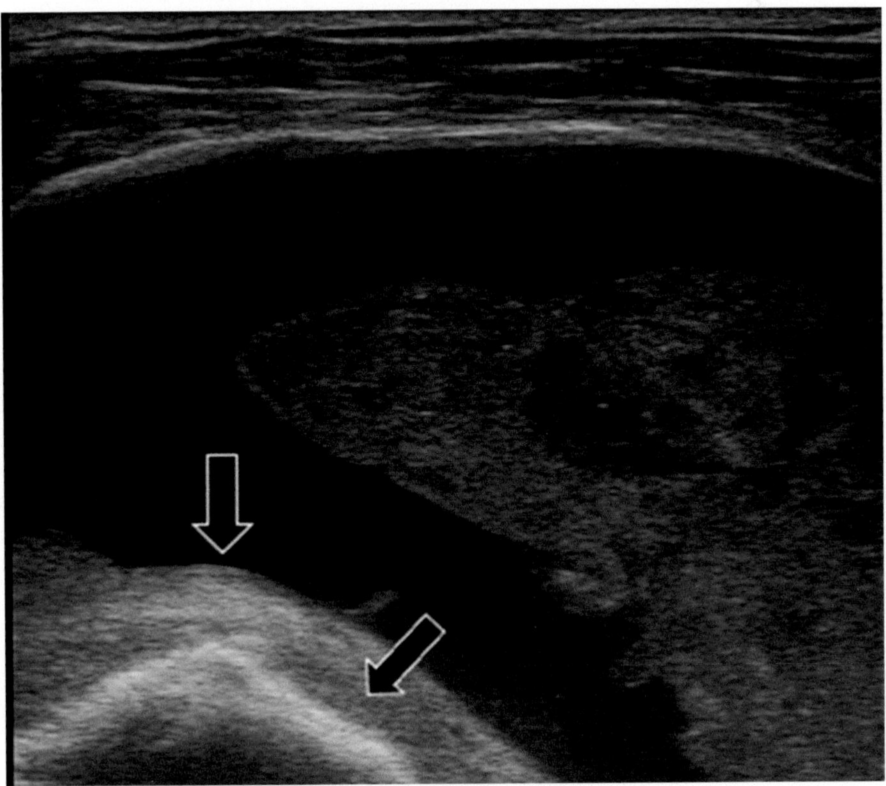

Fig. 2.7   Post-septic shoulder bursitis, with a massive proliferative synovitis accompanied by effusion. Underneath the effusion posterior enhancement artifact (arrows)

21. **Dynamic range**. Using this function varies the range of sound wave amplitudes. A high dynamic range results in minimal compression and creates a smoother image, while a low compression results in a high contrast image. Thus, when a sharper contrasting image is required, e.g., for imaging a nerve in a fascial plane, a low dynamic range should be set.

22. **Elastography** or real-time elastography (RTE) is a relatively new technology that uses the physical principle that tissue compression produces a strain within the tissue. The strain is smaller in harder tissue than in softer. This elastic difference can be visualized so that inelastic areas become dark and softer tissue bright, or red and blue when color-coded.

23. **Three-dimensional (3D)** ultrasound has several advantages over conventional 2D ultrasound, because it is composed of multiple 2D images and unlike 2D ultrasound, it is not dependent on the angle of scanning to the body. Microbubble contrast agents remain in the circulation for a few minutes and result in a marked increase of the ultrasound image.

2.6   How to Optimize Your Image?

Everyone wants to get the best images as possible. Knowledge of how to master the correct machine adjustments for a "perfect" image and to maximize the potential of all the knobs on the machine is not so easy as it sounds. There are a couple of aspects to bear in mind when getting the best images.

First and foremost, a good contact between probe and the skin is necessary. This requires a sufficient amount of coupling gel. Next, it is worthwhile to take a look at the factory machine presets, which are standard settings for a particular indication. Regarding rheumatology, you may forget the usual presets for urology, vascular ultrasound, or ob/gyn, and instead focus on the musculoskeletal (MSK) modality. In addition, the thyroid preset is useful for the examination of the major salivary glands. Thus, for the majority of the joint regions, select MSK. From a practical viewpoint, it is efficient to select these presets, including shoulder, knee etc., when you examine a patient. Depending of the specific pathology of the particular joint region, one has to make adjustment in depth, focus, and sometimes, frequency and gain. In general, it takes quite some time and experience to find your way in image optimization, but it is worth the effort.

Chapter 3
Choosing an Ultrasound System

Ultrasound offers the rheumatologist substantial support in diagnosing and monitoring a variety of musculoskeletal conditions. Thus, when choosing the best system for the office, take plenty of time to research what equipment is available (Fig. 3.1). A list of requirements should usually include the following aspects.

First and foremost, the bread-and-butter of any machine is the quality of the grayscale images. These should be of high-definition so that the operator can be confident of his diagnosis. During scanning, the machine assigns shades of gray to the returning echo signals. The number of shades of gray depends on how many bits of information can be stored for each horizontal and vertical point of image memory. The quality of the images depends on the features of the system's software and hardware. Some manufactures market upgraded models which are more expensive than the older models, yet they contain in essence the same chips and electronics. When considering which system to purchase, a rule of thumb is to look at images that appear on the screen when you scan the palmar side of your own wrist. Small anatomic structures such as the median nerve and the various flexor tendons should be outlined clearly on the system monitor and should be distinct from each other. The monitor should not be too small, but on the other hand the device should also be easy to use. The keyboard is used for entering the patient's data, such as name, and annotations describing the anatomical area that will be scanned. Additional information can be typed on the image using the "Write" function button. Scanned structures can be measured on the monitor, using digital calliper cursors. These callipers can also be used for measuring the cross-sectional area, circumference or volume of a structure, for instance the median nerve. The keyboard should have a logical positioning of the buttons for easy navigation.

Second, careful attention should be paid to the choice of probes. A breadth of transducers is available. Modern probes may offer bandwidths of over 50%. Thus, a probe centred on 12 MHz would cover all frequencies between 6 and 18 MHz, or even around 4 and 20 MHz. This means that in the near field the scanner electronically filters out the low frequencies resulting in higher resolution whereas in the far field the device lets the lower frequencies pass through, giving better penetration. A 10 MHz

© The Author(s), under exclusive license to Springer Nature Switzerland AG 2023

G. A. W. Bruyn and W. A. Schmidt, *Musculoskeletal Ultrasound for the Rheumatologist*, https://doi.org/10.1007/978-3-031-27737-5_3

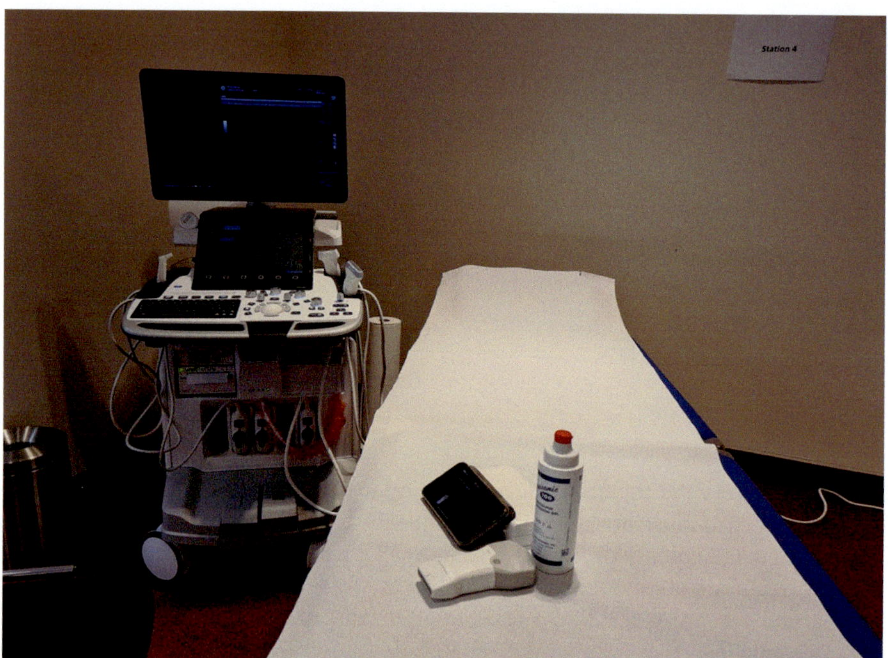

Fig. 3.1 An optimal combination of modern ultrasound machines. On the left, a high-end ultrasound system configured with several probes including a hockey stick, and on the right a handheld pocket-sized probe that includes a convex and linear array scanner and sends the information by Bluetooth to a mobile phone or tablet

linear array probe can be applied to practically all large joints except the hip. To scan down the femoral head in an adult patient, either a lower frequency *curved array* or a linear array probe of lower frequency of about 5 MHz can be used.

Curved array probes that are commonly employed for abdominal ultrasound may be used for hip joint sonography in obese patients and fit better to the anatomy of the groin or arm pit than linear array probes (Fig. 3.2). The width of the transducer, also called footprint, should be taken into account, which is usually about 40–50 mm. A transducer footprint of 40–50 mm is useful for medium-sized to large joints. For scanning small finger joints or toe joints, and small vessels like the temporal artery, a small foot print probe such as the *hockey* stick (e.g., surface area of 26 mm × 10 mm), preferably with a high frequency of up to 25 MHz, is practical, e.g., 6–24 MHz. In conclusion, it is a comfortable luxury to have two to three probes, but, one ultra-broadband linear array probe with a frequency range of 4–20 MHz may adequately serve a rheumatologist too.

All modern machines have a unit capable of visualizing the vascular system. The vascular imaging unit includes color and power Doppler technology. Color Doppler examination is now the non-invasive method of choice for the evaluation of patients

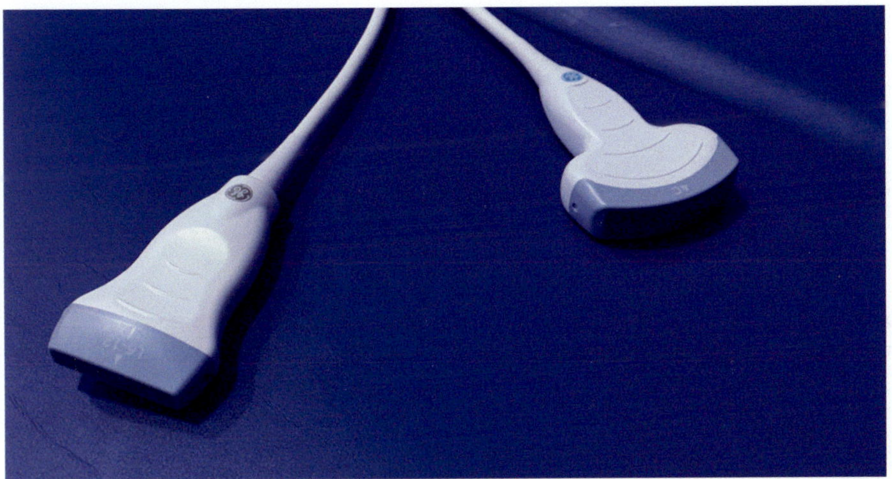

Fig. 3.2 On the left, a linear array probe, and on the right a curved array probe

suspected of deep vein thrombosis. Another application of color Doppler is the assessment of blood flow in arteries, for instance of the temporal artery and its terminal branches, or axillary arteries. Standard examination of arteries is done with a high-resolution transducer of > at least 15 MHz according to the EULAR recommendations on imaging in vasculitis. Particularly hockeystick probes or small footprint probes with >20 MHz frequency provide excellent resolution. Two modalities are required: grayscale imaging and color flow Doppler, both on transverse and longitudinal planes. The two most commonly used imaging techniques to evaluate flow in vessels are color flow mapping and 2D sector scanning. Flow mapping produces a static image of the blood flow within a vessel. Two-dimensional sector scanning produces a sectional image of the vessel's anatomy which is updated many times per second. True simultaneous duplex scanners allow the 2D image to remain in real time while the Doppler beam provides flow information. Power Doppler is useful for the detection of hyperemia with slow flow velocities in joints, tendon sheaths, and entheses and is thus potentially capable of assessing inflammation.

Other relevant aspects are data storage and pricing. The frozen image or sequential real-time images can be recorded and stored in the machine's data storage system. Most machines come with one or several USB ports.

Other components include extras such as elastography, extended panorama view, a biopsy guidance facility, patient records and registration, connection possibilities with the hospital picture archiving and communication system (PACS), and ergonomic design. An interface with the hospital PACS allows images and videos to be safely stored and shared on the hospital network.

Prices for an average complete ultrasound system vary between €30,000 and 70,000, although lower and higher priced systems are available. There are portable

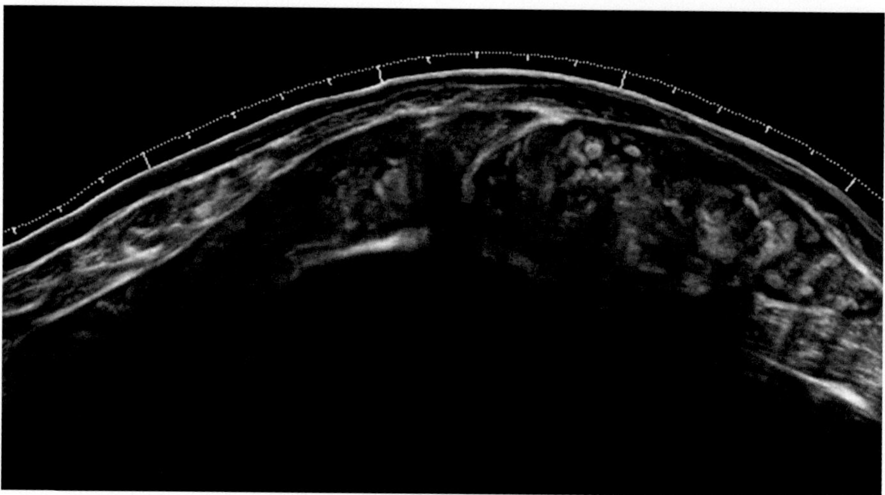

Fig. 3.3 Panoramic view of a subacromial-subdeltoid bursa filled with rice bodies in a patient with rheumatoid arthritis

systems which are affordably priced. These portables may come in a lap top configuration, however more recently improved technology of hand-held probes made it possible to connect wirelessly to your iPhone IOS or Android by an app. Such blue tooth devices improve the availability of ultrasound in the physician's office and at the bedside.

High-end, more expensive, equipment may include modalities such as harmonic imaging, panoramic view (Fig. 3.3), 3D imaging, or shear wave elastography.

Chapter 4
General Sonoanatomy

Ultrasound is a tomographic imaging method like CT and MRI. These imaging methods generate anatomical slices. In CT and MRI, the distance between the slices is variable according to indication and anatomical region. It may be 1 mm, 2 mm, or 4 mm, for instance. For ultrasound, slices are produced continuously comparable with a movie. An anatomical slice provides an overview of only a limited anatomical region. This makes the interpretation of ultrasound images more difficult. Furthermore, ultrasound only depicts the anatomical area between probe and bone surface.

In general, there are two types of scans, the transverse (cross-sectional) scan and the longitudinal scan. Before starting to perform ultrasound, it is essential to orientate and localize anatomical structures on an ultrasound image.

The transverse view is like that of a CT and MRI. Normally, the patient is lying at the right side of the sonographer (Fig. 3.1). The sonographer looks at the patient from caudal. The images can be compared with a transverse cut of a cucumber (Fig. 4.1). The upper part of the image is the anatomic area close to the probe. This is anterior (ventral) if the patient is supine. The lower part is the area distal to the probe. This is posterior (dorsal) if the patient is supine. The left side of the image is the left side from the perspective of the sonographer. This is the right side of the body if the patient is supine. In the past, some sonographers preferred to localize the medial (ulnar, tibial) anatomical area always on the left side of the image and the lateral anatomical (radial, fibular) area on the right side of the image to better compare findings of both extremities.

The longitudinal view generates an image that is like a cucumber which is cut in length (Fig. 4.2). Again, the upper side of the image depicts the area that is close to the probe, and the lower part of the image depicts the area that is distal to the probe. The left side of the image displays the cranial (proximal) anatomical structures, and the right side the caudal (distal) anatomical structures.

© The Author(s), under exclusive license to Springer Nature Switzerland AG 2023

G. A. W. Bruyn and W. A. Schmidt, *Musculoskeletal Ultrasound for the Rheumatologist*,

https://doi.org/10.1007/978-3-031-27737-5_4

Fig. 4.1 Transverse slice of a cucumber. Upper part of image: anterior (proximal to probe), lower part of image: posterior (distal to probe), left side of image: left side seen from the sonographer

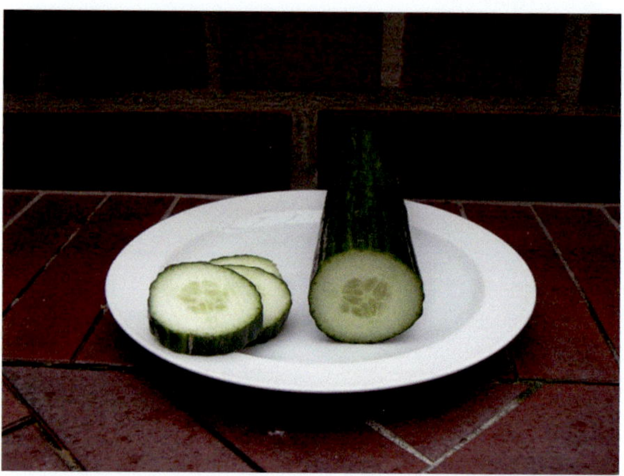

Fig. 4.2 Longitudinal slice of a cucumber. Upper part of image: anterior (proximal to probe), lower part of image: posterior (distal to probe), left side of image: left side seen from the sonographer. Thus, this side represents the proximal (cranial) anatomical structures

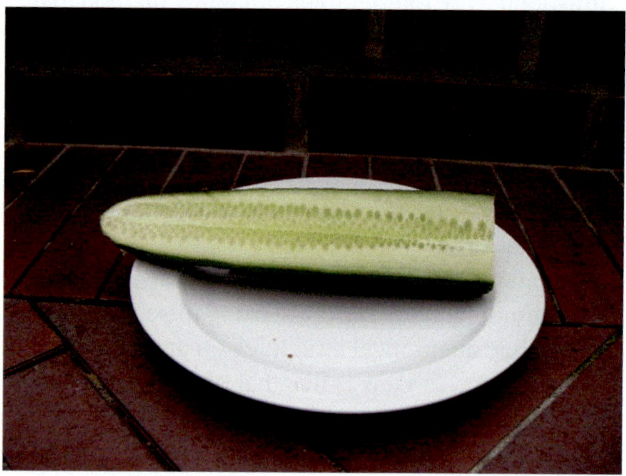

When starting to perform ultrasound, it is important to acquire this "cucumber view". Translated to the image of a tendon, this view is shown in Figs. 4.3 and 4.4 for a transverse plane and in Figs. 4.5 and 4.6 for a longitudinal plane.

Figure 4.5 also shows the sonographic appearance of the most important anatomical structures. Figure 4.6 explains the anatomy.

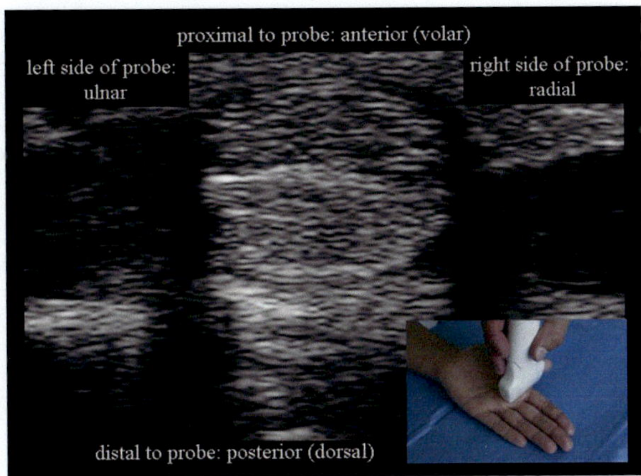

Fig. 4.3 Transverse view of the region proximal to a left MCP 2 joint that explains the localization of anatomical structures in a standardized ultrasound image

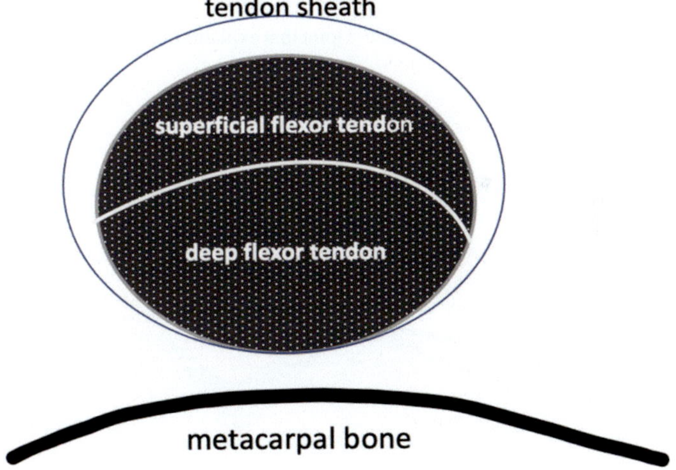

Fig. 4.4 Transverse view of the volar anatomical structures proximal to a left MCP 2 joint ultrasound image

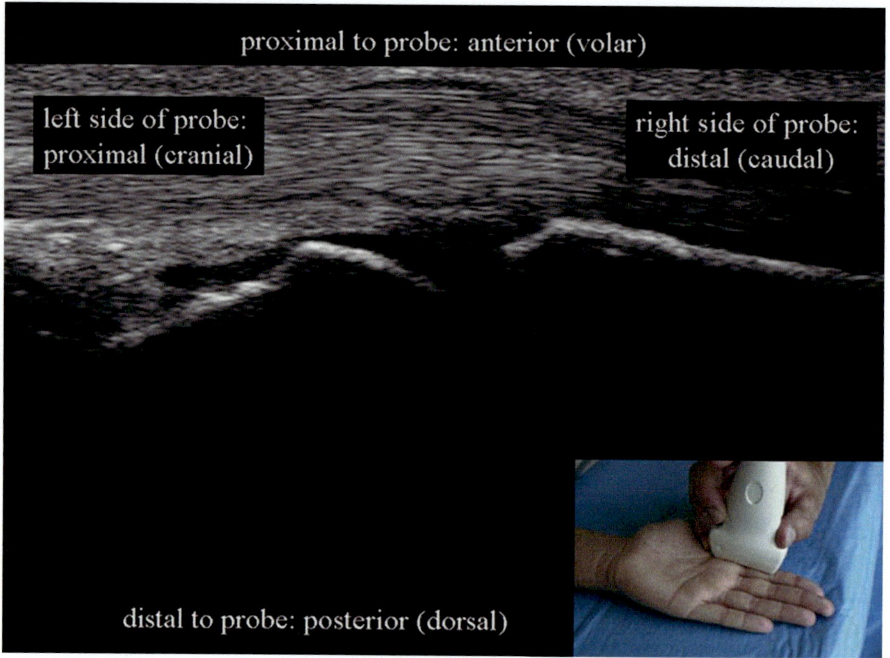

Fig. 4.5 Longitudinal view of an MCP 2 joint that explains the localization of anatomical structures in a standardized ultrasound image

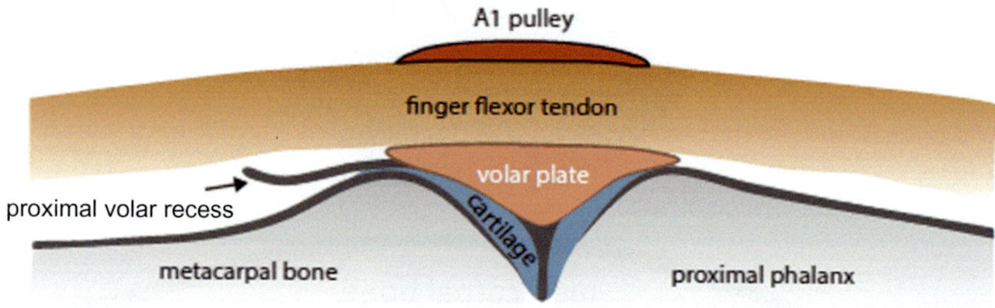

Fig. 4.6 Longitudinal view of the volar anatomical structures of a MCP 2 joint ultrasound image

4.1 Distinguishing Between the Anatomical Structures

Bright structures like bone are referred to as "hyperechoic", dark structures such as muscle as "hypoechoic", and black structures representing for instance fluid or cartilage are called "anechoic". Liver or thyroid tissue is referred to as "midechoic or isoechoic".

1. **Bone surface**. Bone surface is hyperechoic with posterior acoustic shadowing. Ultrasound does not provide any information on anatomical structures that are localized below an intact bone surface.
2. **Cartilage**. Hyaline cartilage is anechoic. It is localized directly adjacent to the bone surface. Its surface is regular. Degenerated cartilage may become hypoechoic or midechoic with an irregular surface. Fibrocartilage, e.g., meniscal or labrum cartilage, is slightly hyperechoic.
3. **Synovium** is hypoechoic to midechoic tissue within a joint. In joints of healthy persons, it usually does not exhibit Doppler signals. Nevertheless, ultrasound equipment with a high sensitivity to flow signals may also show minor flow in joints of healthy individuals.
4. **Synovial fluid** is anechoic material within a joint. It is displaceable and compressible but does not exhibit Doppler signals.
5. **Joint capsule** The joint capsule is the tendon- or ligament like tissue that forms the frontier between the hypoechoic synovium, anechoic synovial fluid, or anechoic cartilage and periarticular structures, the latter often consisting of midechoic connective tissue.
6. **Connective tissue** is midechoic and slightly irregular.
7. **Subcutaneous fat** is also hypoechoic and slightly irregular.
8. **Tendons** are characterized by a fine internal fibrillar pattern. They are slightly hyperechoic if localized parallel to the probe. If the tendon is not parallel to the probe, it becomes hypoechoic or anechoic as the ultrasound waves are not reflected to the probe (anisotropy). On transverse scans, tendons show a granular appearance.
9. **Nerves** have a mixed ultrasound appearance, with a hyperechoic rim corresponding to the epineurium, and hypoechoic fascicles. On transverse scanning, nerves show a honeycomb appearance, with hypooechoic fascicles. Compared to tendons they are slightly hypoechoic, and their structure is more dotted and less fibrillar (see Wrist, Standard Scans 7-7 and 7-10).
10. **Muscles** are usually hypoechoic. Muscles are usually hypoechoic but sometimes mid- or hyperechoic according to the orientation or the probe. Fine intramuscular hyperechoic lines represent the epi- and paramysium, thicker hyperechoic lines represent septae and investing fascia.
11. **Bursae** are hypoechoic or anechoic depending on the structures that prevail in the bursae.
12. **Ligaments** appear like tendons. They are hyperechoic with a fibrillar structure. If they consist of several layers, the fibrillar pattern may run in different directions.

In Chaps. 5–12, scans relevant for musculoskeletal ultrasound in rheumatology are presented; they are organized into different anatomical sections. The format is logical and systematic, i.e., the Standard Scans show the normal anatomy, and scanning techniques are described in detail. These are followed by ultrasound scans of pathologies commonly seen in rheumatology practice. Chapters 13–15 give detailed information on the use of ultrasound in vasculitis, salivary glands, lymph nodes, and the pleura.

Chapter 5
The Shoulder

5.1 Standard Scans of the Shoulder

5.1.1 Transverse View of the Biceps Tendon (Standard Scan 5-1)

The patient is seated upright on a low revolving stool. A right-handed sonographer should sit directly in front of the machine with the patient is slightly to the right. When examining the right shoulder, the patient should face the examiner, and the patient's back should be directed towards the ultrasound machine; for the left shoulder, the patient should face the machine. Alternatively, the examiner may sit or stand behind the seated patient while the patient is facing the ultrasound machine.

The patient's arms rest on the thigh with the palm of the hand facing upward (supination) and the elbow flexed at 90°. The probe is placed transversely and anteriorly over the shoulder. The shoulders are usually examined bilaterally.

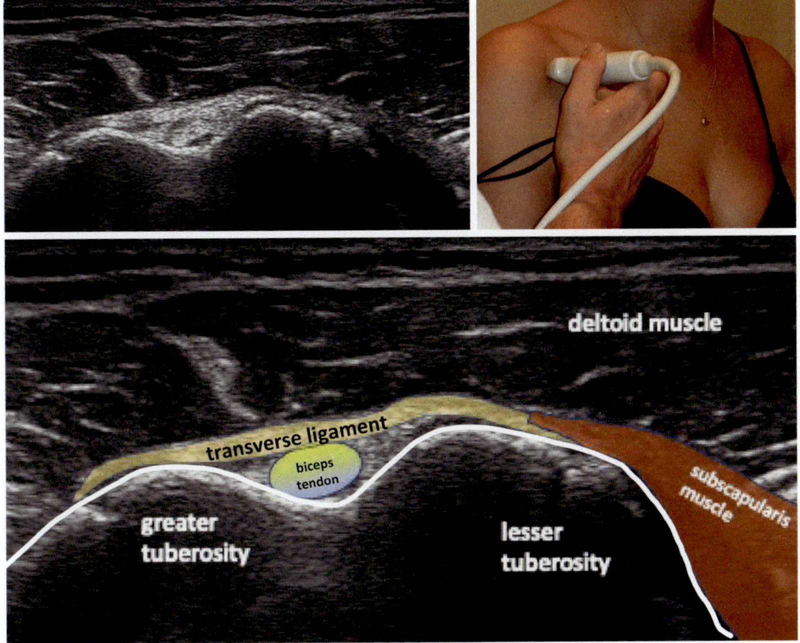

© The Author(s), under exclusive license to Springer Nature Switzerland AG 2023
G. A. W. Bruyn and W. A. Schmidt, *Musculoskeletal Ultrasound for the Rheumatologist*,
https://doi.org/10.1007/978-3-031-27737-5_5

The long head of the biceps tendon is the landmark of anterior shoulder scans. The transverse or axial sonogram locates the biceps tendon within the bony bicipital groove of the humerus. On normal ultrasound the tendon has a bright appearance. The transverse humeral ligament is located anterior to the tendon and straps the tendon down. Medially to the biceps tendon, the subscapularis tendon and muscle are present whereas the supraspinatus tendon is lateral. When shifting the probe upwards and directing the distal end of the footprint downwards and 45° medially along with pulling the arm posteriorly with the elbow adjacent to the body, the rotator cuff interval becomes visible (Scan 5.1.12). Sitting on top of the long head of the biceps tendon, the coracohumeral ligament can be distinguished, and at the medial border of the biceps tendon, the superior glenohumeral ligament.

What is normal?

The mean transverse diameter of the biceps tendon is 5.0 ± 2.1 mm (2.1–8.8 mm). A minimal amount of physiological fluid may be present around the tendon.

5.1.2   Longitudinal View of the Biceps Tendon (Standard Scan 5-2)

The longitudinal or sagittal view of the biceps tendon is obtained by rotating the probe by 90°. The position of the patient and the examiner remains the same as in the first Standard Scan of the transverse bicipital view, Standard Scan 5-1. The tendon should be depicted parallel to the probe because of anisotropy. This is achieved by applying more pressure on the distal end of the probe.

Then, the probe should be shifted slowly downwards towards the musculotendinous junction. The parallel arrangement of the fibrillar pattern of the long head of the biceps tendon, located within the bony bicipital groove, is easily visualized. The long head of the biceps tendon should be followed distally, where it disappears into the musculotendinous junction and the biceps muscle (*).

What is normal?

The mean sagittal diameter of the long biceps tendon measured at the end of the rotator cuff is 2.6 mm (1.2–4.0 mm). A slight fluid collection at the distal end of the bicipital sheath is physiological.

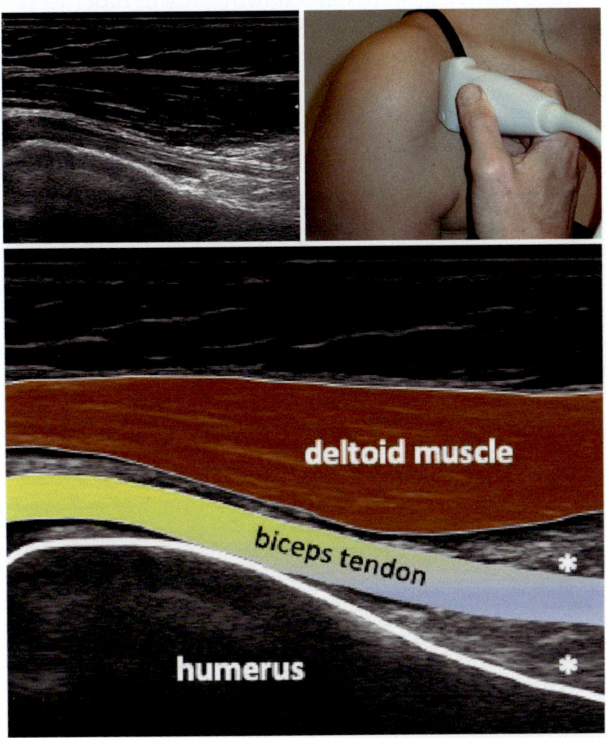

5.1.3   Anterior Transverse View of the Shoulder (Standard Scan 5-3)

This scan is performed with the shoulder in a neutral position and the lower arm supinated, with elbow flexed. The probe is positioned obliquely and transversely with respect to the axis of the body and longitudinally to the tendons of the rotator cuff.

This scan is intended to examine the subscapularis and the medial anterior part of the supraspinatus tendon. Firstly, the biceps tendon is identified within the bicipital groove; then, the subscapularis tendon is detected medially inserting to the lesser tuberosity. To examine the full length of the subscapularis tendon the arm should be rotated externally. In this scanning position, the insertion of the subscapularis tendon on the lesser tuberosity appears beak-shaped. Some fibers run across the bicipital groove and merge with fibers of the supraspinatus tendon to form the transverse humeral ligament. The tendon moves smoothly with the surrounding structures when examined dynamically.

The examination is then continued while rotating the arm internally. Thus, lateral of the biceps tendon, the supraspinatus tendon is identified inserting at the greater tuberosity. Overlying the rotator cuff, a thin hypoechoic line between two hyperechoic lines represents the subacromio-subdeltoid bursa. The examination is continued by shifting the probe slowly upwards and downwards in order to scan more of the insertion of the supraspinatus tendon. Anteflexion of the shoulder results in a smaller window to delineate the rotator cuff within the anterior scans. Anteflexion or scanning below the rotator cuff may lead to a false diagnosis of a rotator cuff tear or a thinned rotator cuff.

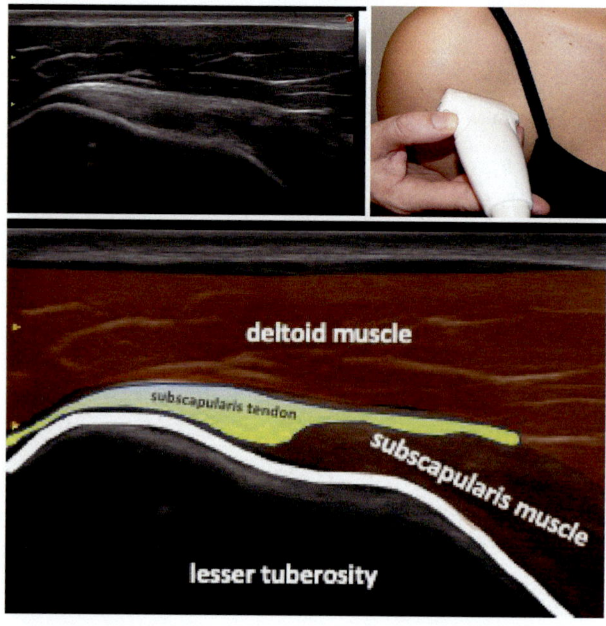

5.1.4   Anterior Longitudinal View of the Shoulder (Standard Scan 5-4)

The probe is placed longitudinally to the axis of the body and transversely to the tendons of the rotator cuff. Both the subscapularis and the supraspinatus tendons should be examined in the longitudinal and in transverse planes, as depicted here. This is important for identifying all abnormalities such as rotator cuff tears and calcifications. Tears or calcifications need to be visualized in both planes. It is very important to shift the probe zigzag-wise through all areas of the rotator cuff between the mentioned Standard Scans in order to see all the anatomy.

At the start of the examination the arm is held in a neutral position, with elbow flexed and palm directed upwards. Medially to the biceps tendon the subscapularis tendon is found. It inserts at the lesser tubercle. In order to have a complete view of the subscapularis tendon, the arm of the patient is then rotated externally as fast as possible.

What is normal?

The subscapularis tendon appears as hyperechoic fiber bundles. The darker areas between them correspond to subscapularis muscle tissue. They must not be confused with rotator cuff lesions.

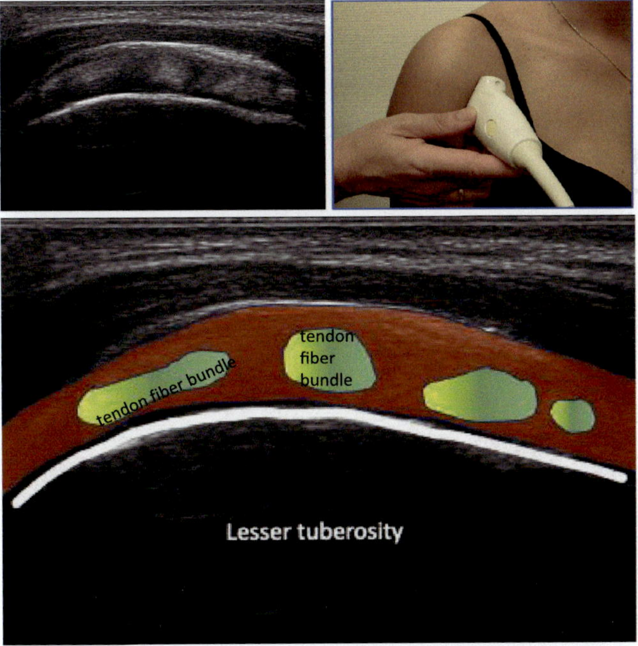

5.1.5   Lateral Transverse View of the Shoulder (Standard Scan 5-5)

This scan starts with the arm in a special position, the Crass or modified Crass position. The Crass position is achieved by placing the hand as high as possible on the back, or at least on the buttock. In this way the supraspinatus tendon is pulled out from below the acromion. The probe is positioned laterally to the position shown in Standard Scan 5-4. Lateral to the biceps tendon, the supraspinatus tendon is identified. The sonogram shows a transverse view of the supraspinatus tendon. Overlying the supraspinatus tendon, the subacromial-subdeltoid bursa is visible as a thin hypoechoic layer between two parallel curvilinear hyperechoic lines, representing the bursal-muscle interfaces. The examination is performed starting with the biceps tendon at the medial side and gradually sweeping the probe laterally and upwards and downwards in order to visualize the entire supraspinatus tendon. As mentioned earlier, to allow an optimal view of the supraspinatus tendon the examination should not be performed too inferiorly or with the shoulder in adduction.

What is normal?

The supraspinatus tendon looks like a regular arc. The mean transverse diameter of the supraspinatus tendon measured 2 cm lateral of the biceps tendon is 4.6 mm (2.7–6.5 mm).

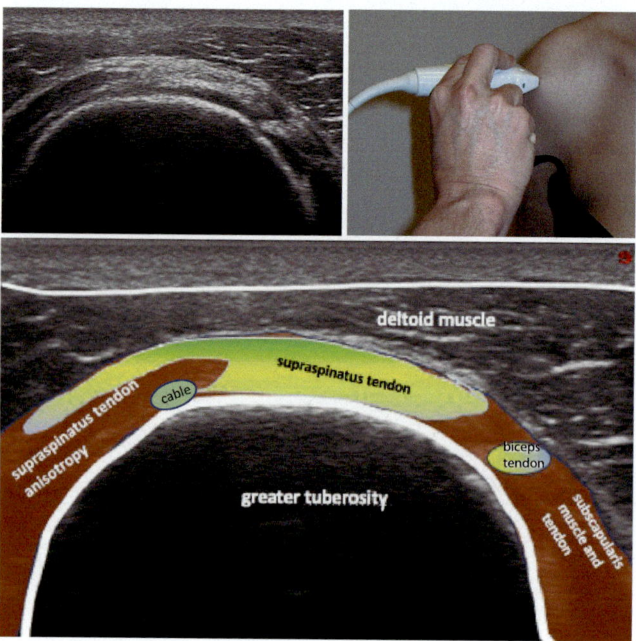

5.1.6   *Lateral Longitudinal View of the Shoulder (Standard Scan 5-6)*

The probe is placed identically to the previous position but rotated by 90°, so that the supraspinatus tendon can be visualized where it attaches to the greater tuberosity. The arm should be rotated internally and adducted, by asking the patient to hold the arm behind their back (Crass position). This scan, together with the previous scan, is important for identifying pathology of the rotator cuff, which usually involves the supraspinatus tendon. Rotator cuff tears should be visualized in two planes. Also, calcifications may be present in distal areas of the rotator cuff. Sometimes they have larger diameters in the longitudinal plane than in the transverse plane. Using this scan, it is also possible to test for impingement. By lifting the internally rotated arm, the rotator cuff should completely disappear under the acromion.

What is normal?

The supraspinatus tendon is seen as a beak-shaped structure protruding from under the acromion and attaching to the greater tuberosity.

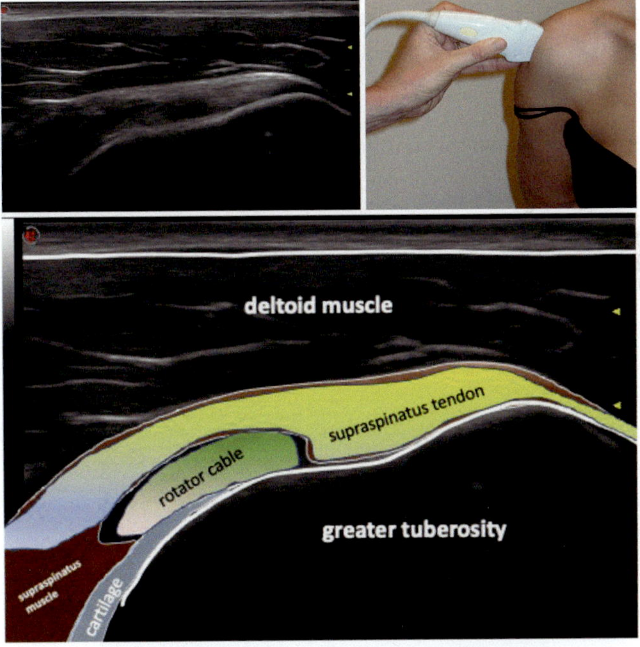

5.1.7   Posterior Transverse View of the Shoulder (Standard Scan 5-7)

Ultrasound examination of the posterior part of the shoulder visualizes the posterior recess of the glenohumeral joint, the posterior glenoid labrum, the hyaline cartilage on top of the humeral head, the bone underlying the cartilage and the infraspinatus tendon inserting at the greater tubercle. When shifting the probe downwards, the smaller tendon of the teres minor muscle becomes visible.

The fibrocartilaginous posterior labrum is easily identified as a sharply triangular shaped hyperechoic structure partially capping the anechoic hyaline cartilage of the humeral head.

The transverse view also allows scanning for erosions of the humeral head. Larger cortical defects, such as the Hill-Sachs lesion, are the result of trauma or recurrent dislocation of the humeral head. With external rotation of the arm smaller effusions of the glenonohumeral joint become visible. Without this maneuver they are often overlooked. Again, the probe should be shifted cranial to caudal (or vice versa). When sweeping a bit medially, the spinoglenoid notch can be seen. Through the notch, the suprascapular nerve and artery pass from the supraspinatus fossa to the infraspinatus fossa. The artery is below, the nerve on top, separated by the spinoglenoid ligament.

In obese patients the posterior joint space and the glenoid labrum may be located quite far away. Therefore, low frequencies down to 4 MHz may be needed.

What is normal?

The diameter between humerus and joint capsule (a) in external rotation is 2.0 mm (0–30 mm).

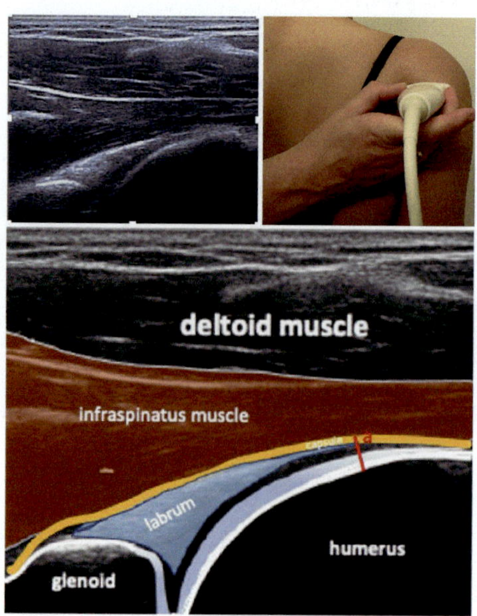

5.1.8 *Posterior Longitudinal View of the Shoulder (Standard Scan 5-8)*

The longitudinal view of the posterior shoulder is conducted in the same way as the transverse view, with the probe rotated by 90°. Maneuvering the arm externally and internally allows visualization of erosions of the humeral head. Particularly with external rotation small effusions can be seen in the second plane.

More distally, the trapezoid shaped teres minor muscle becomes visible. A strong fibrous septum (arrow) distinguishes the infraspinatus muscle from the teres minor muscle. Although the transverse scan is more important than the longitudinal posterior scan, both scans should be performed to assess all structures in two planes.

What is normal?

Two separate rounded structures corresponding to the tendons of infraspinatus and teres minor tendons should be visible near the insertion at the greater tuberosity. The muscle bellies of the infraspinatus and the teres minor muscle are separated by a fibrous fascia (arrow).

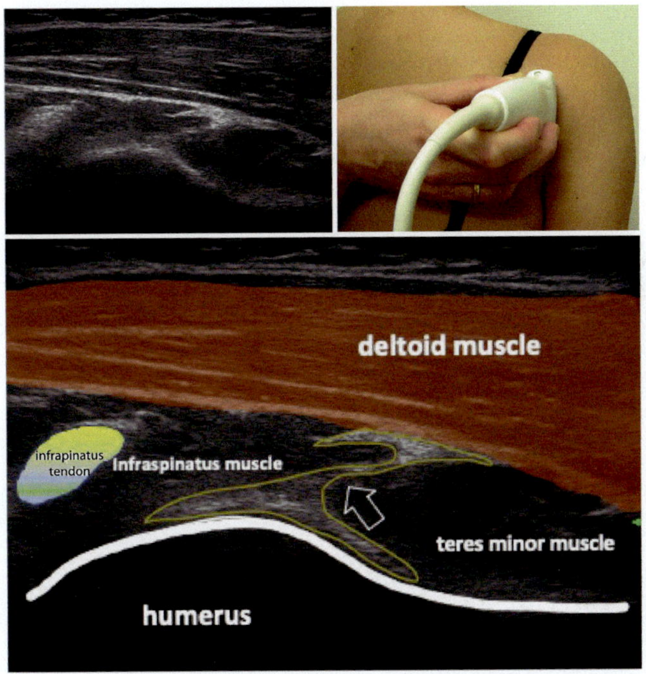

5.1.9   Acromioclavicular Joint View of the Shoulder (Standard Scan 5-9)

The acromioclavicular (AC) joint is one of the two synovial articulations of the shoulder. The end of the clavicle rides higher than the acromion and is readily palpated. In between the two bones, the acromioclavicular ligament and the joint capsule can be found. The AC joint is best scanned from above in the longitudinal plane along the long axis of the distal clavicle. Inflammation of the AC joint can mimic rotator cuff disease, because the supraspinatus tendon and subacromial bursa run directly underneath. Effusion of the AC joint, which produces the "geyser" phenomenon, may be caused by a tear in the underlying bursa and inferior capsule of the AC joint, or by synovitis of the AC joint itself. However, the most common pathology of the AC joint is osteoarthritis, often complicated by calcium pyrophosphate deposition disease (CPPD). Sonographic signs of osteoarthritis are joint space narrowing, hypertrophic spurs and synovial thickening. Subluxation of the AC joint may occur in trauma or in severe osteoarthritis. The joint space is widened and usually a step-off sign is present between acromion and clavicle, with the clavicle lower than the edge of the acromion.

What is normal?

The mean intra-articular distance between bone and joint distance is 1.7 mm (0.9–3.1 mm) medially and 2.5 ± 1.7 mm laterally. The width of the acromioclavicular joint space is 5.2 mm (1.9–8.5 mm).

Osteophytes are common in persons aged >50 years.

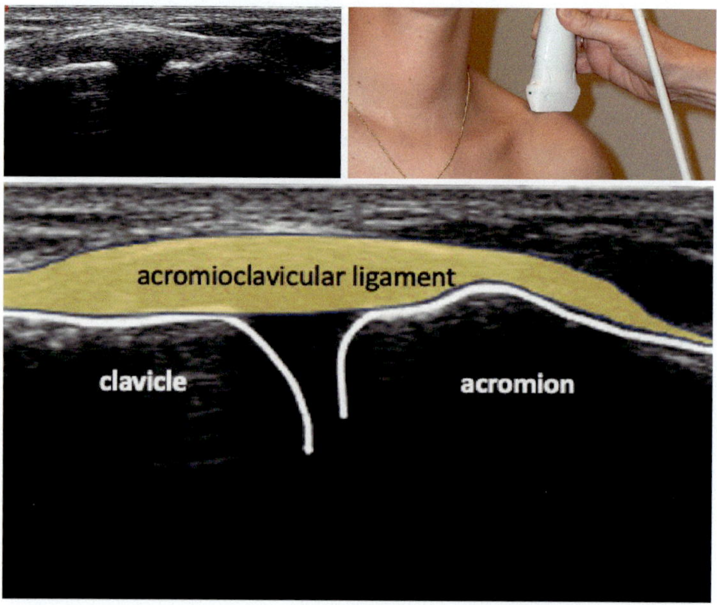

5.1.10   Axillary View of the Shoulder (Standard Scan 5-10)

The capsule of the glenohumeral joint is reinforced in the superior, anterior and posterior areas by the glenohumeral ligaments and the tendons of the rotator cuff muscles. The capsule is, therefore, relatively tight, allowing only fluid collection in its recesses. The shoulder recesses are the axillary recess, the (anterior) subscapular recess and the posterior recess.

The axillary view gives information on the presence of fluid in the axillary recess of the glenohumeral joint. Second to the posterior transverse view with external rotation, the axillary scan is the most sensitive maneuver to detect effusion or synovitis of the glenohumeral joint. The patient is asked to raise the arm to about 90° and move the hand across the chest to the top of the opposite shoulder or to the head if this is more comfortable. The probe is positioned in the longitudinal axis in the arm pit. The ultrasound image shows a longitudinal view of the humeral head and the joint capsule. This scan may not be possible in the presence of a frozen shoulder. If elevation is impaired, the patient can try to lift the arm with 60° internal rotation (arm in front of chest) to obtain enough elevation of the arm to perform this scan.

Pathological findings should be confirmed by a corresponding transverse scan.

What is normal?

The mean distance between humerus and joint capsule at the middle of the concavity of the humeral head and neck is 2.2 mm (0.6–3.8 mm).

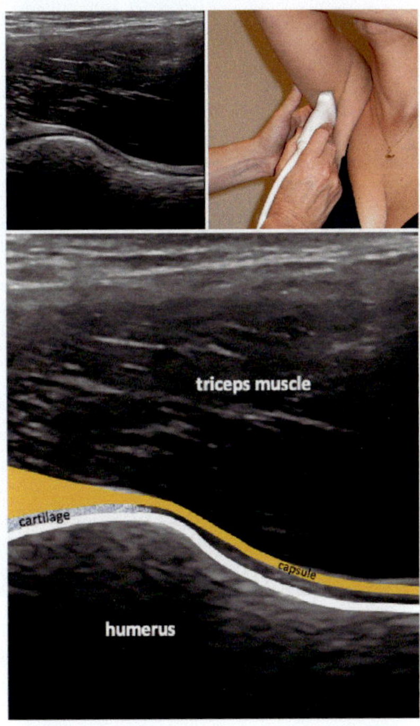

5.1.11   View of the Sternoclavicular Joint (Standard Scan 5-11)

Strictly speaking, the sternoclavicular (SC) joint is not part of the shoulder. However, pathology of this joint may mimic shoulder disease. The most common pathology is osteoarthritis (OA), where ultrasound may show irregular bony contours, effusion, joint space narrowing and hypertrophic spurs. Synovitis particularly occurs in SAPHO syndrome and in spondyloarthritis. Subluxation may be found in patients with the hypermobility syndrome. The patient may sit or lie down. The proximal probe end is about 45° oblique to the lateral end. Pathological findings should be confirmed in a plane 90° to this scan.

What is normal?

The mean sternoclavicular joint, bone-capsule distance measured at the medial sternoclavicular joint oblique to the cranial lateral end of the sternum is 0.9 (0–2.2) mm.

The mean sternoclavicular joint bone-capsule distance at the lateral sternoclavicular joint measured obliquely to the medial end of clavicle is 1.5 (0–3.1) mm.

The mean width of the sternoclavicular joint space is 8.2 (2.9–13.5) mm. The surface of the clavicle and sternum is normally regular.

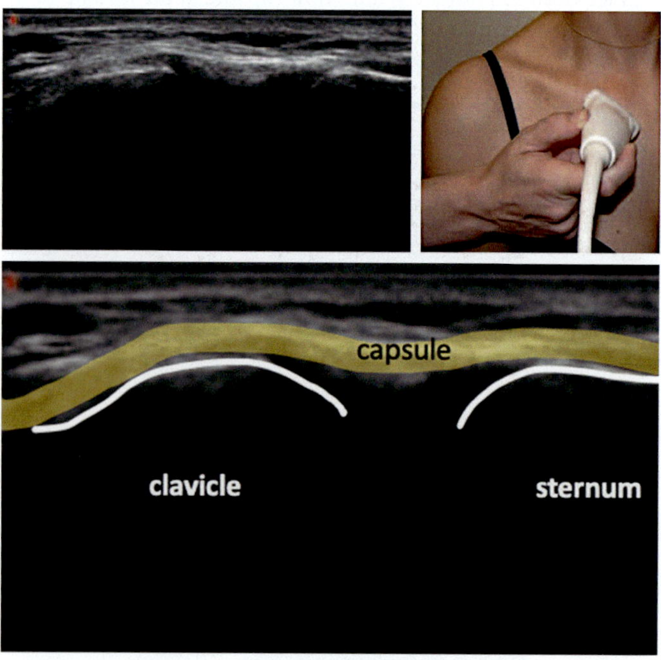

5.1.12   The Rotator Cuff Interval View (Standard Scan 5-12)

The starting patient position is the same as in Standard Scan 5-3. Then, the shoulder is brought into maximal retroversion with the elbow flexed and slight supination of the hand adjacent to the body. Tracing the long head of the biceps tendon in a superior direction above the bicipital groove while rotating the distal pole of the probe footprint 45° downwards medially, the cartilage layer of the humeral head becomes visible, indicating the entrance of the glenohumeral joint. This point relates to the most distal part of the rotator interval, where the long head of the biceps tendon is wrapped around by a fibrous sling consisting of the coracohumeral ligament (chl) and the superior glenohumeral ligament medially (sghl). The coracohumeral ligament splits in a lateral (lchl) and a medial part (mchl). The triangular area demarcated by the coracoid process and the insertions of supraspinatus and subscapularis tendons is called the rotator cuff interval. To the lateral side of the biceps tendon, hyperechoic fibers at the undersurface of the supraspinatus tendon can be distinguished consistent with the rotator cable which is an extension of the coracohumeral ligament.

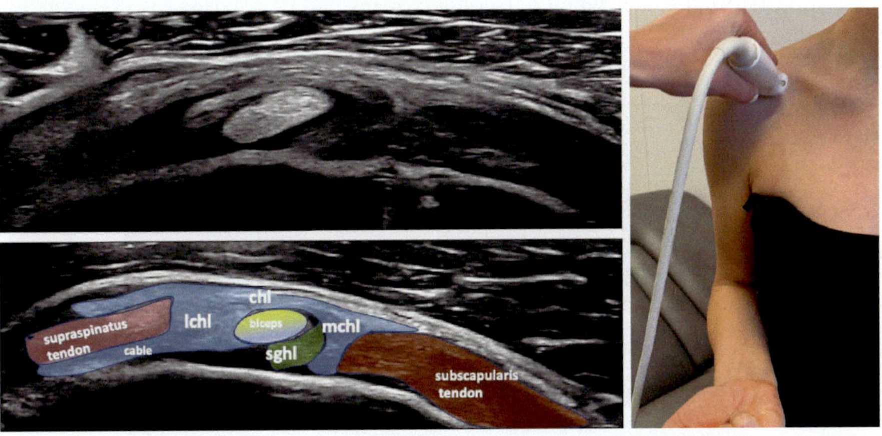

5.1.13   Ultrasound-Guided Injection
of the Subacromial-Subdeltoid Bursa

The rheumatologist should always face the monitor, so that, when holding the probe and introducing the needle, he has a direct view on the screen. The subacromial —subdeltoid bursa can be reached using an anterior, lateral or posterior approach. The glenohumeral joint can best be reached using a posterior approach, as the joint space is hard to visualize anteriorly.

Anterior approach to the bursa. The probe should be aligned with the transverse axis of the body, i.e., the long axis of the subscapularis tendon, while the patient is seated (or semisupine) with the arm in slight external rotation. The prescan should include the deltoid muscle, the rotator cuff, and the convex contour of the humeral head. The needle should be introduced laterally to the probe. The introduction of the needle can be directly visualized in real time. The needle appears as a bright line as long as it is kept parallel to the probe. The needle tip should ideally be identified as a moving deflector. The needle should be manipulated so that its progression can be followed on the screen. The needle tip should be followed into the subdeltoid bursa. Aspiration is often easier when a T-connector instead of a syringe is connected to the needle.

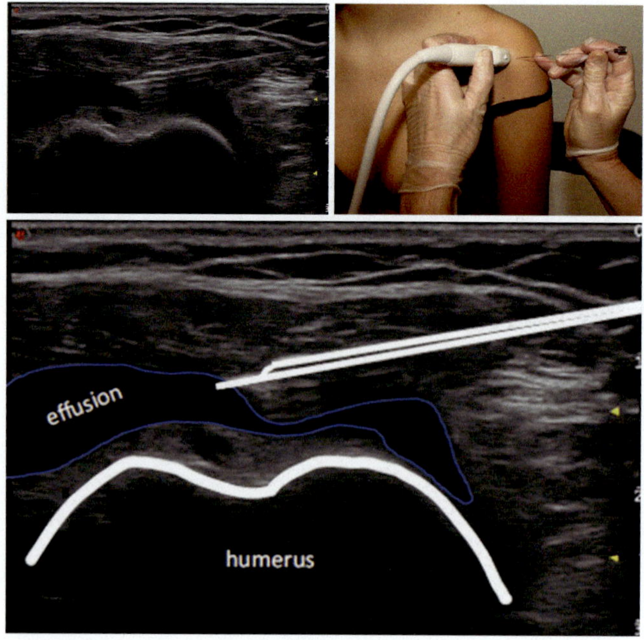

5.1.14   *Ultrasound-Guided Injection of the Glenohumeral Joint*

The glenohumeral joint can best be approached posteriorly, as the joint space is hard to visualize anteriorly.

Posterior approach to the joint. The probe should be aligned in a transverse scan with regard to the body, i.e., a longitudinal view of the infraspinatus muscle and tendon, while the patient is seated (or semisupine) with the arm in slight external rotation. The prescan should include the deltoid muscle, the infraspinatus tendon, the convex contour of the humeral head and the posterior glenoid labrum. A 5 cm long needle should be introduced medially or laterally to the probe. The introduction of the needle can be directly visualized in real time, while the needle appears as a bright line. It is usually not possible to have the probe completely parallel to the needle. The needle tip should ideally be identified as a moving deflector. Since the joint space is deeper than the bursa, the inclination of the needle insertion relative to the skin is steeper than the angle in the previous scan. The needle tip should be followed into the joint. The penetration of the joint capsule by the needle is felt as a transient resistance, followed by a slight sensation of vacuum suction. An option is to inject air into the joint for confirmation, which will give rise to bright bubbles.

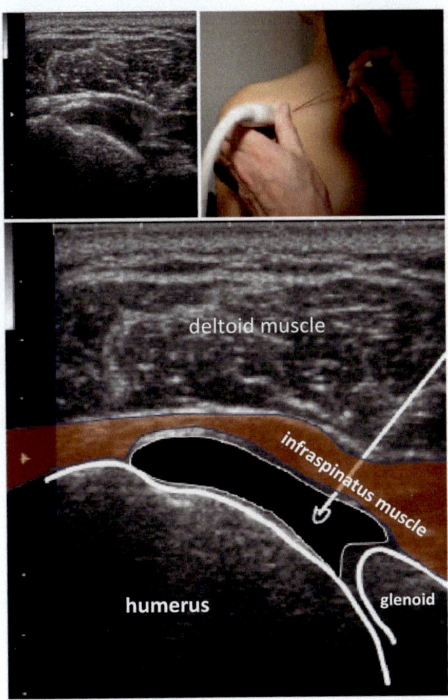

5.1.15   *Ultrasound-Guided Injection of the Long Biceps Tendon Sheath*

Fluid within the biceps tendon sheath is commonly seen. Usually, it is related to fluid within the glenohumeral joint, yet ultrasound may point to other diagnoses, including biceps sheath tenosynovitis or biceps tendinopathy. Thus, administering injectate into the biceps sheath will not only spread along the sheath itself, but will also pass into the glenohumeral joint cavity. The patient may be seated similar to 5.1.1, but for injections, a (semi) supine position may be preferred. Depending of the amount of visible fluid, the biceps tendon sheath may either be injected proximally in the bicipital groove, or at the end of the biceps tendon sheath near the myotendinous junction. The injection should be performed in plane, holding the probe in an axial plane.

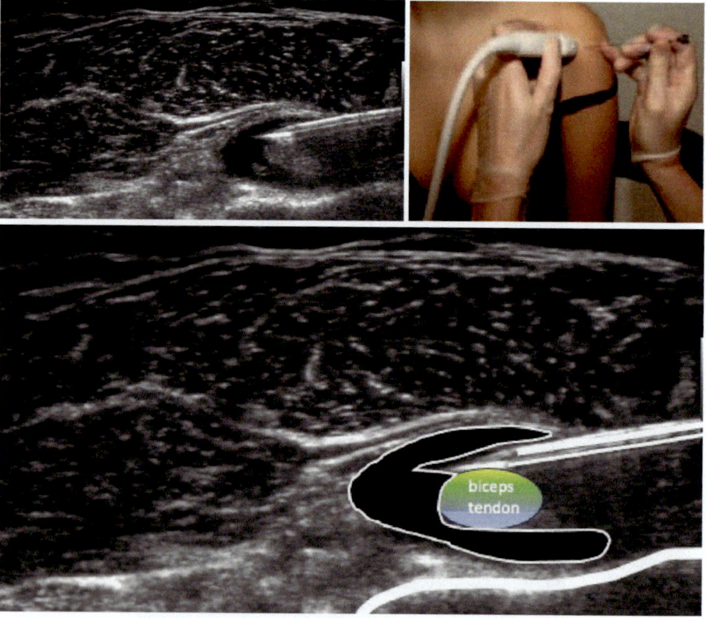

5.1.16 *Ultrasound-Guided Injection for Suprascapular Nerve Block or Posterior Labrum Cyst Aspiration*

The supascapular nerve can be blocked either at the suprascapular notch or at the spinoglenoid notch (Figure **a**). Suprascapular nerve compression is commonly the result of impingement by the transverse scapular ligament or a labrum cyst, respectively. A labrum cyst may arise when joint fluid leaks through a torn postero-superior glenoid labrum (Figure **c**). These labrum cysts may balloon in loci minoris resistentiae, like the spinoglenoid notch, impinging the distal branch of the nerve and resulting in atrophy of the infraspinatus muscle belly. Impingement of the suprascapular nerve in the superiorly located scapular notch by a thickened ligament not only leads to chronic shoulder pain, but also to atrophy of both the supraspinatus and infraspinatus muscle bellies.

a. *Nerve block of the suprascapular nerve in the suprascapular notch.* With the patient seated, the ultrasound-guided injection of the superior scapular notch is performed with the probe in a coronal position over the suprascapular fossa. Superficial to the fossa, the trapezius and supraspinatus muscles are identified. Deep to the supraspinatus muscle, the bony contour of the notch is identified. The depth should be adjusted, as the nerve, accompanied by the artery, just saddle on top of the bony surface. Use Doppler mode to visualize the artery. Injection should be done in plane.

b. *Nerve block of the suprascapular nerve in the spinoglenoid notch.* Ultrasound-guided block of the nerve in the spinoglenoid notch is done in a slightly oblique axial plane, starting with a transverse scan of the posterior humeral head, the posterior recess, the infraspinatus muscle and the scapular spine. Less depth is necessary compared to the suprascapular notch scan. Use Doppler again to localize the artery, which is on top of the nerve here.

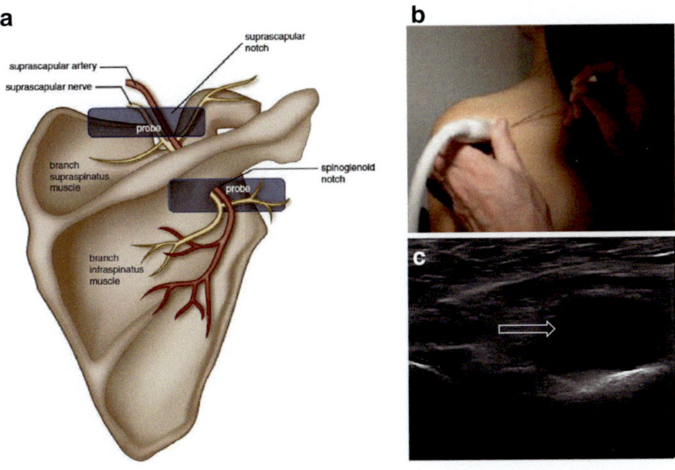

Figure **c** shows a posterior longitudinal scan at the level of the spinoglenoid notch. A labrum cyst (arrow) is visible which can be punctured under ultrasound-guidance (Figure **b**).

5.2   Pathology of the Shoulder

5.2.1   Pathology of the Biceps Tendon 1

Best Scans: Standard Scans 5-1 and 5-2.

In Fig. 5.1, a hypoechoic rim resembling a halo is visible around the biceps tendon (long head) on the transverse scan. The fluid distends the sheath of the biceps tendon (Figs. 5.1 and 5.2) and causes the transverse ligament to pop up. This fluid may represent either synovial fluid from the joint or a genuine biceps tenosynovitis. Compress in order to distinguish between sheath synovitis and synovial fluid spilling over from the glenohumeral joint. Synovial hypertrophy is non-compressible whereas synovial fluid can be balloted away by probe pressure.

Figure 5.2 depicts a longitudinal ultrasound scan of the biceps tendon showing a hypoechoic fluid collection anteriorly and posteriorly of the tendon.

Figure 5.3 depicts a transverse scan of the anterior shoulder in a patient with polymyalgia rheumatica. Showing a widened long biceps tendon sheath, hypoechoic material around the biceps tendon consistent with tenosynovitis is present. Doppler signals reflect the intense inflammation.

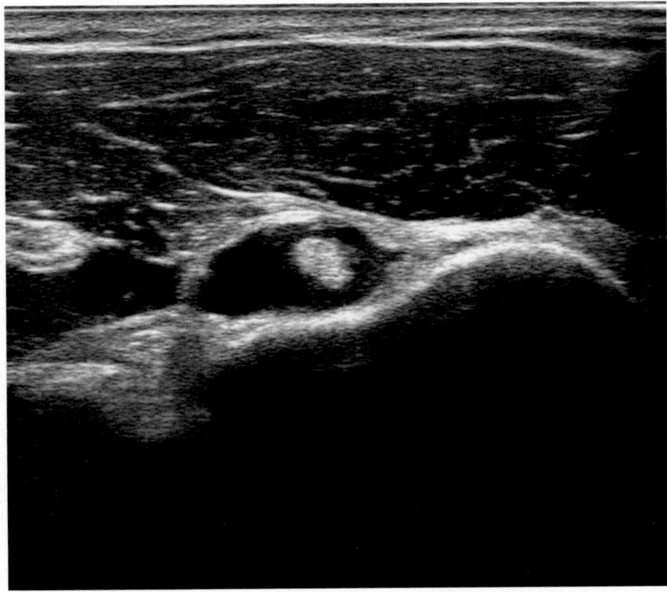

Fig. 5.1 Tenosynovitis, long biceps tendon (transverse scan of biceps tendon)

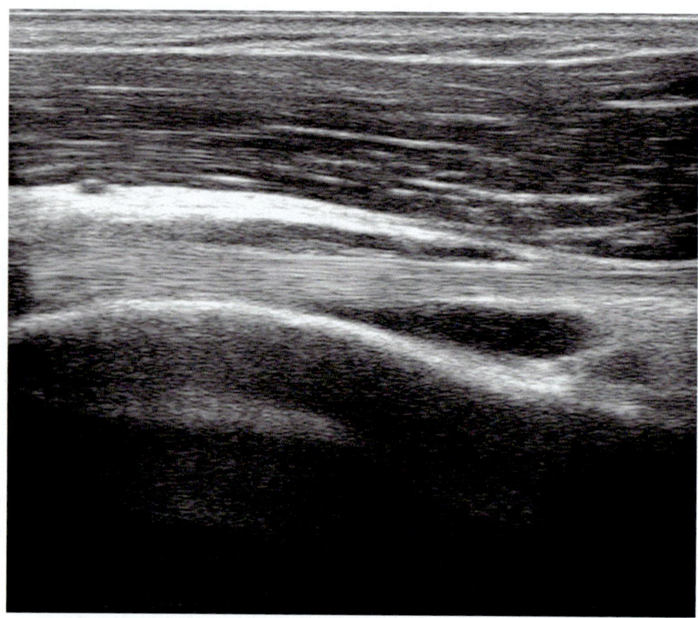

Fig. 5.2 Tenosynovitis, long biceps tendon (longitudinal scan of biceps tendon)

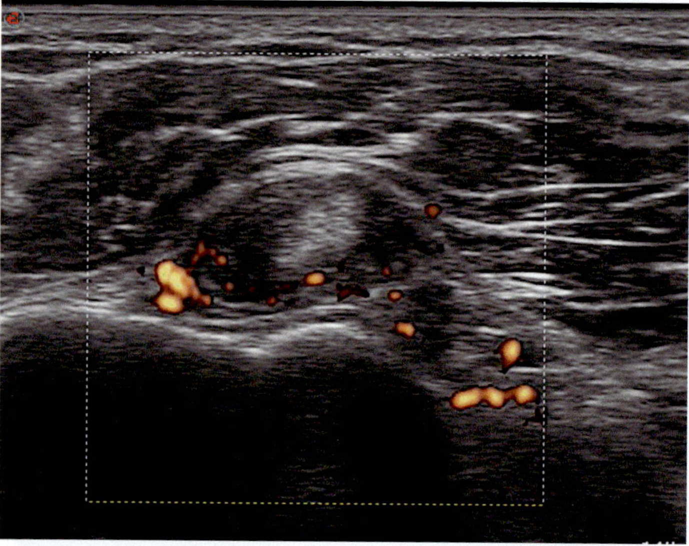

Fig. 5.3 Tenosynovitis of the long biceps tendon (transverse scan of biceps tendon)

5.2.2 *Pathology of the Biceps Tendon 2*

Best Scans: Standard Scans 5-1 and 5-2.

Figure 5.4 is a transverse scan showing the long head of the biceps tendon ($\Rightarrow\Leftarrow$) medial to the bicipital groove. The empty bicipital groove ($\Uparrow$) appears to be filled with isoechoic material corresponding to soft tissue. Most dislocations of the long head of the biceps tendon occur medially.

Figure 5.5 is a longitudinal scan showing anechoic fluid ($\Downarrow$) within the bicipital sheath due to a tear of the long head. There is an associated effusion of the subdeltoid bursa ($\Uparrow$).

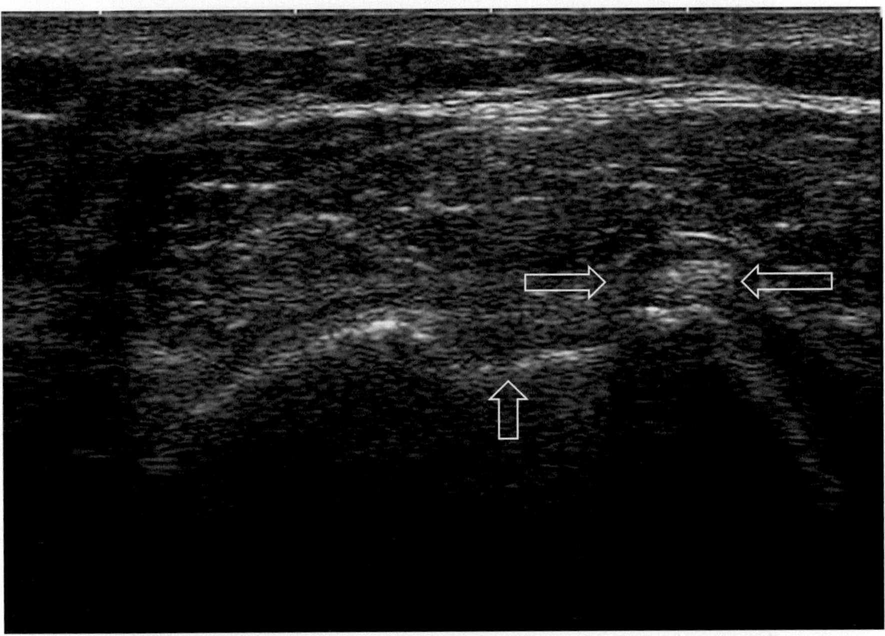

Fig. 5.4 Dislocation of long biceps tendon (transverse scan of biceps tendon)

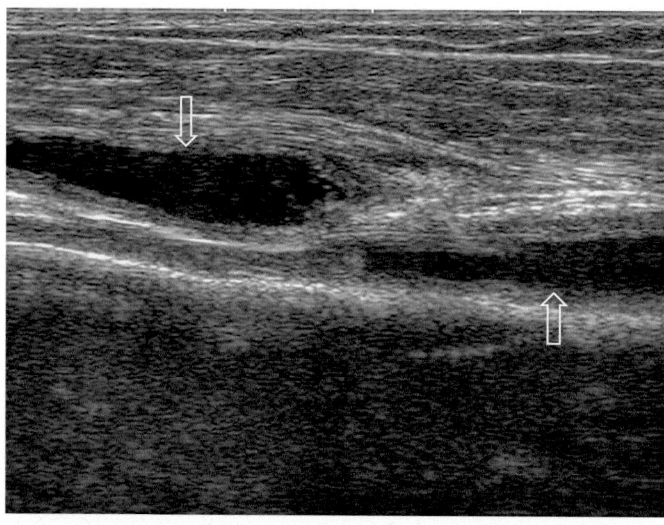

Fig. 5.5 Long biceps tendon tear and subdeltoid bursitis (longitudinal scan of biceps tendon)

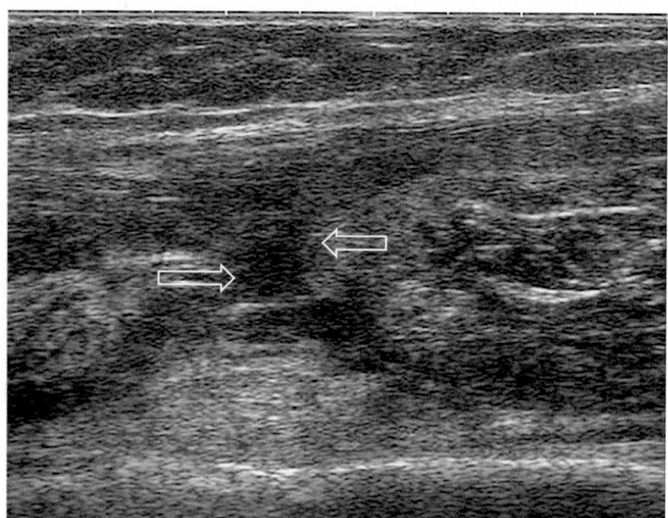

Fig. 5.6 Long head of biceps muscle tear (longitudinal scan of biceps tendon and muscle)

Figure 5.6 is a longitudinal scan of the long head of the biceps muscle close to the musculotendinous junction showing a full-thickness tear. There is a central discontinuity of the muscle with hypoechoic material consistent with a hematoma filling the gap. The two retracted muscle margins are also visible ($\Rightarrow \Leftarrow$).

5.2.3 Subdeltoid Bursitis

Best scans: Standard Scans 5-3 to 5-8.

Figure 5.7 is a longitudinal ultrasound image showing both hypoechoic fluid in the subdeltoid bursa (⇓) and a small quantity of fluid surrounding the long head of the biceps tendon. The bursa is anterior to the tendon.

Figures 5.8 a, b are transverse scans showing a fluid-distended subdeltoid bursa in a patient with rheumatoid arthritis.

Figure 5.9 is an anterior transverse scan showing an inflamed fluid-distended bursa in a patient with polymyalgia rheumatica. The biceps tendon is not visible due to anisotropy (*).

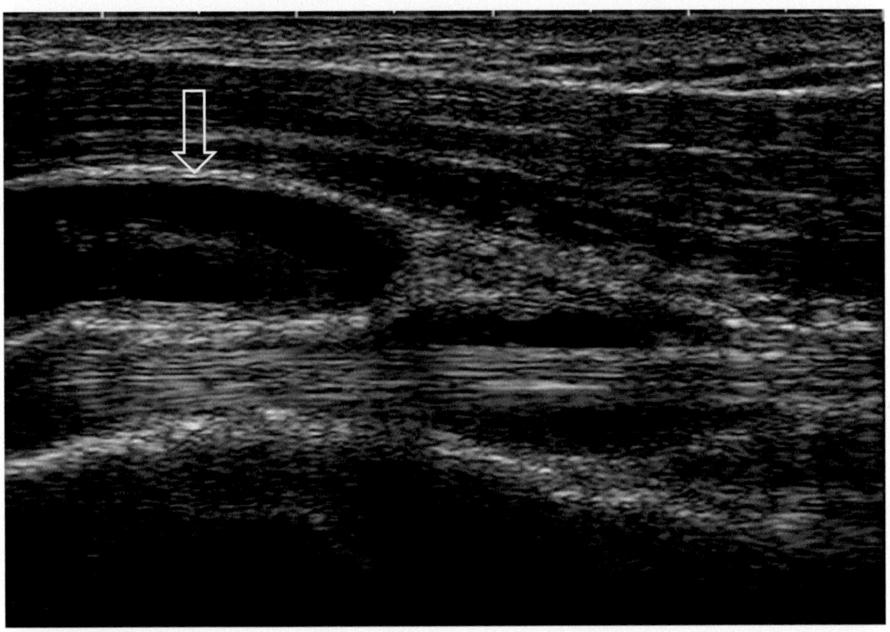

Fig. 5.7 Subdeltoid bursitis and tenosynovitis of the long biceps tendon (longitudinal view of biceps tendon)

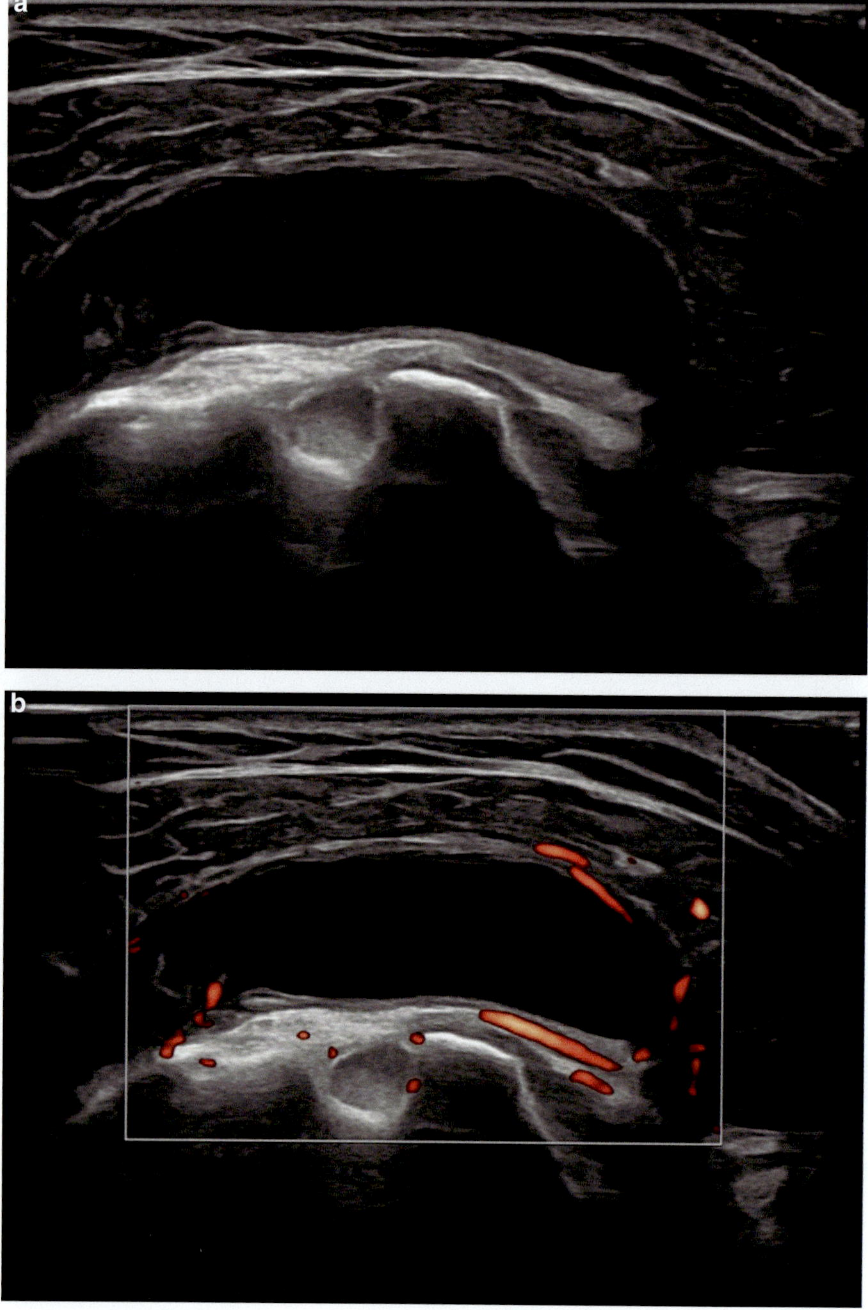

Fig. 5.8 a, **b** Inflammatory subdeltoid bursitis in rheumatoid arthritis (transverse anterior view)

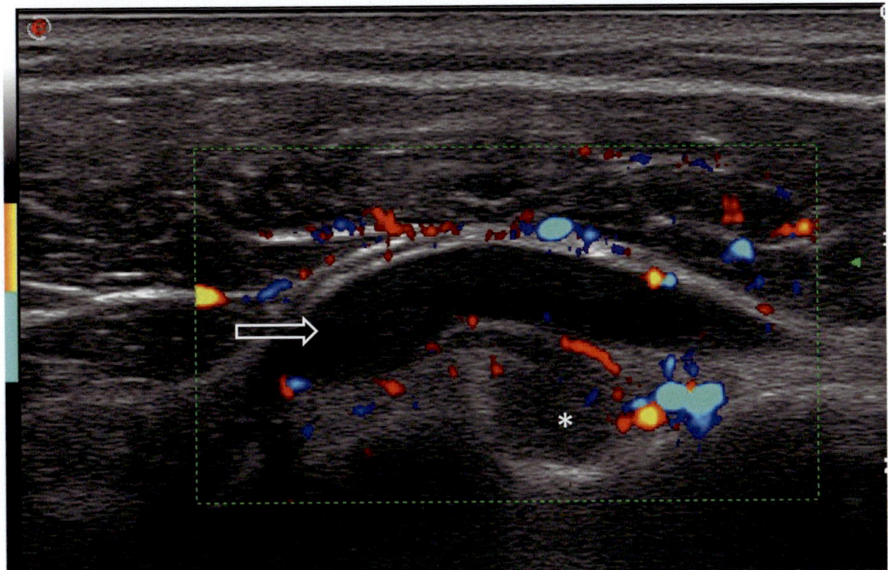

Fig. 5.9 Active subdeltoid bursitis (transverse anterior view)

5.2.4 Crystal Arthropathies

Best scans: Standard Scans 5-3 to 5-8.

Figure 5.10 shows multiple conglomerates of hyperechoic deposits in the hyaline cartilage ($\Leftarrow$) corresponding to chondrocalcinosis. The supraspinatus tendon is inhomogeneous with flattening in the center ($\Downarrow$) due to a tendon tear.

Figure 5.11 shows a massively distended subdeltoid bursa filled with cloudy deposits consistent with urate aggregates ($\Rightarrow\Leftarrow$). In between the cloudy deposits, two fluid-filled vacuoles are present. In addition, urate aggregates are present around the long head of the biceps tendon ($\Uparrow$).

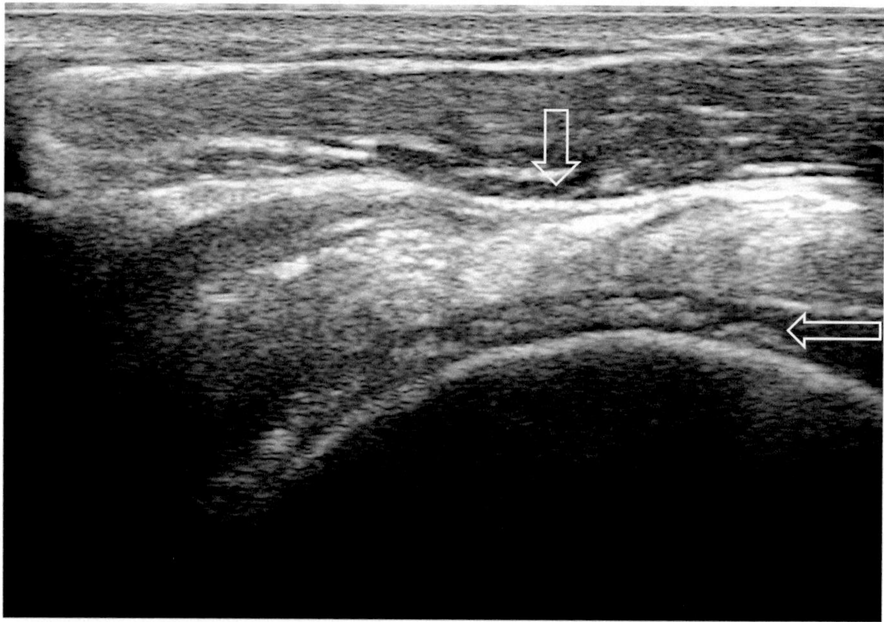

Fig. 5.10 Chondrocalcinosis of the shoulder together with partial tear of the supraspinatus tendon (lateral longitudinal scan)

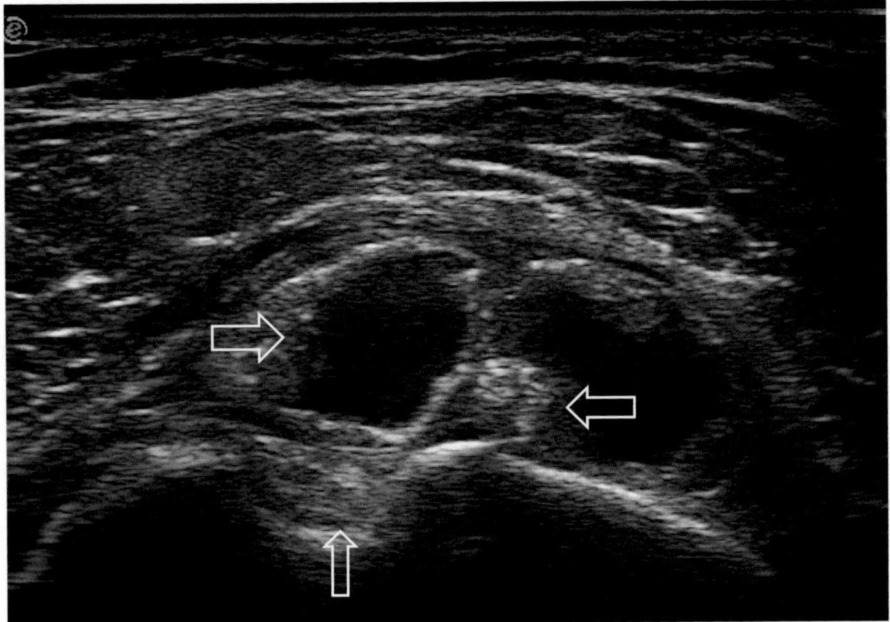

Fig. 5.11 Inflammatory subdeltoid bursitis in gout (transverse anterior scan)

5.2.5　Tears of the Rotator Cuff

Best Scans: Standard Scans 5-3 to 5-8.

In the normal situation, the supraspinatus tendon is found as a tendon deep of the deltoid muscle.

Figure 5.12 shows the humeral head and the deltoid muscle with complete absence of the supraspinatus tendon, leaving a "bald" humeral head, due to a complete retraction of the supraspinatus tendon below the acromion. Large tears as seen on this scan, have the characteristic appearance of the complete absence of the supraspinatus tendon.

Figure 5.13 shows a focal depression (⇊) due to loss of the normal convexity of the superior surface of the supraspinatus tendon, with the deltoid muscle sinking into the gap. This is a full-thickness tear. Rotator cuff tears are sonographically hypoechoic or anechoic as generally fluid—synovial fluid or blood—will fill up the lesion.

Figure 5.14 shows a clear discontinuity of the supraspinatus tendon as an anechoic area (⇒⇐). Of note, there is a communication with a distended bursa (⇊) filled with fluid. This represents a partial thickness tear of the supraspinatus tendon.

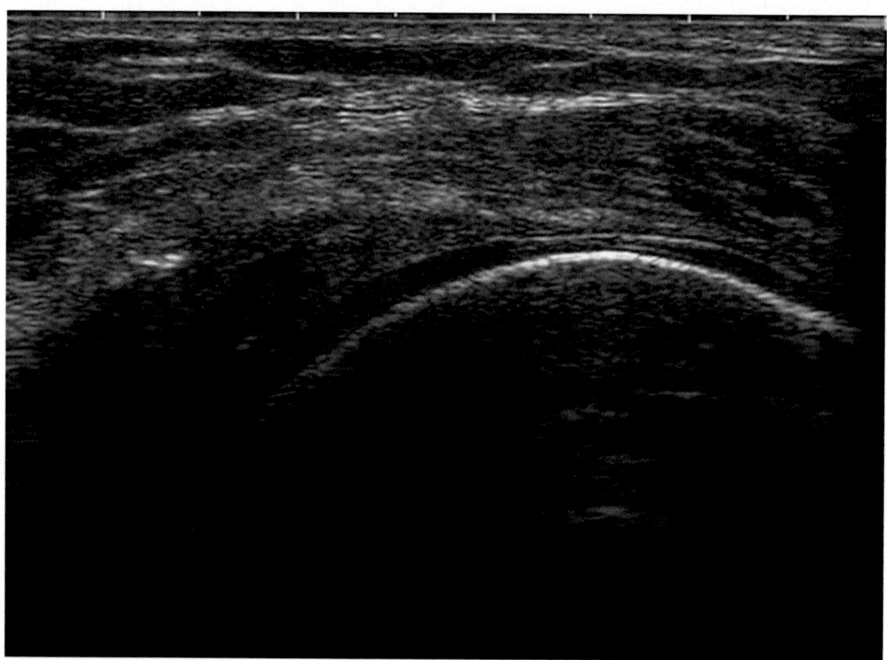

Fig. 5.12 Complete tear of supraspinatus tendon with "bald" humeral head (anterior transverse scan)

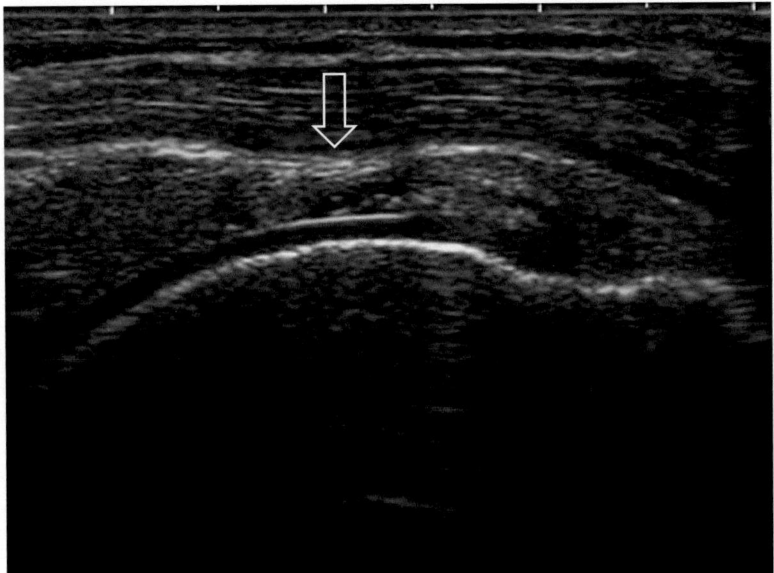

Fig. 5.13 Full-thickness tear of supraspinatus tendon (anterior transverse scan)

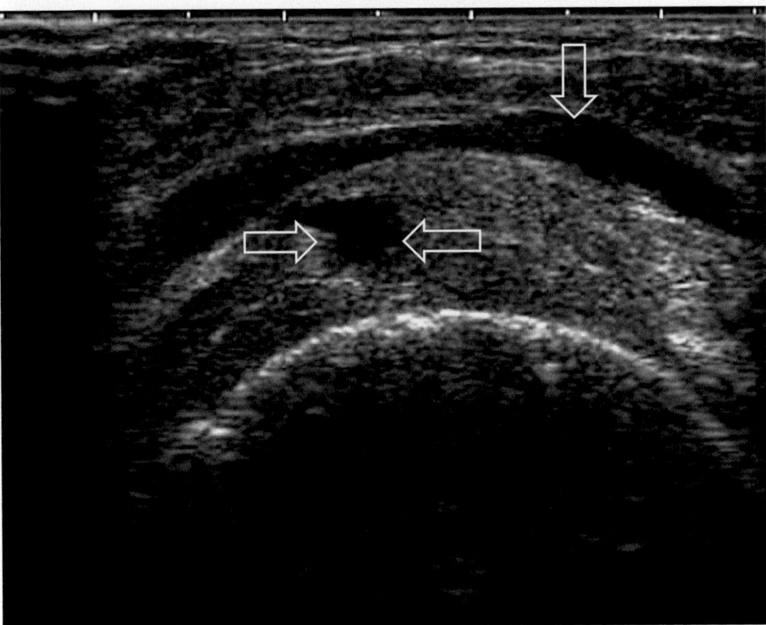

Fig. 5.14 Partial thickness incomplete tear of supraspinatus tendon and subdeltoid bursitis (anterior transverse scan)

5.2.6   Other Pathologies of the Rotator Cuff

Best Scans: Standard Scan 5-3 to 5-8.

Figure 5.15 shows an erosion with irregular floor of the humeral head (⇑). There is a small depression in the convex superficial surface of the supraspinatus tendon because of a partial thickness tear.

The supraspinatus tendon shown in Fig. 5.16 is thickened and inhomogeneous due to tendinitis. The sagittal diameter is 10.4 mm (normal < 6.5 mm). The dark areas (⇑) represent a partial tendon tear that does not reach the deltoid border of the tendon.

Figure 5.17 shows a well demarcated hyperechoic structure (⇒⇐) in the subscapularis tendon with an acoustic shadow. This represents a calcification. The pitfall of a single hyperechoic focus is that this may be confused with a rotator cuff tear.

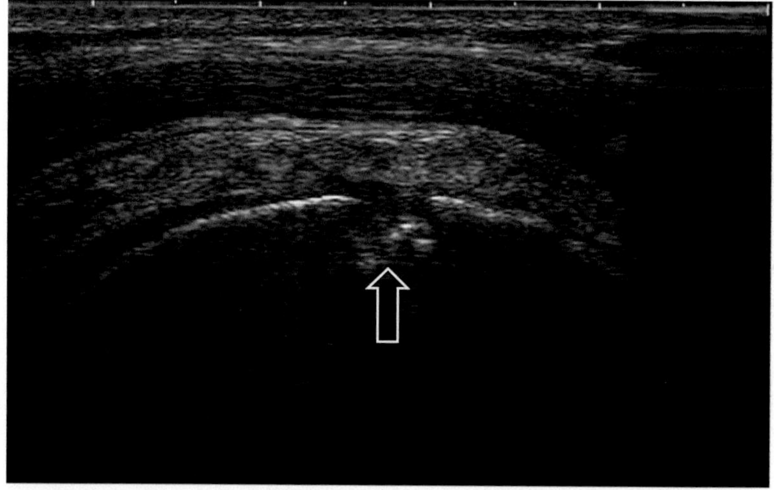

Fig. 5.15 Supraspinatus tendon with an erosion of the humeral head and partial tear (anterior longitudinal view)

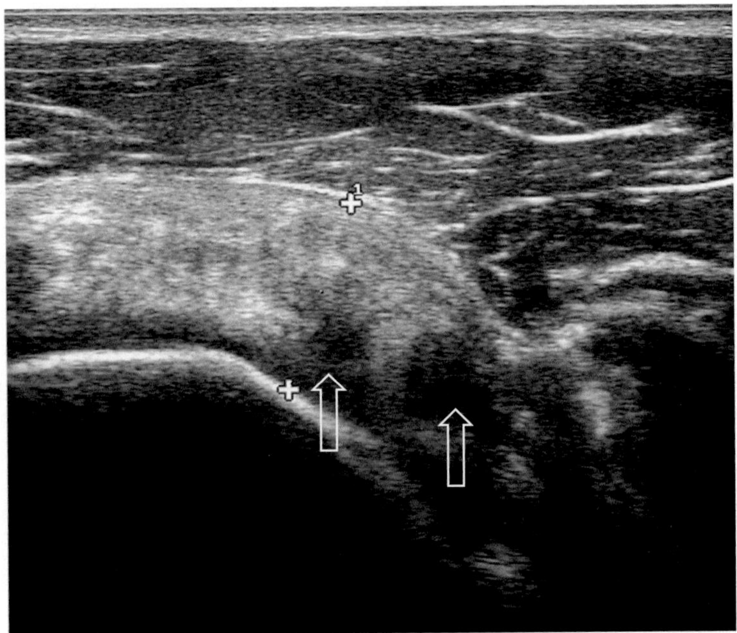

Fig. 5.16 Tendinitis with an inhomogeneous, thickened and partially torn supraspinatus tendon (anterior transverse view)

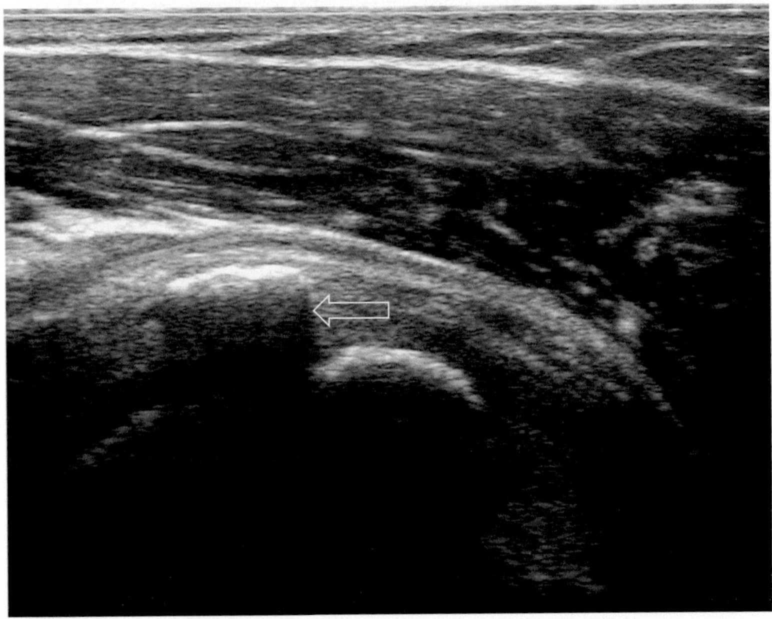

Fig. 5.17 Calcification of the subscapularis tendon (anterior longitudinal view)

5.2.7   Glenohumeral Joint Synovitis and Effusion

Best Scans: Standard Scans 5-3, 5-7, 5-8 and 5-10.

There are two accessible recesses of the glenohumeral joint with ultrasound. In the transverse scan of the posterior recess, fluid can be observed in the posterior glenohumeral joint (Fig. 5.18). Elevation of the joint capsule of more than 3 mm from the humeral head is a strong indicator of effusion or synovitis (+…+) if the shoulder is externally rotated. The capsule is localized just below the infraspinatus tendon or muscle. This ultrasound image depicts a large effusion that is visible even in internal rotation.

In Fig. 5.19, a small quantity of hypoechoic material (⇓) is seen in the glenohumeral joint in this transverse posterior sonogram. This material may represent either effusion or synovitis. The glenoid labrum is absent. Furthermore, there are osteophytes (⇑) and erosions (⇐) at the humeral head. After recurrent luxation this is called Hill-Sachs lesion.

Figure 5.20 shows hypoechoic material in the axillary recess that indicates synovitis. The joint capsule (⇓) is slightly elevated so that it is not any more parallel to the humeral head and neck. This image also shows osteophytes at the humeral head (⇑) that represent osteoarthritis of the glenohumeral joint.

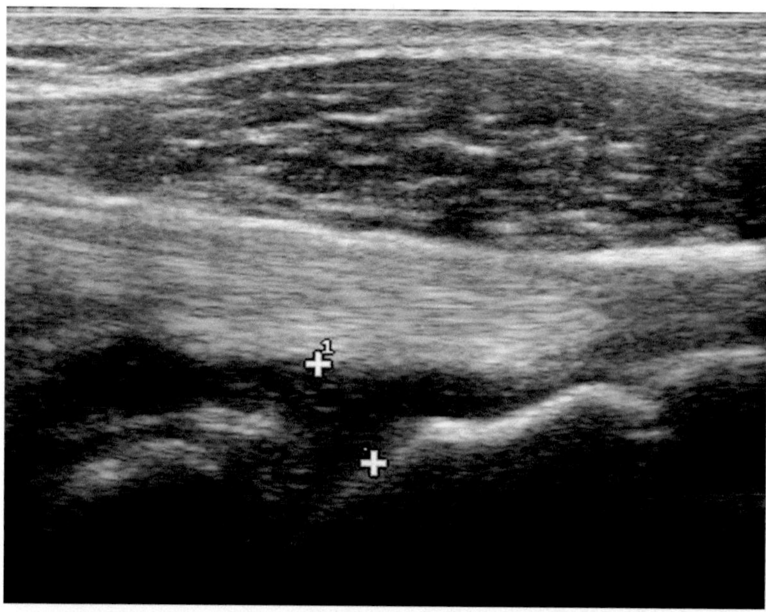

Fig. 5.18   Large effusion of the glenohumeral joint (posterior transverse scan)

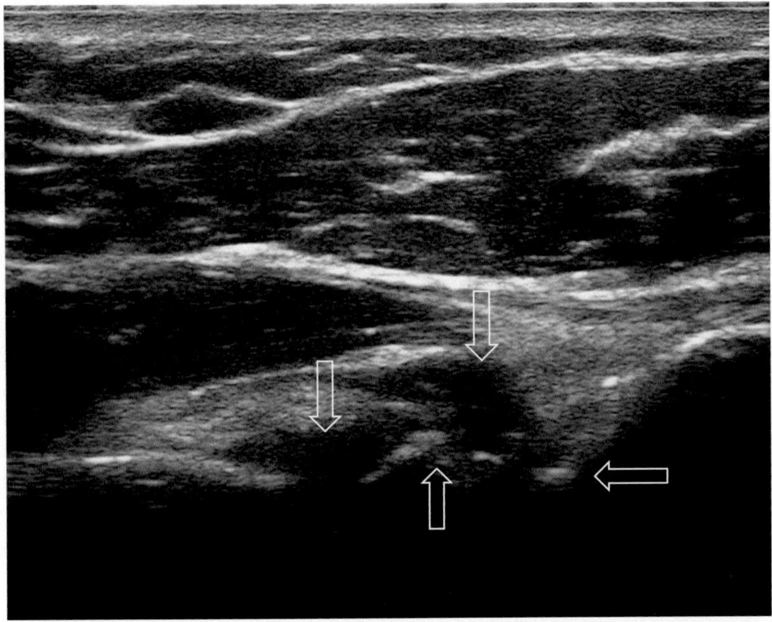

Fig. 5.19 Glenohumeral joint with small effusion, osteophytes, erosions, and destroyed glenoid labrum (posterior transverse scan)

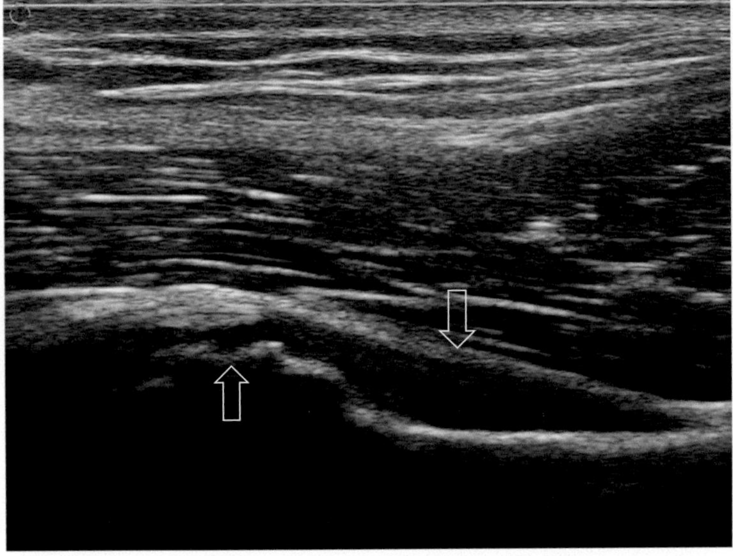

Fig. 5.20 Synovitis at the axillary recess with osteophytes of the humeral head (axillary scan)

5.2.8   Pathologies of the Acromioclavicular and Sternoclavicular Joints

Best Scans: Standard Scans 5-9 and 5-12.

Figure 5.21 shows a marked elevation of the superior joint capsule of the right acromioclavicular joint with thickened synovium. This sign is called the "geyser" phenomenon. Slight bony irregularities represent minor osteoarthritis.

Figure 5.22 shows the relationship of the rotator cuff and the acromioclavicular joint. The distance between the distal margins of the acromion and the clavicle is markedly increased due to a tear of the acromioclavicular ligament. In this patient, there might be an associated tear of the much stronger coracoclavicular ligament. An effusion with hyperechoic dots is present in the AC joint which corresponds with a subacromial bursa. The supraspinatus tendon is visible at the bottom of the effusion.

In SAPHO syndrome, the sternoclavicular joint is often inflamed. Synovitis may also occur in other rheumatic diseases. Figure 5.23 shows a markedly elevated capsule of the sternoclavicular joint due to synovitis in a patient with SAPHO syndrome. In chronic synovitis of the sternoclavicular joint, the bone surface is often more irregular.

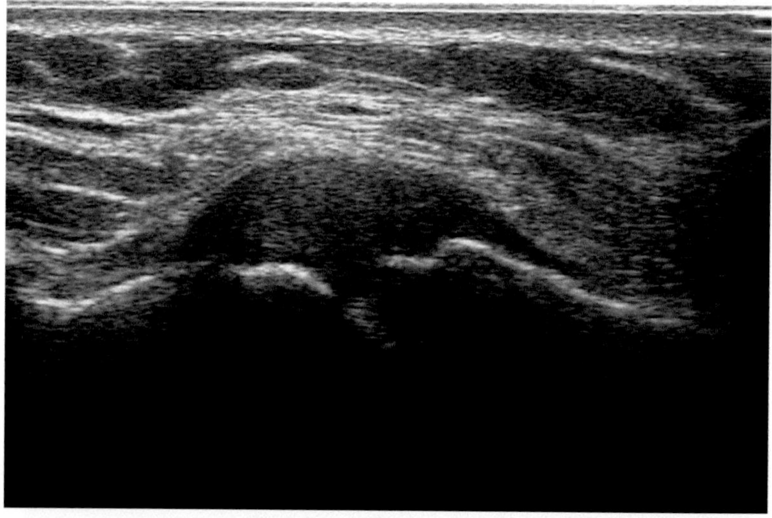

Fig. 5.21 Synovitis of the acromioclavicular (AC) joint, aka geyser sign (acromioclavicular joint view)

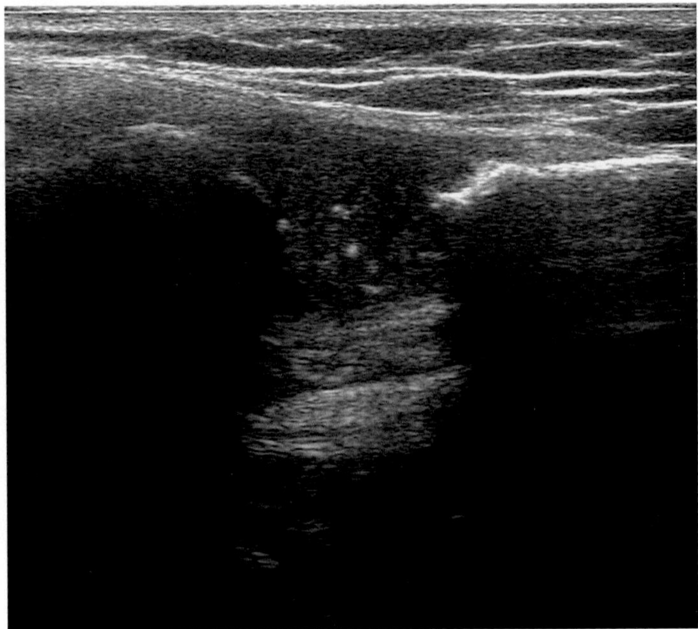

Fig. 5.22 Luxation of the AC joint with effusion and tear of the AC ligament (acromioclavicular joint view)

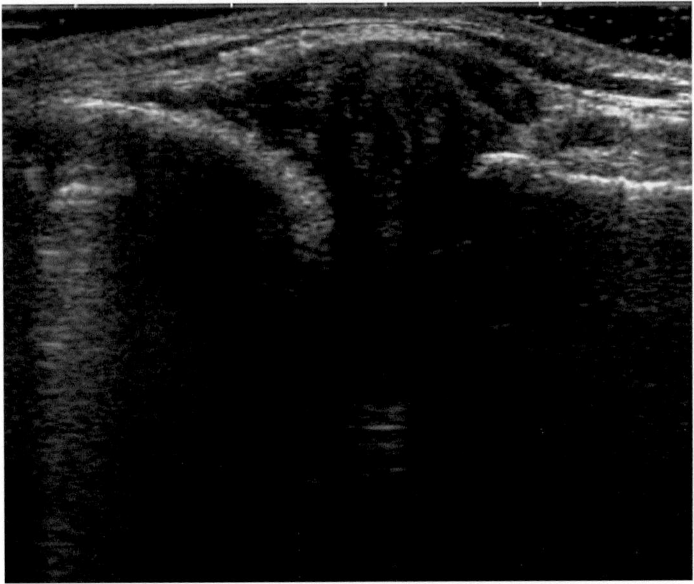

Fig. 5.23 Synovitis of the right sternoclavicular joint. The clavicle is on the left side. The sternum is on the right side (sternoclavicular joint view)

Chapter 6
The Elbow

6.1 Standard Scans of the Elbow

6.1.1 Anterior Longitudinal View of the Humeroulnar Joint (Standard Scan 6-1)

The ultrasound examination of the elbow starts with the longitudinal view of the anterior side of the humeroulnar joint, holding the probe longitudinally to the axis of the arm.

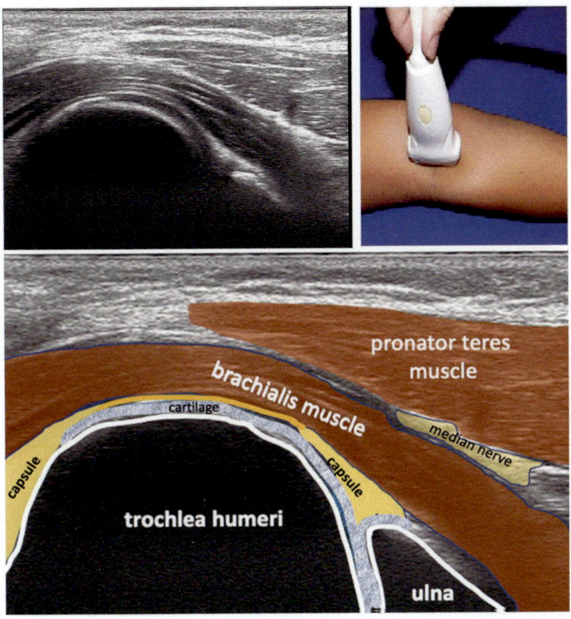

© The Author(s), under exclusive license to Springer Nature Switzerland AG 2023
G. A. W. Bruyn and W. A. Schmidt, *Musculoskeletal Ultrasound for the Rheumatologist*,
https://doi.org/10.1007/978-3-031-27737-5_6

The patient is sitting on a stool or is supine with the elbow completely extended and supinated.

In the middle of the image, the humeral trochlea is located covered by hyaline cartilage; at the distal pole of the articulation the coronoid process of the ulna is visualized. Cranial to the trochlea, the coronoid fossa containing fat tissue is visible. Anterior to the joint, the brachialis muscle is found. It inserts distally at the ulnar tuberosity.

What is normal?

Normally no fluid is visible in the coronoid fossa. The coronoid fossa contains a fat body.

6.1.2   Anterior Longitudinal View of the Humeroradial Joint (Standard Scan 6-2)

The probe is continuously shifted radially from Standard Scan 6-1. The patient's and the examiner's position remain the same as with the previous view. The anterior side should be well exposed by full extension of the elbow.

This view shows the capitulum humeri and the head of the radius. The joint capsule extends cranially far along the capitulum humeri into the radial fossa. It can be seen at the very left end of the ultrasound image and the anatomic drawing. The joint capsule attaches distally at the radial head not far from the joint. Between the humerus and the radius, we can detect the capsule, fat tissue and a fibrocartilaginous meniscus-like synovial fold. Anterior to the joint, the brachioradialis muscle is visible. Directly anterior to the radial shaft, the supinator muscle can be visualized.

What is normal?

The hyaline cartilage covering the capitulum can be easily seen. The synovial fold exhibits a V-form. The radial fossa contains fat tissue. Distance between the bone of the radial fossa and the capsule: 1.8 mm (0–3.7 mm).

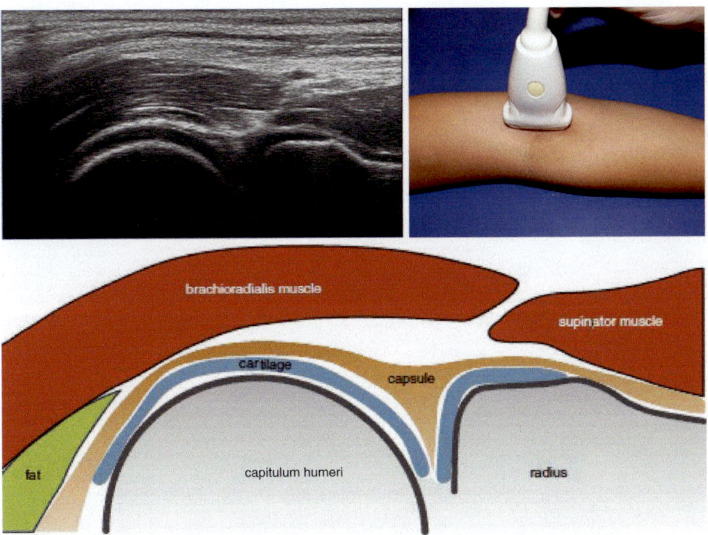

6.1.3   Anterior Transverse View of the Elbow (Standard Scan 6-3)

The position of the patient and the examiner remain the same as in Standard Scans 6-1 and 6-2. The probe is rotated by 90°. On the left side of the screen the capitulum humeri is found, while on the right side the trochlea humeri is visible.

Both humerus and joint capsule have a similar hyperechoic appearance as the joint capsule of the elbow is strong and rather thick. The capsule runs directly parallel to the bony contour of the capitulum and the trochlea. The anechoic region between capsule and bone represents cartilage.

If effusion is present, hypoechoic fluid will lift the capsule, particularly in the fossae. This can be seen when the probe is shifted proximally.

Two portions of the distal biceps tendon (in the top center of this transverse anterior view) can also be examined. Both attach further distally at the ulnar aspect of the bicipital tuberosity on the radius. The long head inserts proximally and the short head of the distal biceps tendon more distally at the tuberosity. The third aponeurosis-like portion, which is called the lacertus fibrosus, originates from the distal short head and is usually not visible with ultrasound. The median nerve localizes medially to the brachial artery.

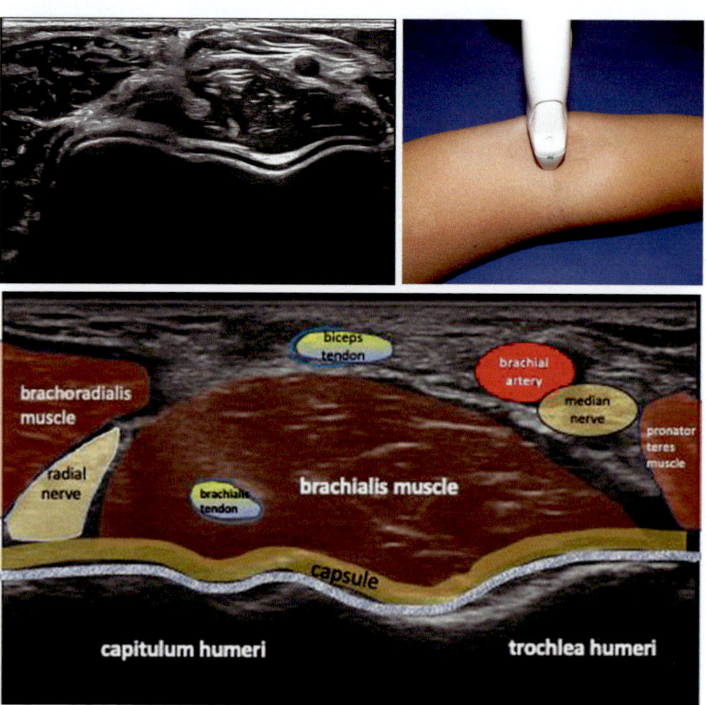

The radial nerve is located between the brachialis and the brachioradialis muscles. Mostly the nerve has already just divided into its superficial branch (lateral) and its posterior interosseous branch (medial) at the level of the elbow. The pronator teres muscle may be seen on the right side of this scan if the probe would be shifted more medially.

What is normal?

The capsule follows the contours of the hyaline cartilage. Bone capsule distance between bone and joint capsule at the ulnar side: 1.0 mm (0.5–1.5 mm). This is usually equivalent to the thickness of the hyaline cartilage.

6.1.4 Posterior Longitudinal View of the Elbow (Standard Scan 6-4)

The posterior longitudinal Standard Scan is suitable for examining the three portions of the triceps muscle, their common tendon with its insertion on the olecranon, the olecranon fossa, and the posterior joint space. Musculoskeletal pathology seen on this standard scan includes particularly joint space effusion. The probe may be shifted distally in order to visualize olecranon bursitis or triceps tendon enthesitis.

In order to obtain an optimal exposure of the joint space and the olecranon fossa, the long axis view is done with the elbow flexed by 90°. The hand may rest on the examination couch. The elbow can be flexed and extended in order to detect small amounts of fluid in the joint.

The humerus and the olecranon fossa with its fat pad are visualized. Posterior to the humerus a long axis view of the triceps muscle is obtained, coursing distally towards its insertion on the olecranon. The bony olecranon is easily identified.

What is normal?

With the elbow flexed, ultrasound allows identification of as little as 1–3 ml of fluid posteriorly. The bone-joint capsule distance at the bottom of the olecranon fossa (a): 1.9 mm (0–3.9 mm).

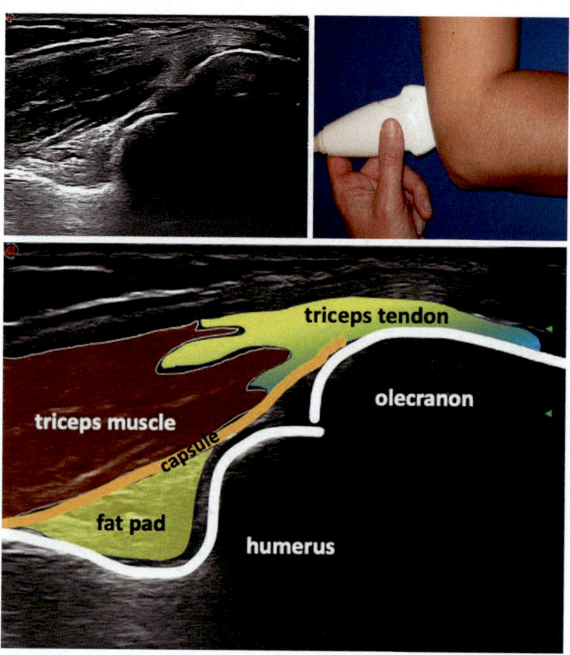

6.1.5 Posterior Transverse View of the Elbow (Standard Scan 6-5)

Rotating the probe by 90° yields the short axis posterior view. Patient and the elbow remain in the same as with the longitudinal view.

In the transverse view, the two humeral epicondyles are visible on each side of the screen. In the middle, the olecranon fossa is filled with fat tissue. Posterior to the fossa, the triceps muscle or its tendon is identified. The medial head of the triceps tendon is the deepest part of the triceps muscle, it has a shorter tendon part than the other heads and a further distal insertion on the olecranon.

This standard scan can be extended distally and ulnarly for examining the ulnar nerve, which runs in the ulnar groove next to the medial epicondyle (Standard Scan 6-8). The probe can also be shifted distally over the olecranon for olecranon bursitis and, further distally, rheumatic nodules.

What is normal?

Small amounts of physiological fluid may be present at the bottom of the fossa as mentioned on the previous page.

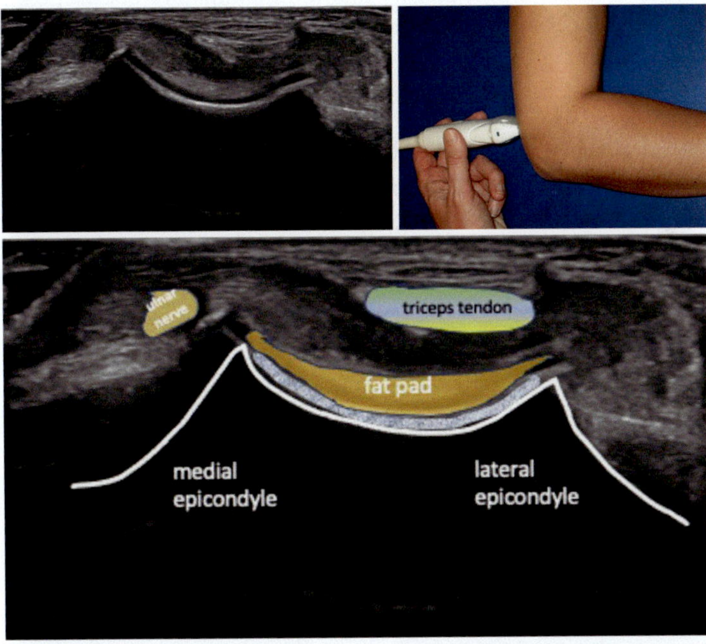

6.1.6   Lateral Longitudinal View of the Elbow (Standard Scan 6-6)

The long-axis view of the lateral aspect, together with standard scan 6-2, is the standard position for the examination of the origin of the common extensor tendon at the lateral epicondyle, the humero-radial joint and the lateral collateral ligament. The patient is seated with the elbow resting on the table. The examination may be easier with varying degrees of flexion of the elbow up to 90°.

The common extensor tendon is composed of different muscle slips, which usually cannot be reliably separated. The common extensor origin is identified as a triangular shaped, slightly hyperechoic structure comprising four superficial extensor muscles, i.e., the extensor carpi ulnaris, the extensor digiti minimi, the extensor digitorum communis, and the extensor carpi radialis brevis. Note that the other extensor tendons, i.e., the extensor radialis longus and the brachioradialis tendon, originate more proximally from a lateral ridge on the humerus. The fibers of the lateral radial collateral ligament (RCL) are coursing deep to the common extensor tendon. This Standard Scan is also suitable to visualize the annular ligament around the radial head.

The extensor tendon insertion may become inflamed both in common overload conditions such as "tennis elbow" and in inflammatory disease, e.g., spondyloarthritis. The hypoechoic origin correlates to edema, and power Doppler shows increased perfusion in enthesitis.

What is normal?

The tendons are homogeneous and slightly hyperechoic. Close to their insertion they may become hypoechoic due to anisotropy. Heel-toe the probe in order to avoid anisotropy. It is important to shift the probe slowly in order to see all parts of the tendons.

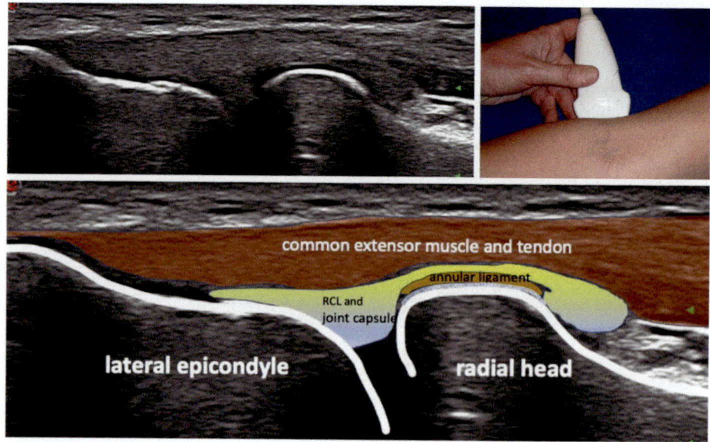

6.1.7 *Medial Longitudinal View of the Elbow (Standard Scan 6-7)*

Standard scan 6-7 is the medial mirror image of the Standard Scan 6-6. The position of the patient is different though, as the elbow is now fully extended and the hand supinated. The medial longitudinal view provides information about the medial epicondyle, which is the humeral site where the common flexor tendon originates.

The standard scan also visualizes the anterior portion of the ulnar collateral ligament (ucl). The ulnar collateral ligament is identified as a tight band-like structure that stretches from the medial epicondyle to the tubercular portion of the coronoid process.

The common flexor tendon origin has a slightly hyperechoic appearance similar to its mirror image on the lateral side. The origin is prone to enthesitis, giving rise to what is known as "golfers elbow".

What is normal?

The ulnar collateral ligament attaches to the coronoid process; the ligament comprises 3 bands: anterior (the most important), posterior and transverse. The superficial surface of the ligament is outlined as a hyperechoic straight line, prone to anisotropy.

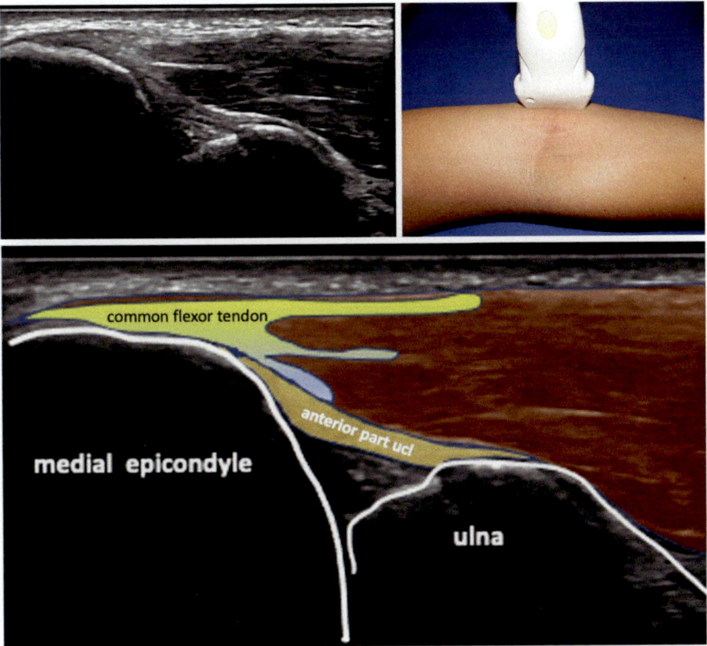

6.1.8   *Transverse View of the Cubital Tunnel of the Elbow (Standard Scan 6-8)*

From the position in Standard Scan 6-5, the probe is shifted more distally and ulnarly so that the distal pole of the probe is seated on the olecranon and the proximal pole on the medial epidcondyle. The ulnar nerve is positioned in the cubital tunnel along the posteromedial aspect of the distal humerus, adjacent to the medial epicondyle. The proximal roof of the cubital tunnel is formed by a thin ligament called Osborne retinaculum. The floor of the tunnel is formed by the posterior part of the ulnar collateral ligament along with the joint capsule of the humeroulnar joint space. In the transverse scan, nerves have a honeycomb-like appearance, with hypoechoic, rounded areas embedded in a hyperechoic background. The hypoechoic structures correspond to the neuronal fascicles that run longitudinally within the nerve, and the hyperechoic background relates to the interfascicular epineurium. The outer boundaries of the ulnar nerve may be poorly demarcated, because of the similar hyperechoic appearance of the superficial epineurium and the surrounding soft tissue and fat tissue.

Testing for ulnar nerve dislocation during flexion can be best performed by putting a wrapped towel beneath the elbow, so that the lower arm can be easily flexed and extended.

What is normal?

A cross-sectional area of ≤ 7 mm^2 is normal, ≥ 9 mm^2 is pathologic, and 8 mm^2 is borderline. There is no difference between the dominant and non-dominant arm.

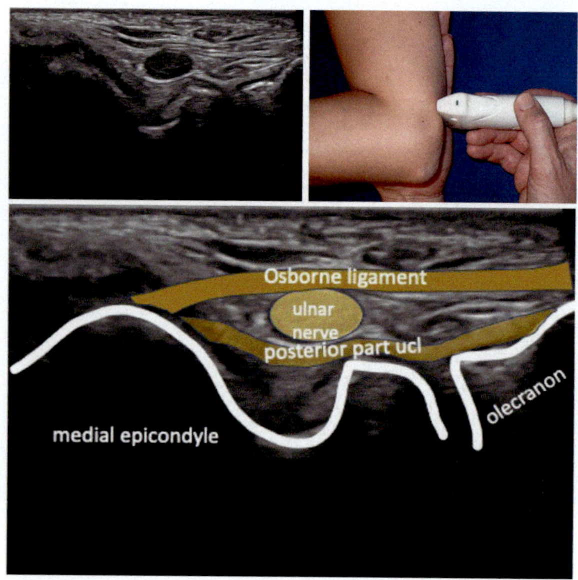

6.1.9   Longitudinal View of the Ulnar Nerve of the Elbow (Standard Scan 6-9)

The position of the arm is the same as in Standard Scan 6-8. The probe is rotated by 90°. In the longitudinal ultrasound plane, all peripheral nerves show a peculiar arrangement made of multiple hypoechoic parallel linear areas separated by hyperechoic bands. Generally, the hypoechoic lines dominate the ultrasound image.

The ulnar nerve passes through the cubital tunnel, which is a bony passage way between the medial epicondyle and the olecranon. The proximal roof of the cubital tunnel is formed by a thin ligament called Osborne's retinaculum. The floor of the tunnel is formed by the posterior part of the ulnar collateral ligament and the joint capsule of the posterior recess. Then, the ulnar nerve curls around the medial humeral condyle at the elbow and courses down the proximal forearm between the two heads of the flexor carpi ulnaris. The distal roof is formed by the thicker arcuate ligament. Then, it descends deep to the muscle of the flexor carpi ulnaris on the surface of the flexor digitorum profundus.

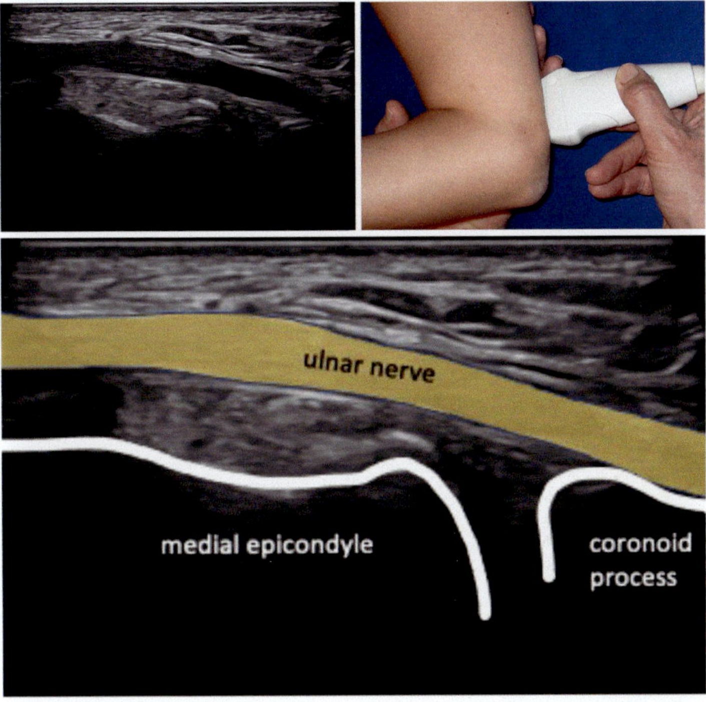

6.1.10   *Ultrasound-Guided Injection of the Elbow*

The longitudinal posterior standard scan is suitable for ultrasound-guided injection of the posterior olecranon fossa as elbow effusions usually extend to this fossa. Alternatively, an effusion can be reached with an anterior approach in the region of the coronoid fossa.

The patient is seated with the elbow flexed by 90° and the hand flat on the examination couch. The probe is aligned with the long axis of the upper arm and the triceps muscle. The prescan should show the triceps muscle and tendon, the fat pad, and the contours of the distal humerus and posterior trochlea, the joint space and the ulnar olecranon. A posterior effusion is clearly visible in the olecranon fossa. After the usual antisepsis, the in-plane introduction of the needle into the posterior joint space under direct visualization is carried out. The needle is introduced posteriorly in the midline at an angle of 45° and directed at the olecranon fossa under direct ultrasound guidance.

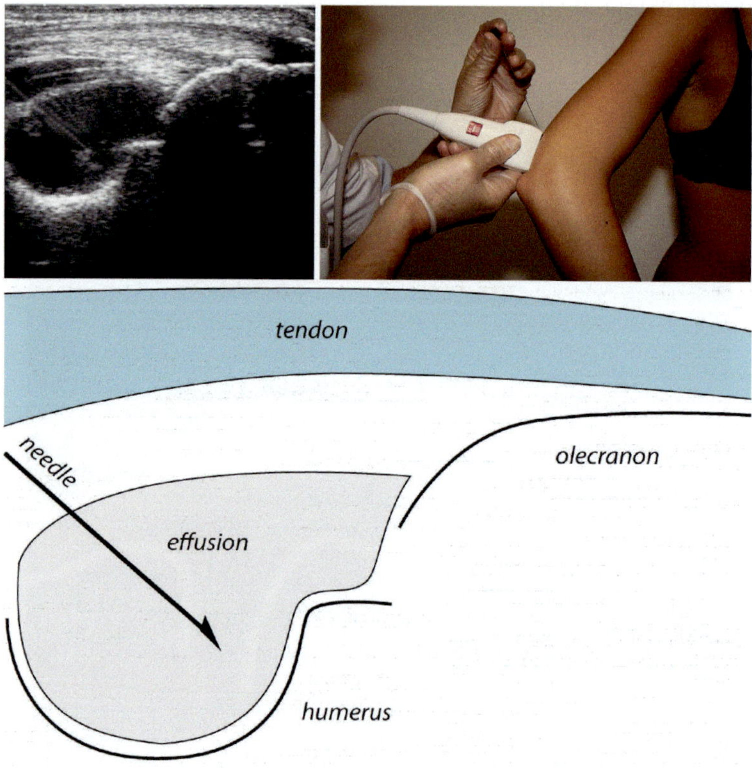

6.2 Pathology of the Elbow

6.2.1 Synovitis of the Elbow

Best scans: Standard Scans 6-1 to 6-5.

Figure 6.1 shows a longitudinal ultrasound image at the anterior radial side of the elbow joint. Small amounts of effusion extend from the joint space into the radial fossa (arrow). The capsule is pushed up by the synovitis at the level of the fossa. The sonographer will miss the effusion if the area of the fossa is ignored.

Figure 6.2 shows an effusion of the right elbow joint in the anterior transverse scan. The effusion elevates the joint capsule at the level of the trochlea and the capitulum humeri closely to the joint space. The hyperechoic line anterior to the effusion represents the joint capsule (⇓). The thinner line anterior to the trochlea represents the interface between the synovial fluid and cartilage (⇑). Smaller effusions can be seen only when shifting the probe more proximally to the fossae.

Figure 6.3 is a posterior longitudinal scan showing a large effusion in the olecranon fossa with elevation of the posterior soft tissue. The amount of effusion can be estimated by the amount of fluid in the olecranon fossa. In this case, the fossa is completely filled. Synovial proliferation is present closely to the posterior joint capsule (⇓).

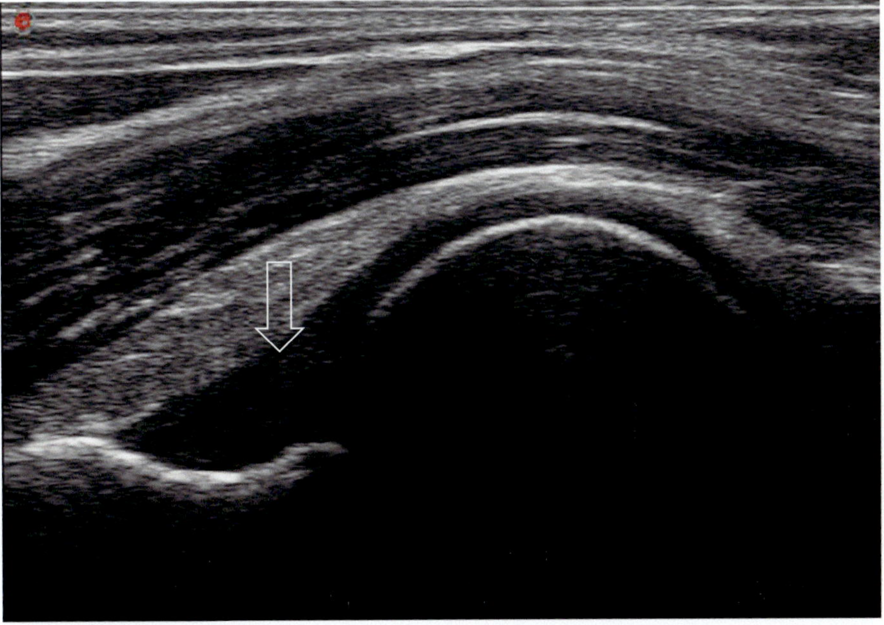

Fig. 6.1 Small effusion in the radial fossa (anterior longitudinal view at the level of the humero-radial joint)

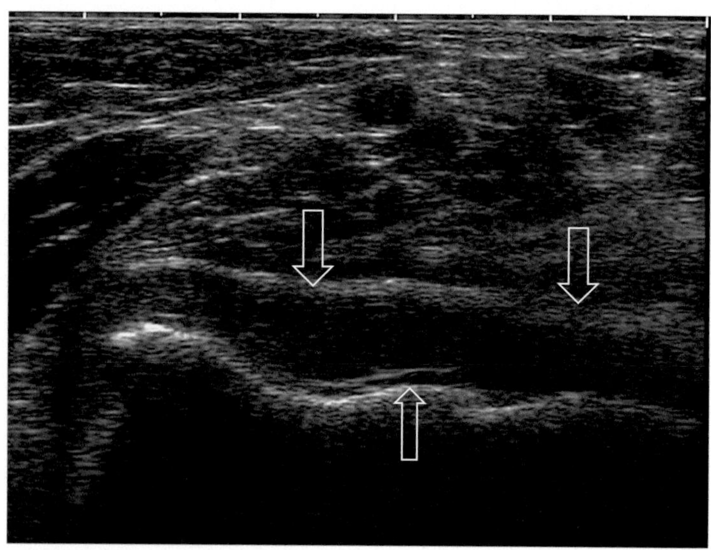

Fig. 6.2 Large effusion of the elbow joint (anterior transverse view)

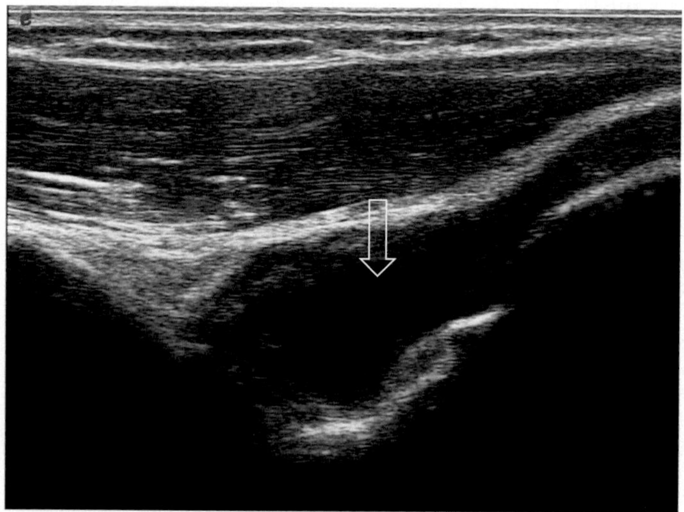

Fig. 6.3 Effusion and synovitis in the olecranon fossa (posterior longitudinal view)

6.2.2 *Enthesitis, Tendinopathy and Bursitis of the Elbow*

Best scans: Standard Scans 6-6 and 6-7.

Figure 6.4 is a longitudinal ultrasound image of the lateral region of the elbow. A calcific deposit localizes within the common extensor tendon close to its insertion (⇓). It is sometimes difficult to distinguish between tendon calcifications, osteophytes, and loose bodies. Osteophytes (enthesophytes) are usually connected to the bone. A loose body is usually intra-articular. Loose bodies and calcifications typically have no connection to the bone. On the other hand, a similar image may be seen if trauma has caused an avulsion of bone at the tendon insertion. Therefore, the image should only be evaluated in conjunction with history and clinical assessment. In lateral epicondylitis, the deep fibers of the common extensor tendon are involved, which belong to the extensor carpi radialis brevis tendon.

Figure 6.5 shows a hypoechoic, dark, inhomogeneous common extensor tendon insertion due to inflammation. Power Doppler ultrasound shows increased blood flow, indicating acute enthesitis.

Figure 6.6 shows a transverse sonogram of the olecranon bursa that is filled with hypoechoic material which may represent cell debris, hematoma, fibrin clots, pus, or other material. There is only a tiny spot of anechoic fluid (⇓) that may be aspirated under ultrasound guidance.

Figure 6.7 shows a longitudinal scan of a hypoechoic thickened triceps tendon, whose echotexture is completely destroyed by deposition of hyperechoic material, consistent with calciumpyrophosphate (CPP) crystals.

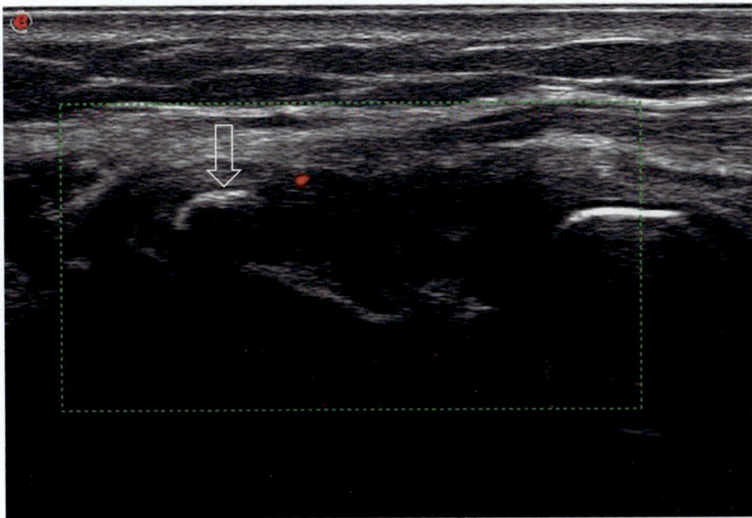

Fig. 6.4 Calcifying enthesopathy at the radial humeral epicondyle (longitudinal lateral view)

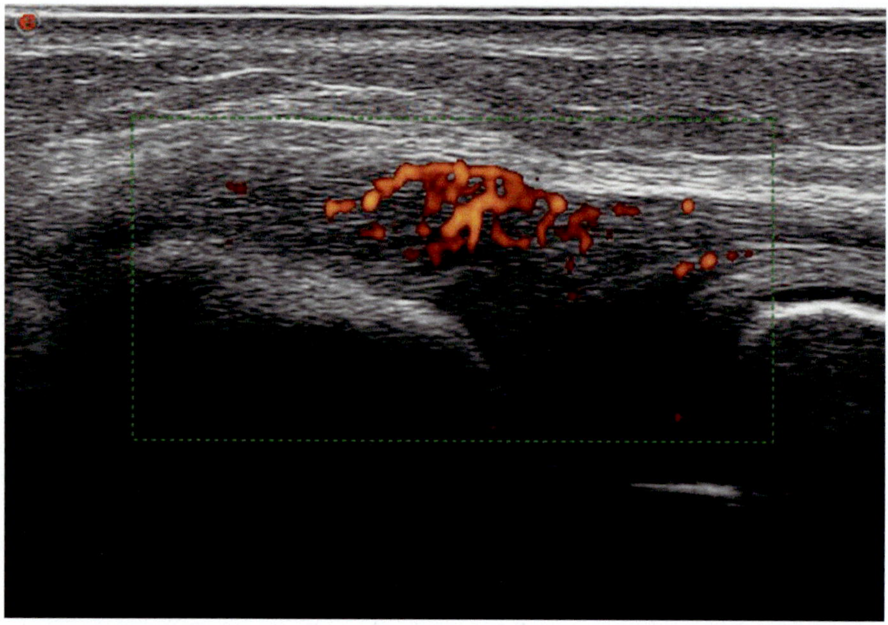

Fig. 6.5 Enthesitis with increased perfusion of the extensor tendons at the radial humeral epicondyle (longitudinal lateral view)

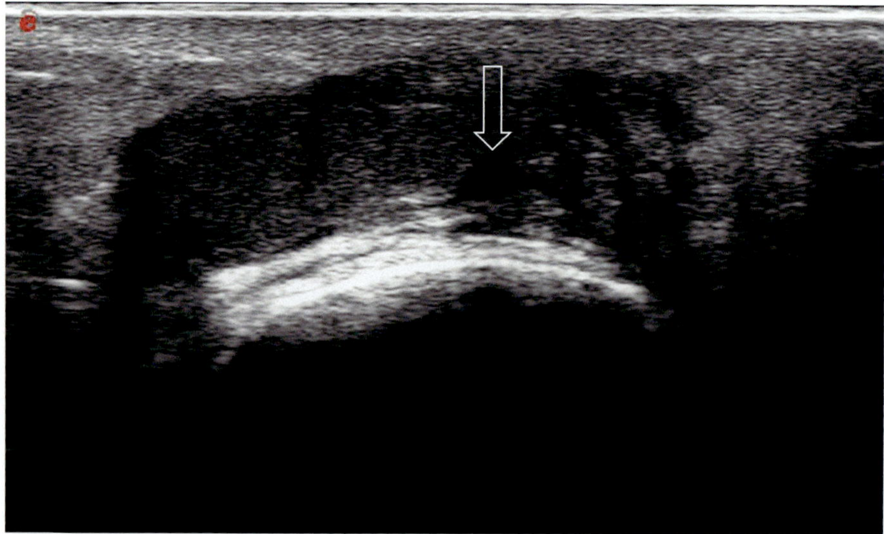

Fig. 6.6 Olecranon bursitis (transverse distal posterior view)

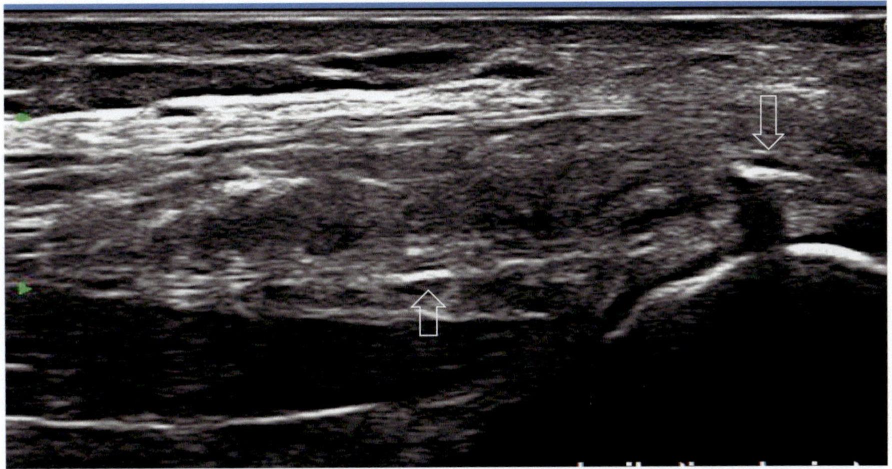

Fig. 6.7 Triceps tendinitis (longitudinal posterior view)

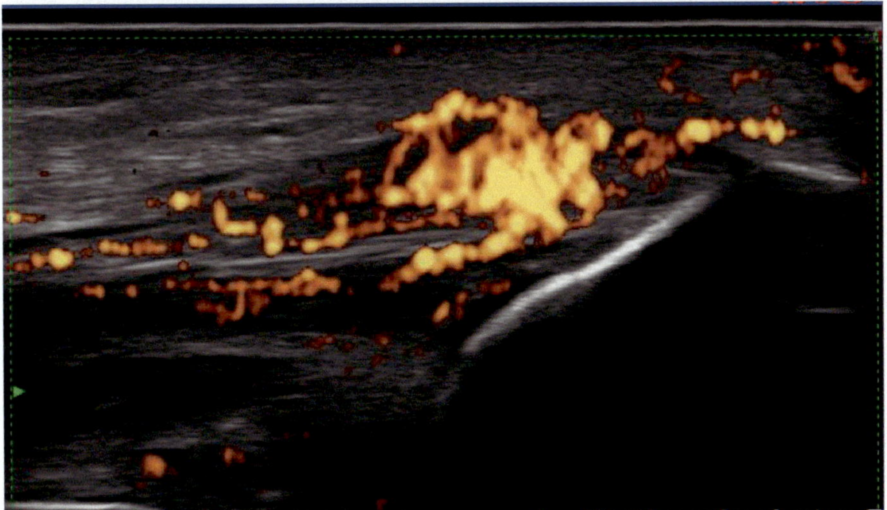

Fig. 6.8 Triceps tendinitis with increased perfusion (longitudinal posterior view)

Characteristic of calcium pyrophosphate deposition disease are the bright, hyperechoic punctate and linear bands with posterior shadowing (⇑⇓).

Figure 6.8 is an example of the strong inflammation caused by the calciumpyprophosphate crystal deposits in the tendon. Differential diagnosis is with gout, which may result in a similar ultrasound image.

6.2.3   *Cubital Tunnel Syndrome and Rheumatoid Nodules*

Best scans: Standard Scans 6-8 and 6-9.

Figure 6.9 is a longitudinal ultrasound image showing a hypoechoic swollen ulnar nerve in the cubital fossa between the medial epicondyle and the olecranon. The nerve is indicated by the arrows ($\Downarrow\Uparrow$).

Figure 6.10 shows a transverse scan with a hypoechoic swollen ulnar nerve ($\Rightarrow$). The cross-sectional area is 10 mm^2 (7 mm^2 on the healthy side). The ulnar nerve in this patient is entrapped due to large synovitis of the elbow with effusion that extends to the medial posterior areas of the joint ($\Leftarrow$).

Cubital tunnel syndrome is the result of inflammation of the ulnar nerve manifested by an enlarged, hypoechoic appearance on ultrasound due to edema. Dynamic imaging during flexion of the elbow may reveal medial subluxation of the ulnar nerve in some individuals, but without signs of ulnar neuropathy. Repeated periods of subluxation may cause neuritis.

Figure 6.11 Rheumatoid nodules (arrows) are a classic extra-articular feature of rheumatoid arthritis overlying the posterior aspects of proximal ulna and other pressure locations such as the occiput, sacrum, knee, or the Achilles tendon. Sonographically, rheumatoid nodules appear as hypoechoic oval structures, with clear demarcation from the surrounding tissue. Power Doppler usually reveals no or minor blood flow.

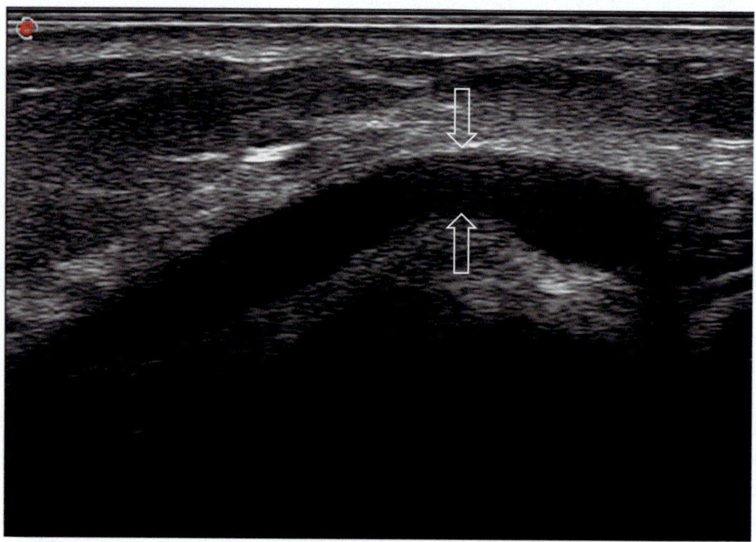

Fig. 6.9 Hypoechoic swelling of the ulnar nerve in primary cubital tunnel syndrome (longitudinal view of the ulnar nerve)

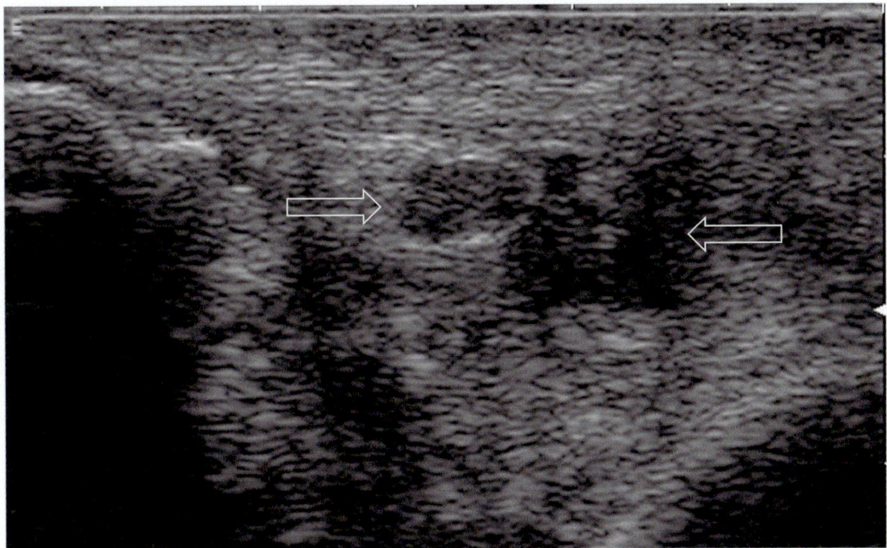

Fig. 6.10 Hypoechoic swelling of the ulnar nerve in cubital tunnel syndrome due to synovitis of the elbow (transverse view of the ulnar nerve)

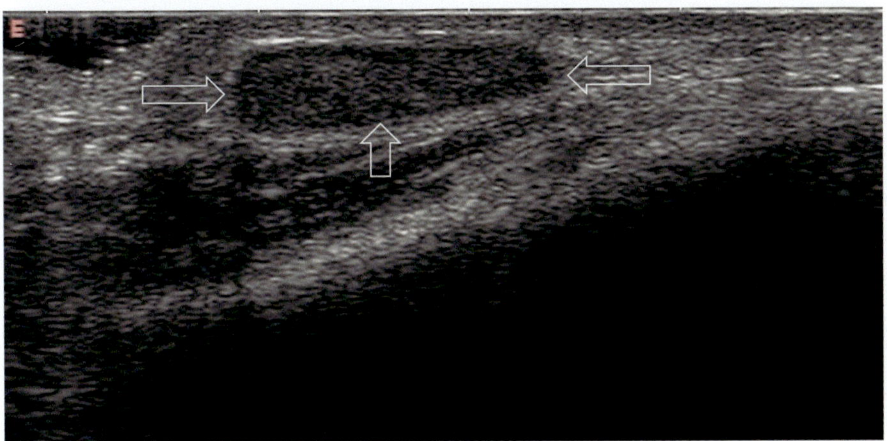

Fig. 6.11 Rheumatic nodule localized typically at the proximal posterior aspect of the ulna (longitudinal distal dorsal view)

Chapter 7
The Wrist

7.1   Standard Scans of the Wrist

7.1.1   *Dorsal Midline Longitudinal View of the Wrist (Standard Scan 7-1)*

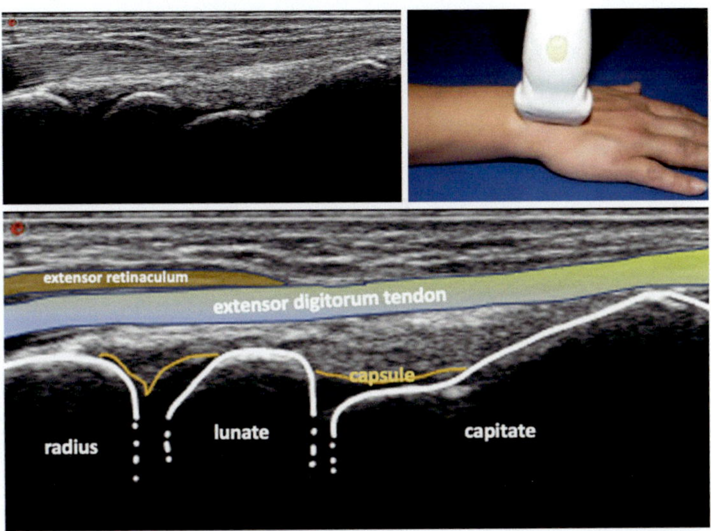

During examination of the wrist and hand, the examiner sits opposite the patient. The hand is placed in a neutral position on a flat surface. It may be extended and flexed for dynamic examination of the joints and tendons. The examination of the

© The Author(s), under exclusive license to Springer Nature Switzerland AG 2023
G. A. W. Bruyn and W. A. Schmidt, *Musculoskeletal Ultrasound for the Rheumatologist*,
https://doi.org/10.1007/978-3-031-27737-5_7

wrist starts with a longitudinal scan of the dorsal midline area of the wrist. This scan provides information on the radiocarpal joint and the midcarpal joint. At the first carpal bones row in the midline, the lunate bone is visible. Further distally, at the second row, the large capitate bone is seen in this scan.

The extensor retinaculum extends from ulnar to radial across the dorsum of the wrist, preventing the extensor tendons from slipping. The retinaculum defines 6 separate extensor compartments, each of which contains a synovial sheath for the tendons that pass through it. The six compartments are readily seen on transverse scanning (Standard scan 7-5). While the retinaculum is hyperechoic, the underlying extensor tendon sheaths have an hypoechoic appearance.

What is normal?

Tendons show a fibrillar pattern. The bone-capsule distance at the scaphoid is 1.7 mm (0–3.4 mm).

7.1.2 *Dorsal Radial Longitudinal View of the Wrist (Standard Scan 7-2)*

For this view, the probe is swept gently in a radial direction. At the radial side, the radioscaphoid joint is seen. The scaphoid is the second largest carpal bone, conceding only the capitate bone before it. Along with the lunate, the scaphoid covers the complete radial border of the first row. The dorsal bony shape is crescent but shallower than the crescent shape of its ulnar neighbour, the lunate bone. Further distally, the scaphoid articulates with two small bones, i.e., on the far radial side with the trapezium, and between the trapezium and the capitate, with the trapezoid. The trapezoid is the smallest carpal bone. The trapezium articulates with the first metacarpal phalanx.

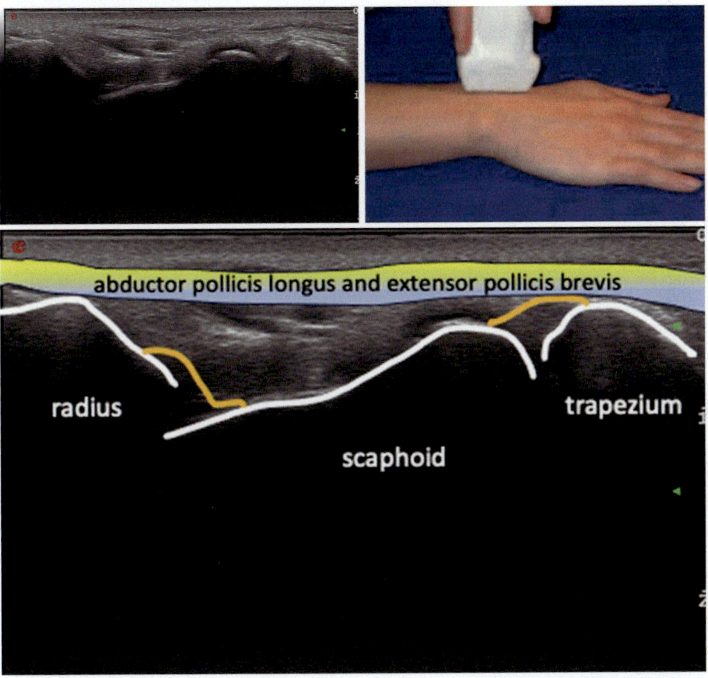

7.1.3　Dorsal Ulnar Longitudinal View of the Wrist (Standard Scan 7-3)

The position of the patient and sonographer including dynamic examination is identical to Standard Scan 7-1 and 7-2. The probe is shifted continuously in an ulnar direction. This scan provides information on the ulno-carpal aspects of the wrist.

An articulation exists between the distal ulna and the distal radius, which is called the distal radio-ulnar joint (DRUJ). Synovitis may occur at the DRUJ. Since there is no joint space strictu sensu between the ulna and the carpal bones at the ulnar side, i.e., the triquetrum and the pisiform bone, spacing material need to be in place. Thus, this area is filled by a fibrocartilaginous disc between the ulna and the lunate, a triangular shaped meniscoid structure and multiple ligaments.

The probe is shifted continuously from the first scan to this position. The wrist may be extended and flexed for dynamic examination of the wrist and the tendons. The distal end of the ulna occupies a smaller area than the radius. When shifting the probe from the radial to the ulnar aspect, the ulna appears with the lunate, then the triquetrum. The distance between the ulna and these midcarpal bones becomes longer when the probe is shifted ulnarly. If synovitis of the DRUJ is present, it extends over the ulna. This scan is also useful to detect erosions of the caput ulnae and the triquetrum.

What is normal?

The distance between ulna and joint capsule at the most dorsal point of the ulna is 0.8 mm (0–1.6 mm).

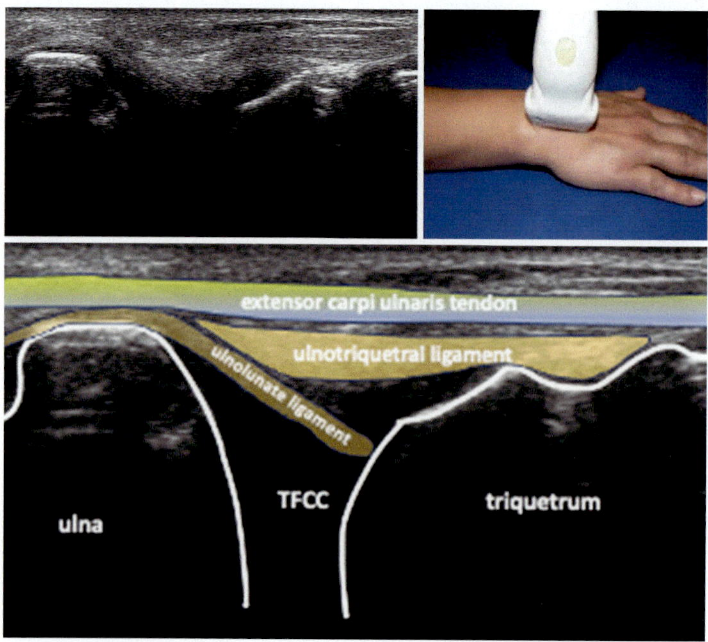

7.1.4 Dorsal Transverse View of the Wrist (Standard Scan 7-4)

The positions of patient and sonographer are identical to the previous scans. The probe is rotated by 90° in order to be transverse to the position in Standard Scan 7-1. It is moved from the radial and ulnar area distally to the midcarpal region.

The transverse dorsal scan gives the best view of all the compartments of the extensor tendons. The sonogram shows, from the radius to the ulna, the second, third, fourth and fifth compartments. The radial side of the hand locates the first compartment, which contains the tendons of the abductor pollicis longus and the extensor pollicis brevis muscles (1a, 1b, respectively). These two tendons are inflamed in the condition termed "De Quervain tenosynovitis". The second compartment comprises the tendons of the extensor carpi radialis longus and brevis muscles (2a, 2b). These tendons run radially to the dorsal tubercle (also called Lister's tubercle) of the distal radius. Lister's tubercle functions as a pulley for the next tendon, the extensor pollicis lonus tendon, as this tendon changes course for its mechanical action. The third compartment (3) contains the tendon of the extensor pollicis longus muscle, compartment four (4) contains the tendons of the extensor digitorum and extensor indicis muscles, and in the fifth compartment the tendon of the extensor digiti minimi muscle is found (5). Compartment three lies directly medial to the distal tubercle of the radius, compartment five overlies the DRUJ.

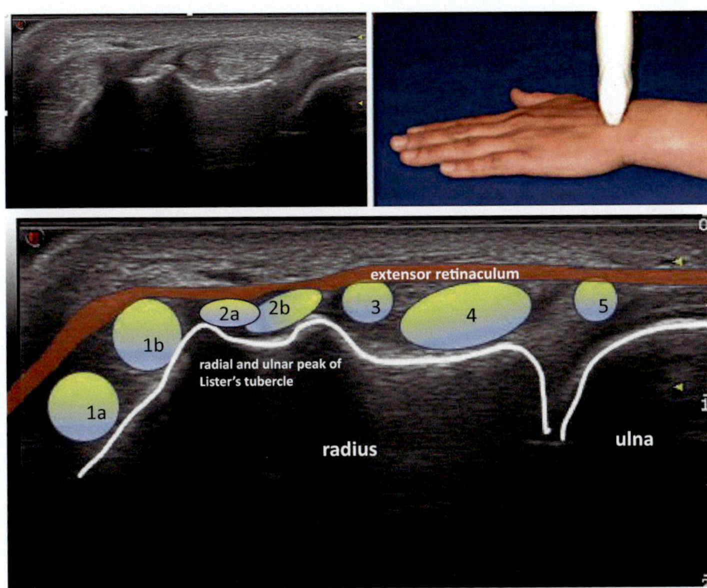

More distally, the ligament between the scaphoid and the lunate can be assessed.

What is normal?

In most persons, Lister's tubercle consist of a single bony prominence on the dorsal distal radius; however as is demonstrated in this image, there is a double peak in a minority of persons. A small hypoechoic rim representing fluid within the sheaths may be present around the extensor tendons. Veins appear as anechoic, compressible structures. The extensor retinaculum appears as a hyperechoic bowed line, but in longitudinal planes may appear hypo-echoic due to anisotropy.

7.1.5 *Longitudinal View of the Extensor Carpi Ulnaris Tendon (Standard Scan 7-5)*

The position of the arm and hand is the same as that in Standard Scans 7-1 through 7-3. The probe is shifted continuously from the position in Standard Scan 7-3 to the ulnar side. The extensor carpi ulnaris tendon occupies the sixth extensor compartment and is in a bony groove adjacent to the styloid process of the ulna. The fibrillar hyperechoic appearance of the tendon is clearly visible on the longitudinal ultrasound scan. It overlies the ulno-carpal area, which is occupied by the triangular fibrocartilage complex (TFCC).

As the extensor carpi ulnaris tendon usually changes its direction at the wrist, one has to be aware of anisotropy and small physiologic hypoechoic areas around the tendon. It is important to investigate the full length of the tendon.

The triangular fibrocartilage complex (TFCC) can be examined in this longitudinal plane. It originates from a groove at the base of the ulnar styloid process and inserts by a broad base along the medial portion of the end of the radius. The fibrocartilage is interposed between the ulna and the carpus, forming an intra-articular disc.

What is normal?

The TFCC appears as a triangular structure with a mixed echogenicity.

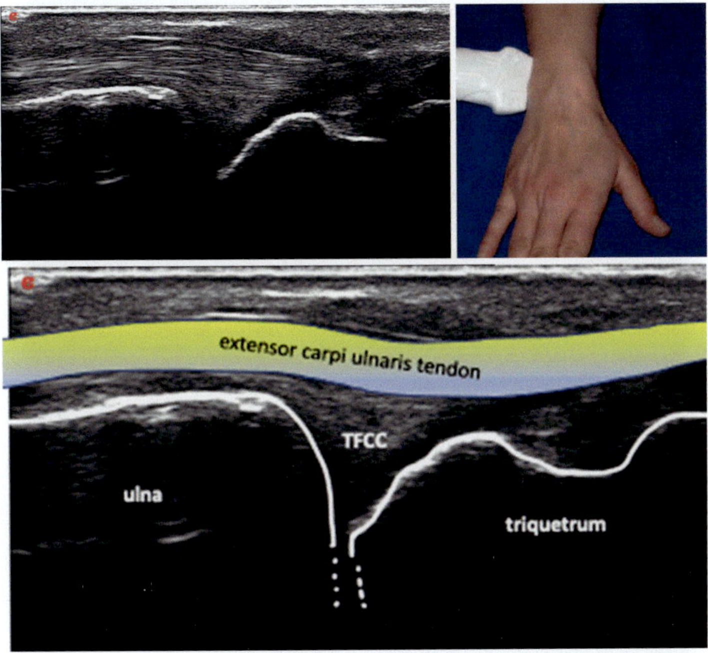

7.1.6   Transverse View of the Extensor Carpi Ulnaris Tendon (Standard Scan 7-6)

This scan is the transverse homologue of Standard Scan 7-4. The position of the arm and hand is similar to the position of the previous scans. The probe is shifted along the extensor carpi ulnaris tendon from an area proximal of the caput ulnae to an area distal to it.

This scan evaluates the extensor carpi ulnaris tendon which is frequently involved in inflammatory rheumatoid diseases. It is also used to search for erosions of the ulnar head. The tendon of the extensor carpi ulnaris muscle is located at the ulnar side of the ulna in a dedicated bony groove.

What is normal?

A hyperechoic layer around the tendon indicates the retinaculum. In addition, a variable amount of tenosynovial fluid is usually present around a normal tendon. The normal diameters directly distal to the head of the ulna are as follows: transverse diameter of the exensor carpi ulnaris tendon 5.4 mm (2.8–8.0 mm), sagittal diameter 2.7 mm (0.6–4.8 mm) and hypoechoic rim 1.2 mm (0.2–2.2 mm).

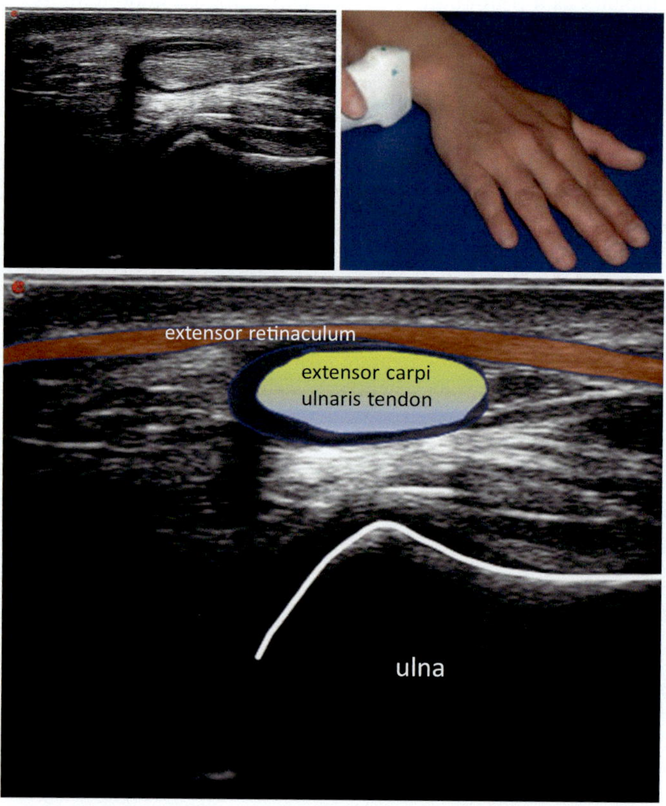

7.1.7 *Volar Midline Longitudinal View of the Wrist (Standard Scan 7-7)*

The forearm should rest on a flat surface. The wrist should be in supination. The wrist may be dynamically examined by flexion and extension maneuvers. The probe is placed in the midline of the wrist and shifted from ulnar to radial or vice versa.

In the midline of the wrist, the distal radius articulates with the lunate. In addition, the median nerve is visible anterior to the flexor tendons. There is a common joint space between the radius, the lunate, and the scaphoid, i.e., the radiocarpal joint, which is among the wrist joints one of the most affected by synovitis.

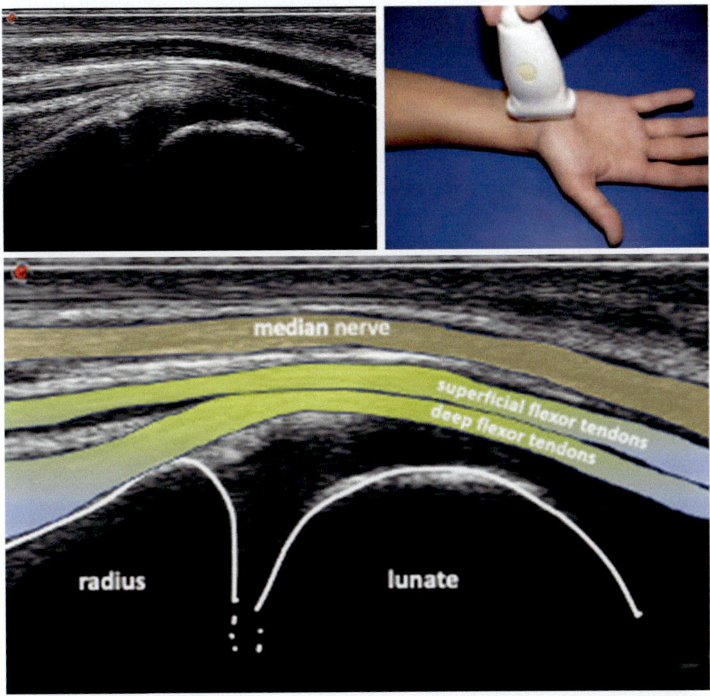

7.1.8 Volar Radial Longitudinal View of the Wrist (Standard Scan 7-8)

From the position in Standard Scan 7.1.7, the probe is swept radially. The forearm stays resting on a flat surface. The wrist should be in supination. The wrist may be dynamically examined by flexion and extension maneuvers.

The lateral distal radius articulates with the scaphoid bone. The tendon of the flexor pollicis longus muscle passes through the radial side of the carpal tunnel towards the thumb. This tendon has a long separate synovial sheath. The flexor carpi radialis tendon runs through the radial side of the carpus, and courses over the tubercle of the scaphoid to subsequently follow its course in a groove of the trapezium. In this scan, the three small thumb muscles, i.e., flexor pollicis brevis, abductor pollicis brevis, and opponens pollicis can be seen originating from the tubercle of the trapezium.

What is normal?

In the longitudinal plane, the nerve runs parallel and anterior to the tendons. It is delineated as a hypoechoic, less fibrillar structure and has continuous hyperechoic anterior and posterior borders, that represent the nerve sheath. Finger tendons, on the other hand, appear as tightly packed echogenic structures with fine parallel internal linear echoes, separated by hypoechoic lines.

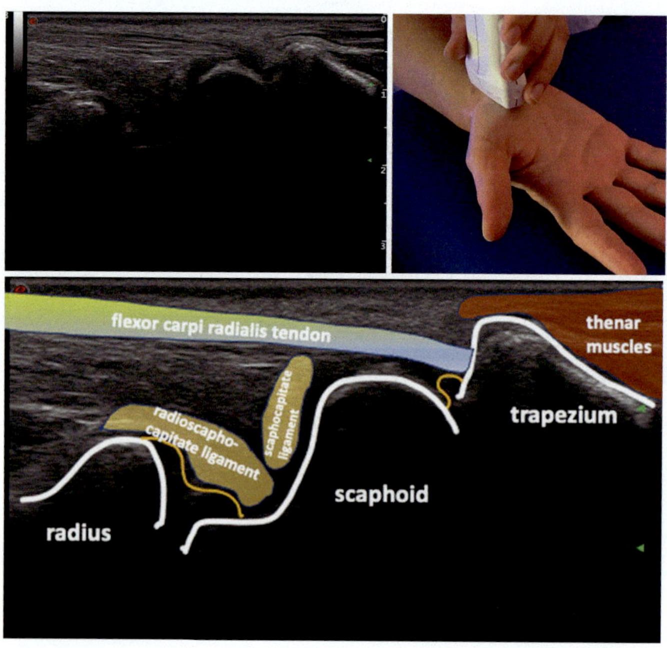

7.1.9 *Volar Ulnar Longitudinal View of the Wrist (Standard Scan 7-9)*

The movement of the probe is continued from the previous scan to this position. The wrist may be extended and flexed for dynamic examination of the joint and the tendons. On the ulnar volar aspect, the bony landmark is the ulnar head and more distally, the triquetrum. Superficial to the triquetrum, the small pisiform bone is visualized, which together with the former make up a synovial-lined articulation, the pisotriquetral joint.

The longitudinal scan shows the flexor carpi ulnaris tendon, inserting at the pisiform bone. Medial to the flexor tendon, the ulnar nerve and artery may become visible in a separate compartment outside the carpal tunnel, the canal of Guyon.

Compared with the nerve, the tendon is hyperechoic, but if the scan head is not in a plane perpendicular to the tendon surface, the tendon will appear hypoechoic due to anisotropy.

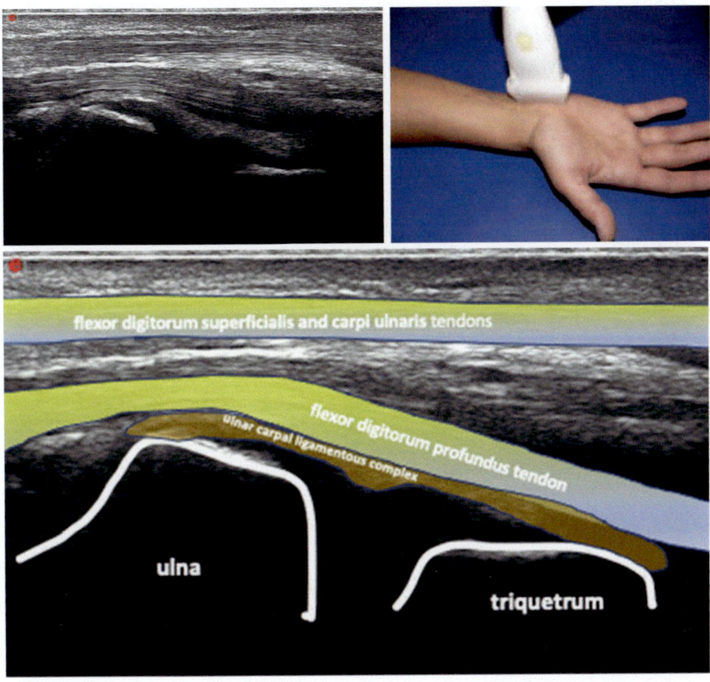

The tendon of the flexor carpi ulnaris muscle is the only wrist flexor tendon without a synovial sheath. The ulnar nerve and ulnar artery run lateral to this flexor tendon in a separate canal called canal of Guyon. The nerve enters the canal medial to the artery and splits in the tunnel into a superfical sensitive branch and a deep motor branch.

What is normal?

The distance between ulna and joint capsule 1 cm proximal of the wrist joint is 1.1 mm (0.1–2.1 mm).

7.1.10   *Volar Transverse View of the Wrist (Standard Scan 7-10)*

The probe is rotated by 90° from the positions in Standard Scans 7-7 and 7-8 and then shifted from an area proximal to the wrist to an area distal to the wrist.

The volar transverse view is the best scan to assess the carpal tunnel. At the proximal carpal tunnel, the radial landmark is the tubercle of the scaphoid, whereas the medial landmark is formed by the ulnar artery and the pisiform. The distal carpal tunnel landmark is formed radially by the trapezium and ulnar by the hamulus (hook) of the hamate bone. The flexor retinaculum is stretched out between these four points.

The median nerve passes through the carpal tunnel to the radial side of the superficial row of flexor digitorum tendons and below the flexor retinaculum.

The flexor carpi radialis tendon (1) does not pass through the tunnel in contrast to the tendons of the superficial finger flexors and the profundus muscles, the tendon of the flexor pollicis longus muscle (2) and the median nerve which do pass through the tunnel. The third and fourth superficialis tendons lie superficial to the second and fifth superficialis tendons (4), and the 4 profundus tendons (5) lie side by side, deep to the second and fifth superficalis tendons (4). The flexor carpi ulnaris tendon courses superficial to the pisiform bone (3).

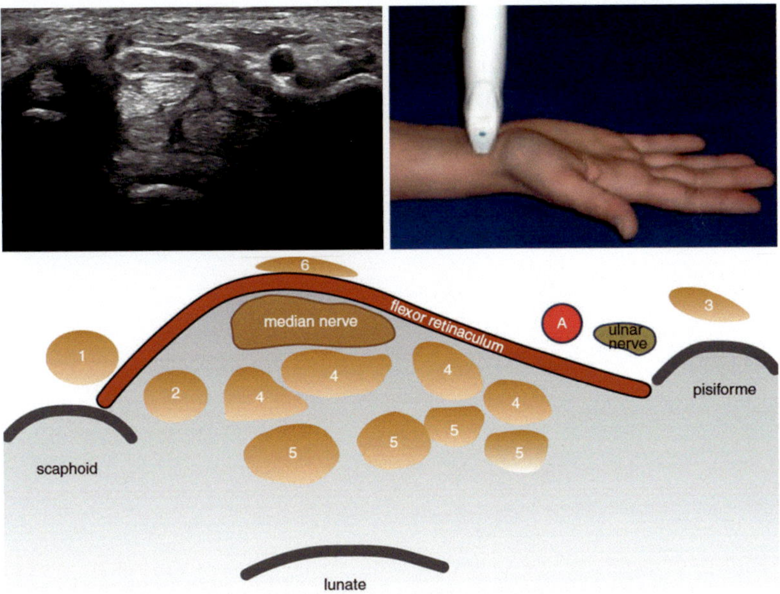

What is normal?

The median nerve is oval or rounded at the entrance of the carpal tunnel. The nerve flattens progressively as it courses through the tunnel. Nerve enlargement can be assessed in the transverse plane at the inlet or the outlet of the carpal tunnel. At the inlet and outlet, the median nerve is considered enlarged if the cross-sectional area >12 mm^2 and >11 mm^2, respectively. A normal nerve has hypoechoic rounded areas embedded in a hyperechoic background. In about 80% of persons, a palmaris longus tendon is present (6).

7.1.11 *Ultrasound-Guided Injection of the Carpal Tunnel*

US-guided injection into the carpal tunnel can be performed either in a plane parallel to the long axis of the arm or transversely to it. Since various important anatomical structures are localized in the carpal tunnel, it is key to check the needle tip in two planes. Cadaver studies have shown that injection of the carpal tunnel can be safely done either by a radial volar or by an ulnar volar approach.

In this case, carpal tunnel syndrome due to flexor tenosynovitis is present. The ultrasound scan is showing the radial approach. The bony landmarks of the carpal tunnel inlet are radially the scaphoid bone and ulnarly the pisiform bone. A prescan showing the median nerve and its immediate radial neighbour within the tunnel, the flexor pollicis longus tendon, is done. Subsequently, the sites of the flexor carpi radialis tendon and the median nerve are marked with a skin marker. The needle is then introduced using a radial window, inserted between the flexor carpi radialis and flexor pollicis longus tendons. The case only shows a transverse scan; however, the exact localization of the needle tip should be checked for in a longitudinal plane.

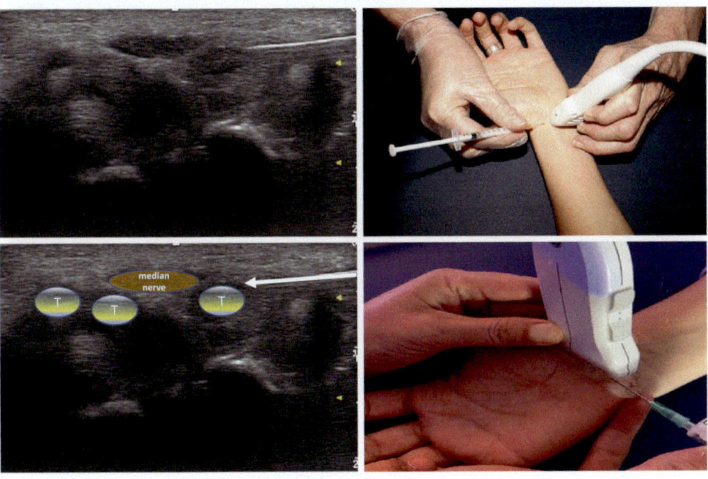

7.1.12 Ultrasound-Guided Injection of the Dorsal Wrist Joint

Ultrasound-guided injection of the wrist is generally performed in a long axis plane. Synovitis of the carpus can be demonstrated both dorsally and volarly, however for injection purposes the dorsal approach is somewhat easier, as there are fewer key anatomical structures present. The patient is comfortably seated with the arm extended on the table. A prescan is performed to identify—from proximal to distal - the radius, scaphoid or lunate bone, and the capitate bone. The probe is positioned in a longitudinal orientation on the target area. Then, the needle is inserted closely to the foot of the probe and directed into the radiocarpal joint space using an in-plane approach. Injection into the extensor tendons should be avoided at all costs.

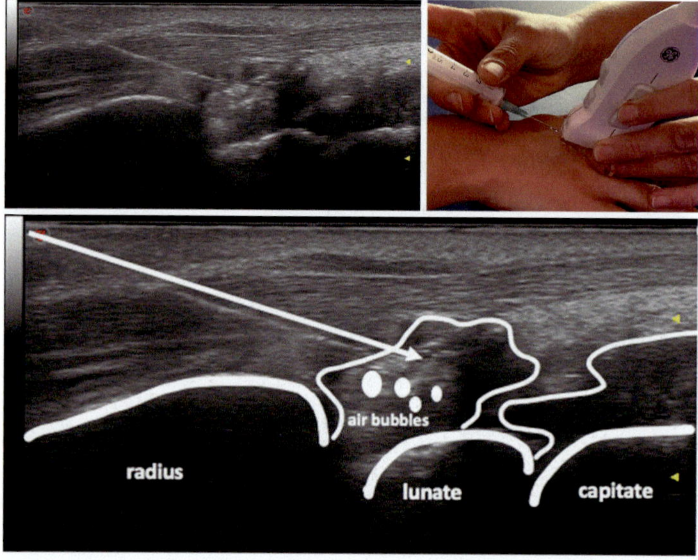

7.1.13 Ultrasound-Guided Injection of the First Extensor Compartment

In tenosynovitis of the first extensor compartment or tenosynovitis of De Quervain, ultrasound can be very useful both for diagnosis and for treatment. Differential diagnosis is with the intersection syndrome and the Wartenberg syndrome. In addition, the first extensor compartment is sometimes divided into two compartments by a retinaculum.

The hand should be placed with the hypothenar on the examination table. The probe should be positioned in a short axis relative to the axis of the wrist plane. Next, the needle should be aligned with the probe to perform an in-plane injection. UItrasound-guidance is important since the radial artery is located just beneath the first extensor compartment.

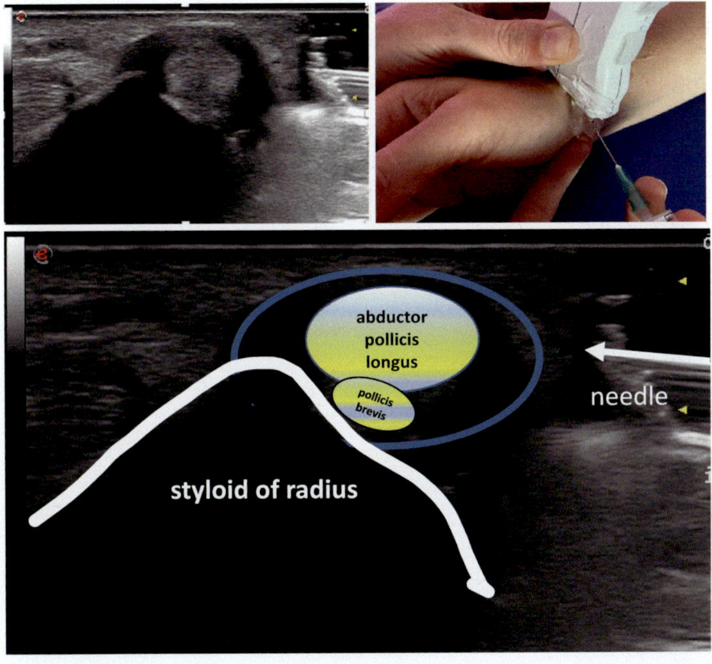

7.2   Pathology of the Wrist

7.2.1   *Synovitis of the Wrist I*

Best Scans: Standard Scans 7-1, 7-2, 7-4, 7-6, 7-7 and 7-8.

Synovitis of the wrist is typically found anteriorly to the carpal bones as shown in Fig. 7.1. It localizes anteriorly to the scaphoid and lunate in the radiocarpal joint (⇓) or ulnocarpal joint and anteriorly to the capitate in the midcarpal joint area (⇑). Both areas are separated by ligaments. In advanced arthritis, these ligaments may be torn, so that these compartments communicate. Synovitis often extends to the radial, ulnar, and palmar sides.

Power Doppler studies show the inflammatory nature of active synovitis (Fig. 7.2). The intensity of power Doppler signals is graded as follows:

Grade 0: no signals

Grade 1: up to 3 signals and <1 confluent signal in one scan

Grade 2: Signals covering <50% of the synovium in one scan

Grade 3: Signals covering >50% of the synovium in one scan.

After steroid treatment, a dramatic reduction in power Doppler signal can be observed. The presence of intraarticular Doppler signals is a strong predictor of erosive disease in RA.

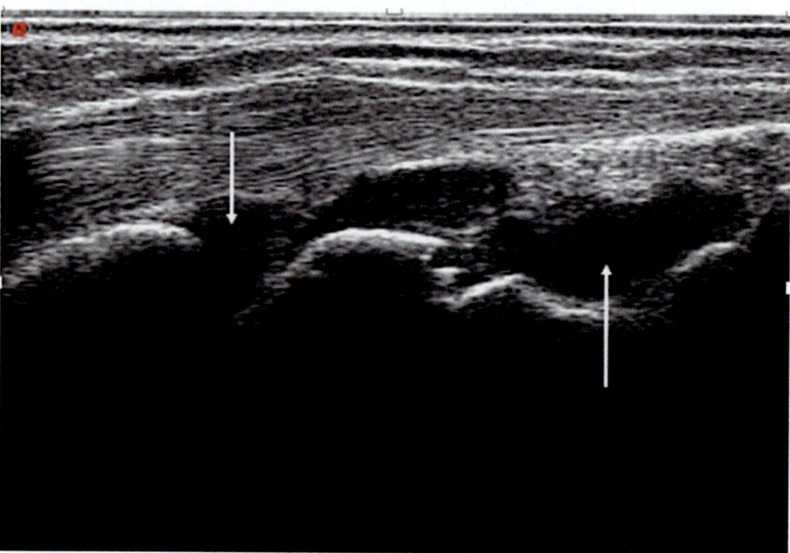

Fig. 7.1   Synovitis of the radiocarpal and the midcarpal joints (dorsal longitudinal view)

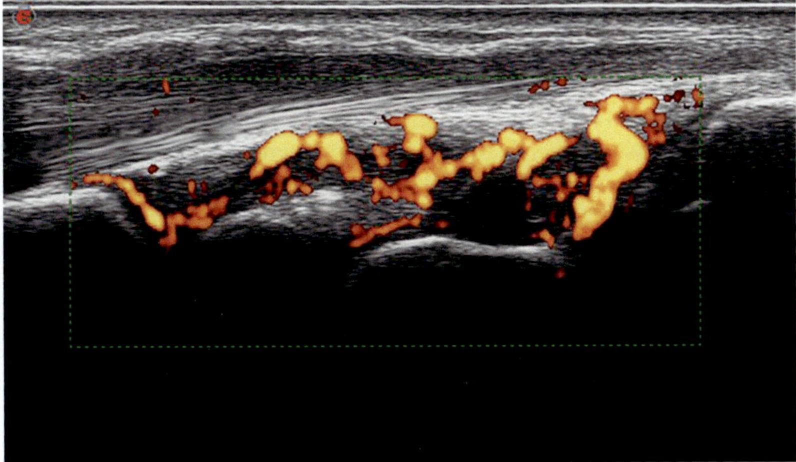

Fig. 7.2 Synovitis with grade 3 power Doppler vascularity of the radiocarpal joint and midcarpal joints (dorsal longitudinal view)

Figure 7.3 shows wrist synovitis (⇓) in a dorsal transverse plane at the level of the lunate and scaphoid. The hypoechoic rim around the extensor digitorum tendons is normal. There is no additional tenosynovitis.

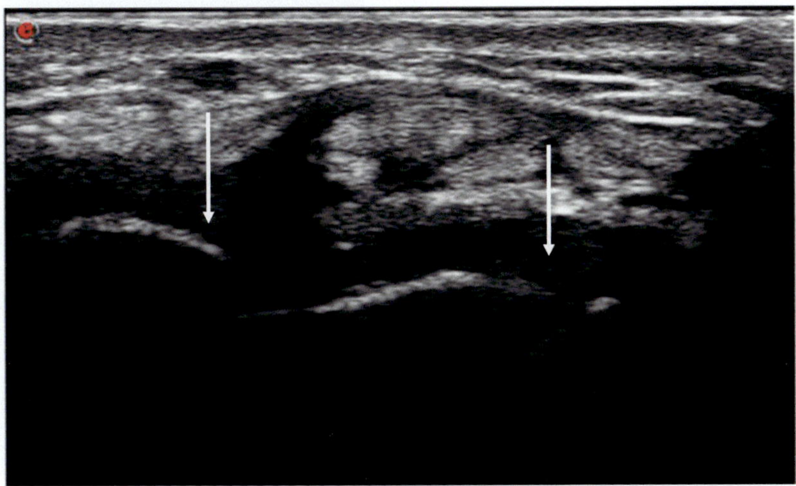

Fig. 7.3 Synovitis of the radiocarpal and ulnocarpal joints (dorsal transverse view)

7.2.2   Synovitis of the Wrist II

Best Scans: Standard Scans 7-1, 7-2 and 7-4.

Figure 7.4a shows a longitudinal sonogram at the level of the joint space between radius and scaphoid showing synovial thickening. There are clearly associated power Doppler signals corresponding to synovial hyperemia (grade 2) at the midcarpal joints. At the radiocarpal joint (wrist), synovitis exhibits only two single signals at the very distal end of the synovium (grade 1). Figures 7.4b and c show active synovitis of the radiocarpal and midcarpal joint space.

Figure 7.5 shows a dorsal longitudinal image of a patient's wrist, with synovitis of the distal radio-ulnar joint, extending both proximally over the ulnar head (⇑) and distally to the triquetrum. There are cortical irregularities but no erosions of the ulnar bone surface.

In Fig. 7.6, there is an effusion of the radiocarpal joint. The fluid extends proximally to the radial head.

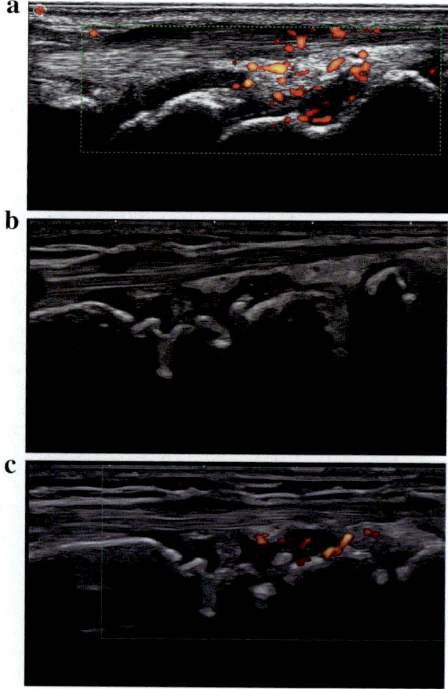

Fig. 7.4 **a** Synovitis of the wrist. The inflammatory activity is higher in the midcarpal region than in the radio-carpal joint (dorsal longitudinal view); **b** Synovitis of the wrist and erosions of the lunate bone in a patient with rheumatoid arthritis (dorsal longitudinal view); **c** Doppler signals in the radiocarpal and midcarpal wrist in a patient with rheumatoid arthritis (dorsal longitudinal view)

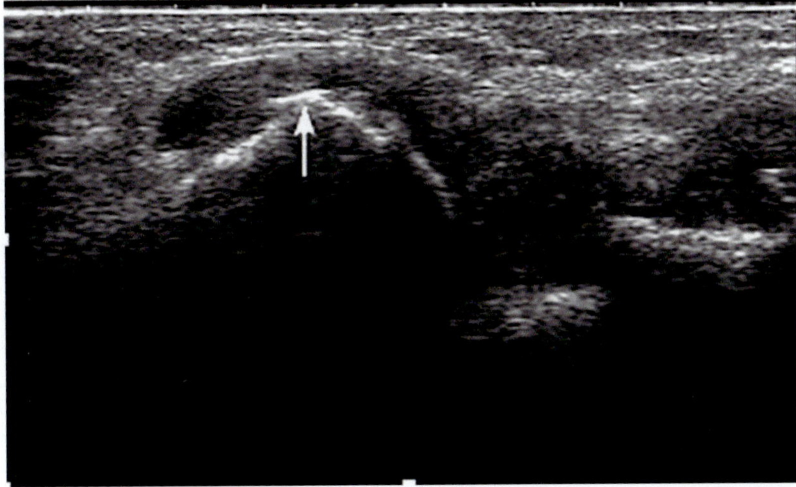

Fig. 7.5 Synovitis of the ulnocarpal joint with bony irregularities of the ulnar head (dorsal ulnar longitudinal view)

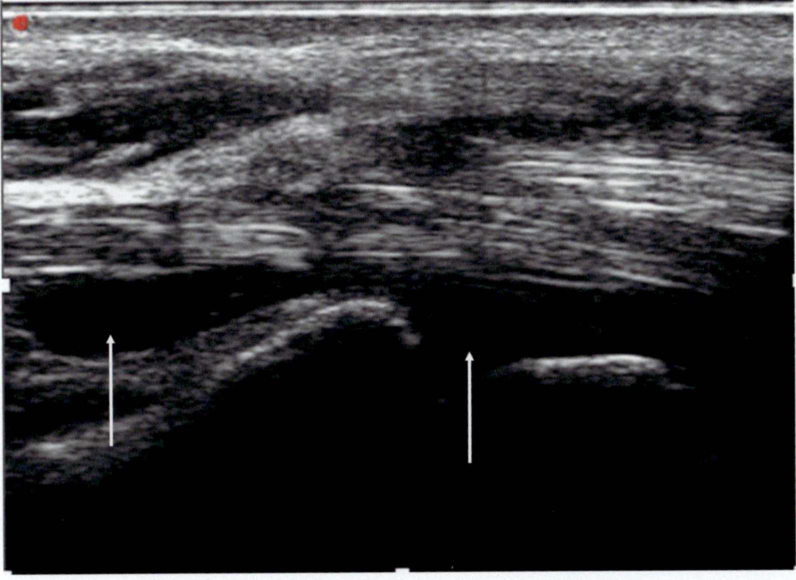

Fig. 7.6 Effusion of the radio-carpal joint (arrows; volar longitudinal view)

7.2.3 *Tenosynovitis of the Wrist I*

Best Scans: Standard Scans 7-1 to 7-8.

In Fig. 7.7, a longitudinal sonogram shows hypoechoic material at the dorsal radiocarpal joint and the midcarpal joints representing synovitis (⇑). In addition, there is hypoechoic material around the extensor digitorum tendons representing tenosynovitis (⇓).

Figure 7.8 shows a transverse sonogram of the extensor digitorum tendons of the right wrist. The ulnar side with the extensor minimi tendon, representing the fifth compartment, is on the left. The extensor digitorum tendons including the extensor indices tendon (fourth compartment) are surrounded by an increased amount of hypoechoic material representing tenosynovitis (**). The hypoechogenicity of the surrounding material enhances the normal echogenicity of the tendons, thus improving their visibility. Further to the right side of the scan, the third compartment with the extensor pollicis longus tendon is seen (*).

Figure 7.9 shows a transverse plane of the sixth compartment, i.e., the tendon of the extensor carpi ulnaris muscle. This sonogram demonstrates tenosynovitis with hypoechoic fluid surrounding the tendon. The cause may be inflammatory disease, trauma, or infection. In addition, there are erosions of the ulnar head.

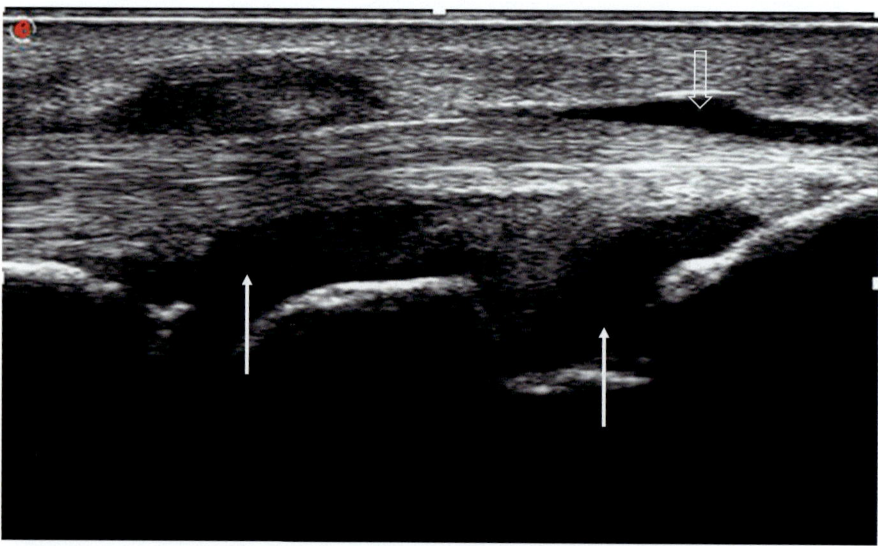

Fig. 7.7 Synovitis of radiocarpal and midcarpal joints and tenosynovitis of extensor digitorum tendons (dorsal longitudinal view)

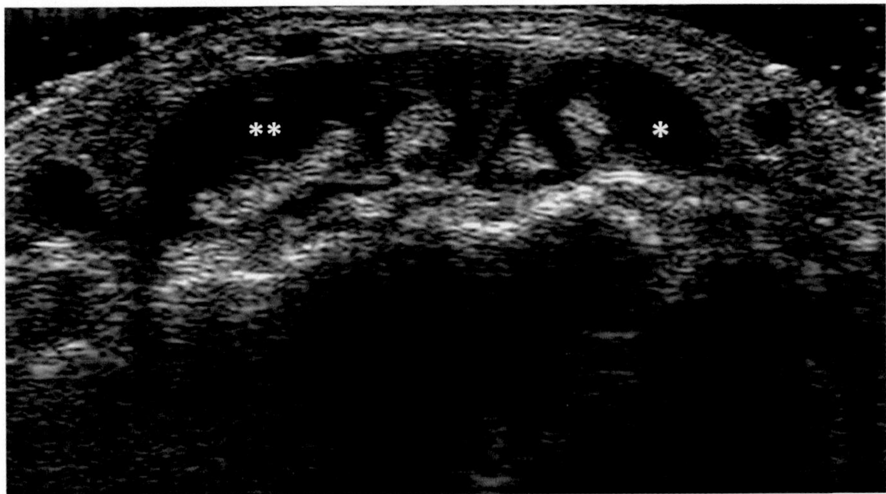

Fig. 7.8 Tenosynovitis of extensor digitorum tendons (dorsal transverse view)

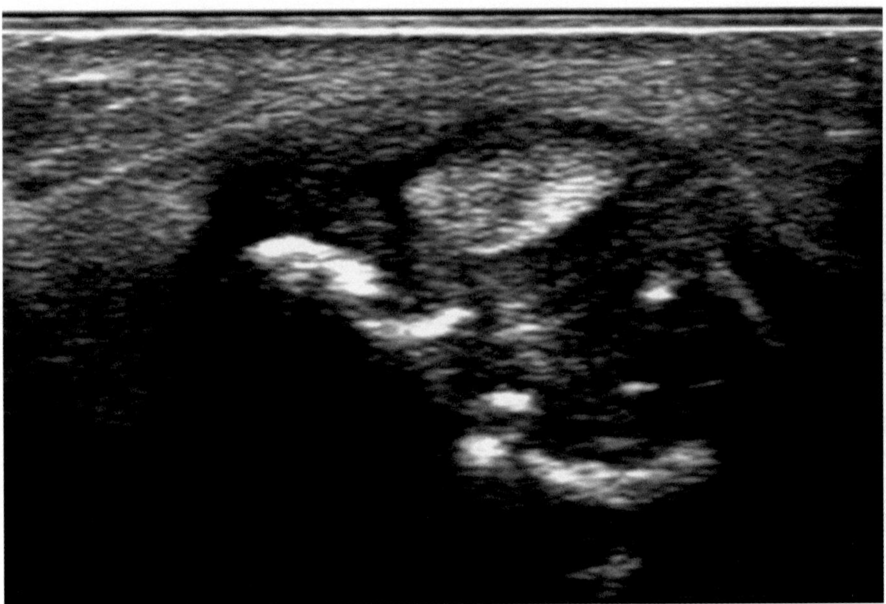

Fig. 7.9 Tenosynovitis of the extensor carpi ulnaris tendon with erosions of the ulnar head (transverse dorsal ulnar view)

7.2.4 Tenosynovitis of the Wrist II

Best Scans: Standard Scans 7-1 to 7-8.

This longitudinal scan of Fig. 7.10 shows tenosynovitis of the extensor carpi ulnaris tendon. The hyperechoic fibrillar echotexture of the tendon is readily recognized. The tendon runs over the ulna, ulnar head, ulnocarpal joint and triquetrum. Hypoechoic material representing tenosynovial proliferation and / or fluid is visualized. The surface of the ulnar head is irregular.

In Fig. 7.11, a volar longitudinal scan shows tenosynovitis of both the superficial (⇓) and deep (⇑) tendons of the flexor digitorum muscles. In addition, there is effusion of the radiocarpal joint that extends proximally over the radial head (⇒).

Figure 7.12 shows a hypoechoic widening of the extensor tendon sheath of the dorsal wrist.

The transverse sonogram of Fig. 7.13 shows the double rows of superficial and deep flexor digitorum tendons separated by fluid (hypoechoic areas) caused by tenosynovitis. Superficial to the flexor tendons, the median nerve is clearly visible. Anterior to the median nerve, the strong flexor retinaculum appears as a hypoechoic band.

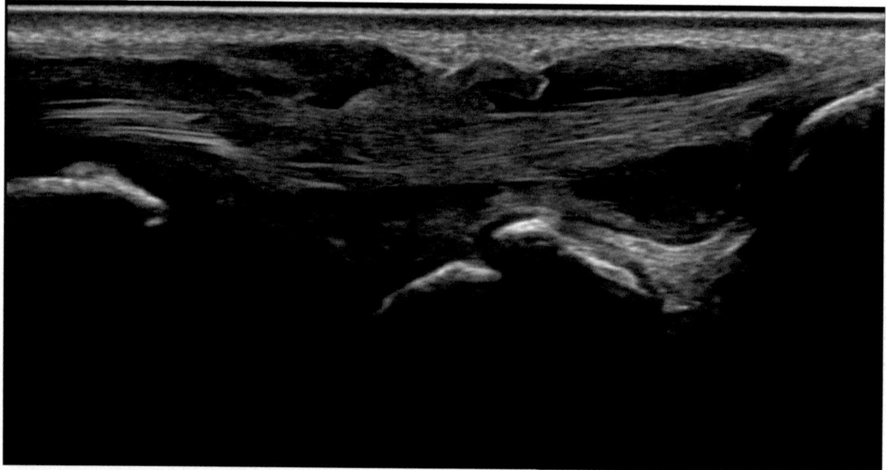

Fig. 7.10 Tenosynovitis of the extensor carpi ulnaris tendon at the wrist (longitudinal dorsal ulnar view)

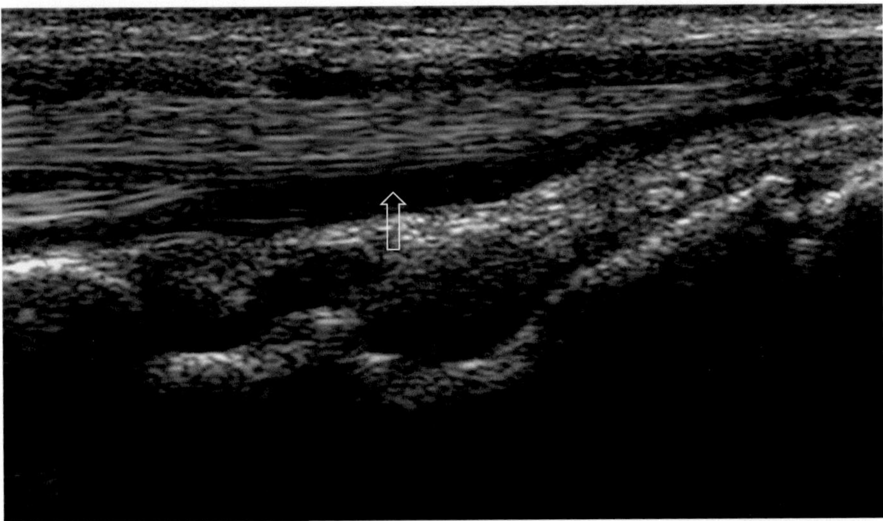

Fig. 7.11 Tenosynovitis of flexor digitorum tendons and effusion of the radiocarpal joint (volar longitudinal view)

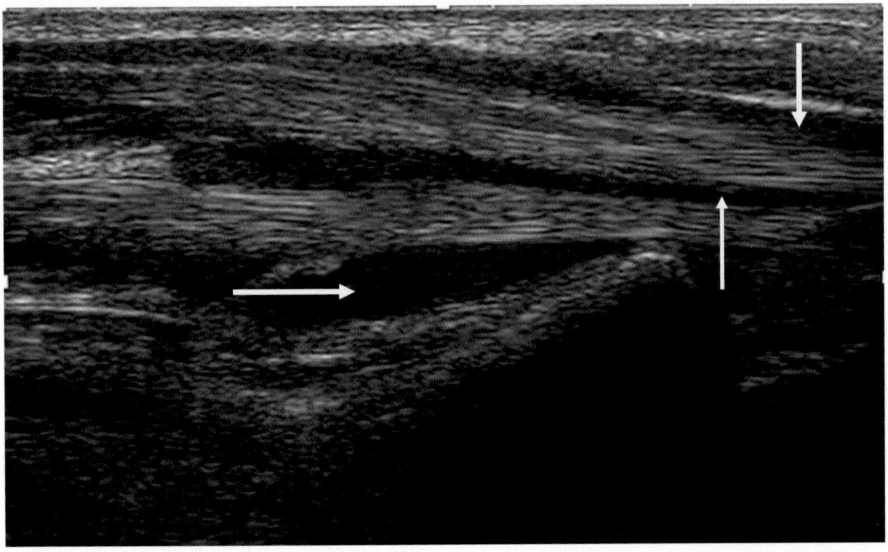

Fig. 7.12 Tenosynovitis of the extensor tendons and wrist effusion (dorsal longitudinal view)

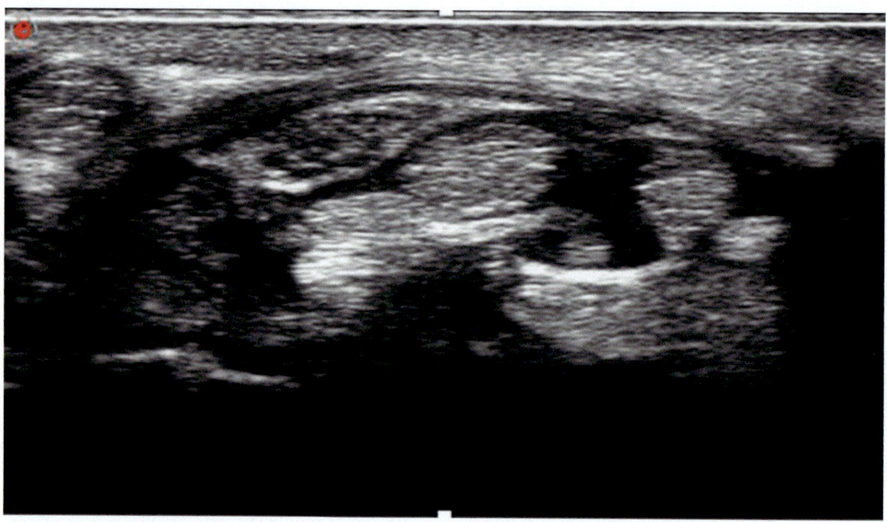

Fig. 7.13 Tenosynovitis of the flexor digitorum tendons in the carpal tunnel with normal median nerve (volar transverse view)

7.2.5 Carpal Tunnel Syndrome

Best Scans: Standard Scans 7-6 and 7-8.

Ultrasound can distinguish between primary and secondary carpal tunnel syndrome. In primary carpal tunnel syndrome, the flexor retinaculum is thickened (about 1.0 mm or more) or the median nerve is altered and no other reason for this can be found. Secondary carpal tunnel syndrome can result from tenosynovitis of the flexor digitorum tendons, wrist synovitis, ganglia or other space-consuming lesions.

Sonographic findings can be divided into qualitative or subjective and quantitative or objective criteria. Subjective findings are hypoechoic enlargement of the nerve at the inlet of the carpal tunnel; volar bulging of the flexor retinaculum; large fluid or soft tissue masses surrounding the tendons; decreased mobility of the median nerve on flexion and extension of the fingers, hand and wrist.

The mean cross-sectional area of the median nerve >12 mm^2 at the inlet of the carpal tunnel seems to have the highest sensitivity and specificity for the presence of carpal tunnel syndrome. Other objective but less specific and sensitive criteria are an increased flattening ratio of the nerve, i.e., transverse diameter divided by the anterior–posterior diameter >4 at the level of the hamate, and volar bulging of the flexor retinaculum >3.1 mm.

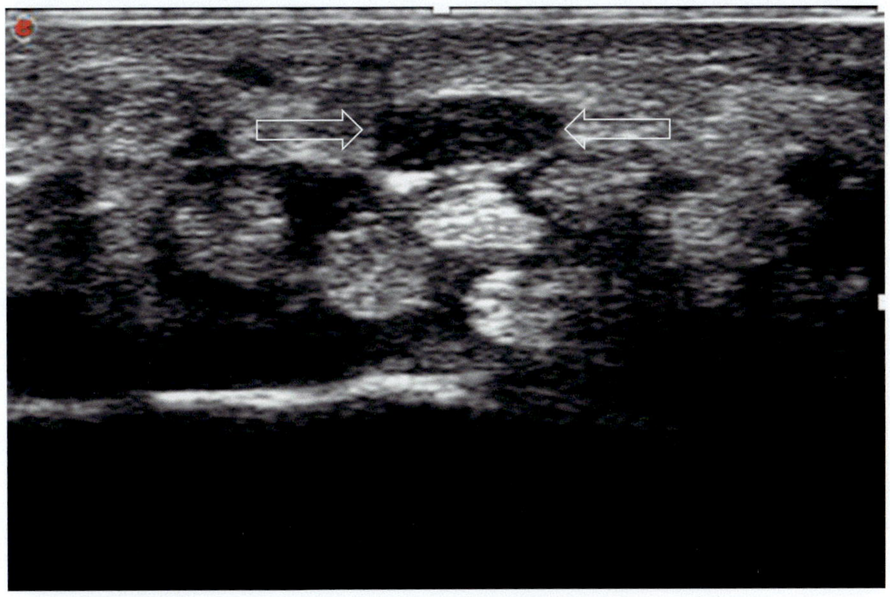

Fig. 7.14 Hypoechoic, enlarged median nerve and tenosynovitis of the flexor digitorum tendons in secondary carpal tunnel syndrome (volar transverse view)

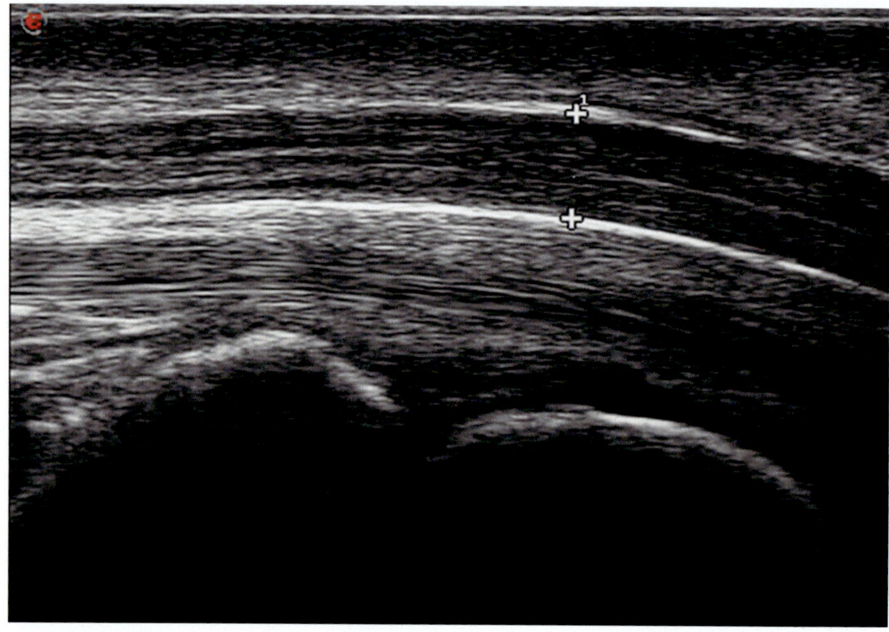

Fig. 7.15 Hypoechoic, enlarged median nerve without any further abnormalities in primary carpal tunnel syndrome (volar longitudinal view)

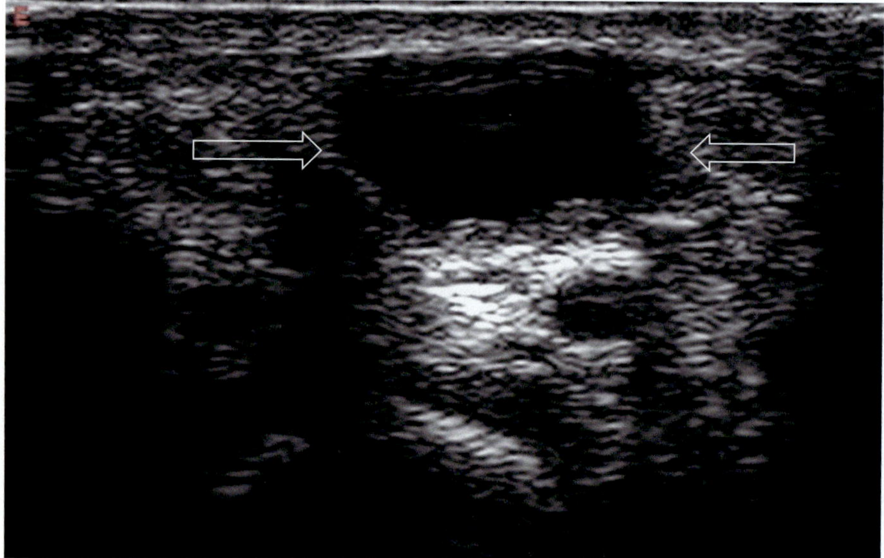

Fig. 7.16 Ganglion at the wrist (volar transverse view)

Figures 7.14 and 7.15 show a swollen, hypoechoic median nerve (arrows), anterior to the flexor tendon. The transverse image delineates tenosynovitis whereas the longitudinal image does not depict any further abnormality suspective of primary carpal tunnel syndrome.

Figure 7.16 shows a ganglion ($\Rightarrow\Leftarrow$), which appears as a well-defined anechoic, non-compressible structure that does not exhibit color Doppler signals. Ganglia often occur at the volar radial aspect of the wrist.

Chapter 8
The Fingers

8.1 Standard Scans of the Fingers

8.1.1 Volar Longitudinal View of the MCP Joints (Standard Scan 8-1)

The patient sits in front of the sonographer with the hand resting on a table or on the thighs. The fingers can be flexed or extended for dynamic examination. The probe is moved as far as possible around the MCP joints. The probe may be moved proximally from the first MCP joint to evaluate the first CMC joint. For examination of the fingers, a high-definition probe with frequencies above 15 MHz and a small foot print is optimal.

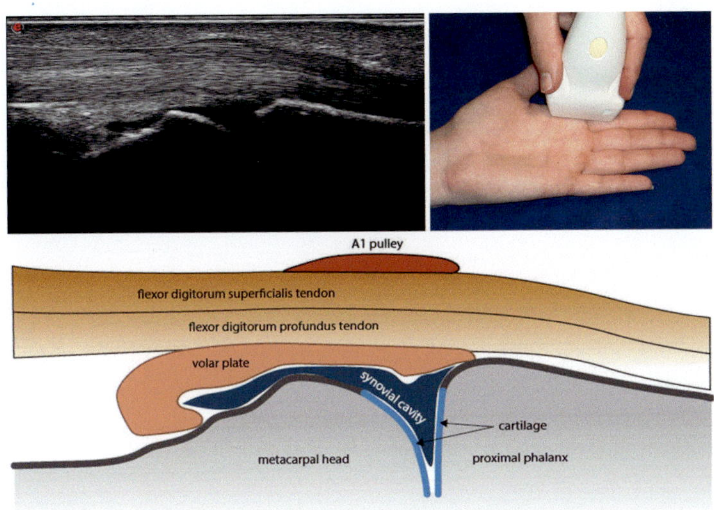

© The Author(s), under exclusive license to Springer Nature Switzerland AG 2023
G. A. W. Bruyn and W. A. Schmidt, *Musculoskeletal Ultrasound for the Rheumatologist*,
https://doi.org/10.1007/978-3-031-27737-5_8

This longitudinal scan shows the flexor tendon of the second finger. It can be applied to all the fingers. The ultrasound image clearly shows the joint space, the thin layer of the anechoic cartilage, the fibrocartilaginous volar plate, the small proximal joint recess, and the capsule. The flexor profundus tendon lies deep to the superficialis tendon in the palm until the superficialis tendon divides in two slips at the level of the distal third of the proximal phalanx between which the profundus continues its course. With high frequency transducers it is easy to distinguish the superficialis and the profundus tendon on either the longitudinal or the transverse scan proximal to the MCP joint. At specific spots, the flexor tendon sheath is reinforced by pulleys. Based on their general appearance, they can be divided into 5 annular pulleys and three cruciate pulleys. The annular A1 pulley, which keeps the flexor tendon close to the palmar plate with finger flexion, is visible as a thin hypoechoic structure anterior to the tendon at the level of the MCP joint. With >20 MHz transducers the pulleys may appear hyperechoic due to their fine fibrillar structure. It is important to shift the probe more proximally to the palmar region and distally towards the PIP joint, particularly when searching for tenosynovitis.

What is normal?

The cartilage rim covering the metacarpal heads should be clearly visible in a normal situation. The mean diameter between the 2nd metacarpal head and the joint capsule is 0.9 mm (0–1.9 mm). Other MCP joints have similar normal values.

8.1.2   *Volar Transverse View of the MCP Joints (Standard Scan 8-2)*

The position of the hand is the same as that in Standard Scan 8-1. Then the probe is rotated by 90° with respect to the previous scan.

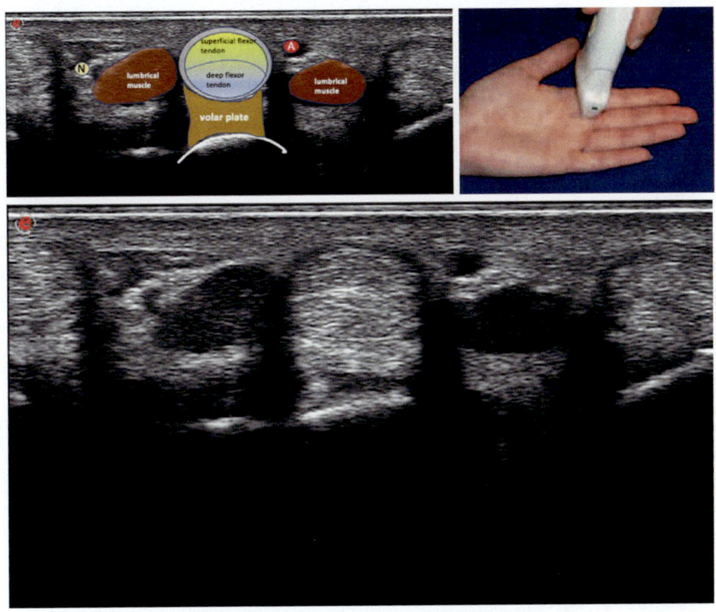

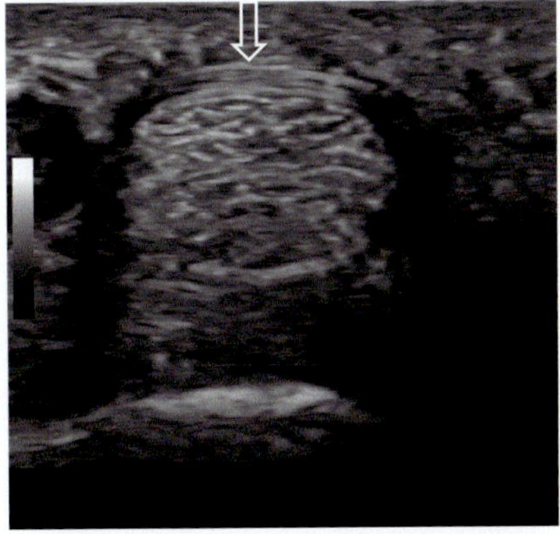

Hyperechoic A1 pulley documented with a 6–24 MHz hockey stick probe adjusted at 24 MHz

With high frequency transducers, the superficial and deep flexor tendons can be differentiated from each other at the distal palm where the former lies superficial to the latter. The flexor tendons of the thumb and fifth digit have separate synovial sheaths. They arise at the level of the wrist and continue to the insertion of the tendon at the distal phalanx. The sheaths for the flexor tendons of the second, third and fourth digits begin at the metacarpal heads and continue over the pairs of tendons to the base of the distal phalanges of digits 2, 3, and 4.

The annular A1 pulley is visible as a hypoechoic structure overlying the flexor tendon, more laterally its appearance is usually hypoechoic due to anisotropy. However, with >20 MHz transducers the pulleys may appear hyperechoic due to their fine fibrillar structure as these provide higher resolution. The pulley inserts on both sides of the tendon into the palmar plate (⇓).

What is normal?

The tendon sheaths contain some hypo-echoic material that is also visible in normal tendons. On transverse scans both lateral sides of the tendon are difficult to assess due to edge shadowing (see Chap. 2). The mean diameter of a normal tendon sheath 1 cm proximal to the second MCP joint is 0.9 mm (0.1–1.7 mm). Diameters are similar for other finger tendons. The transverse diameter of finger flexor tendons is 6.4 mm (3.7–9.1 mm) and sagittal diameter is 3.6 mm (1.4–5.8 mm). The thickness of the A1 pulley slightly increases with age, from 0.11–0.27 mm in children to 0.17–0.35 mm in healthy volunteers over 50 years.

8.1.3 *Dorsal Longitudinal View of the MCP Joints (Standard Scan 8-3)*

This scan also applies to the other fingers as mentioned for the previous scans. The hand is in pronation. As with the previous scans the probe should also be moved to the radial and ulnar aspects as far as possible. The view may be extended proximally and distally. Joint flexion and extension is part of the dynamic examination. In particular, for examination of the cartilage the MCP joint should be maximally flexed.

This longitudinal scan shows an MCP joint from its dorsal side. On top, the hyperechoic parallel lines of the second extensor tendon can be seen.

In contrast to the flexor opponents, the extensor tendons lack a synovial sheath. Deep to the extensor tendon, a small proximal synovial recess may be visible. The dorsal triangular structure contains fibrocartilaginous tissue and is part of the dorsal joint capsule.

What is normal?

Commonly, there is a small cortical depression at the proximal side of the dorsal metacarpal head that can easily be mistaken for an erosion. Osteophytes may occur particularly in the second and third MCP joints in older patients caused by osteoarthritis. Cartilage thickness of the metacarpal head ranges between 0.41 and 1.10 mm in men and between 0.36 and 1.03 mm in women. The mean length of the dorsal synovial recess is 12.1 mm; maximum thickness, 2.3 mm; and thickness over the metacarpal head tubercle, 1.7 mm.

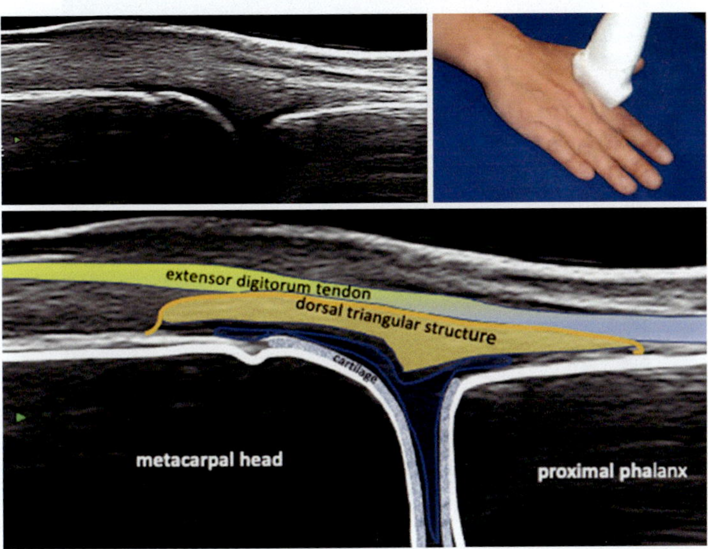

8.1.4   Dorsal Transverse View of the MCP Joints (Standard Scan 8-4)

The position of the hand is the same as that in Standard Scan 8-3. The probe is rotated by 90° with respect to the previous scan.

At the level of the MCP joint the extensor tendon (ET) is stabilized against radial or ulnar subluxation by the sagittal bands of the extensor hood. The extensor tendon has no direct contact with the dorsal side of the synovial cavity, it is separated from it by a fibrocartilaginous structure. This dorsal fibrocartilaginous structure is attached to the joint capsule and along with the sagittal bands complements the stabilization of the extensor tendon over the metacarpal head. Distally from the MCP joint, the transverse ultrasound scan shows the central slip of the extensor tendon (arrows), with medially and laterally to it, the two collateral bands (*).

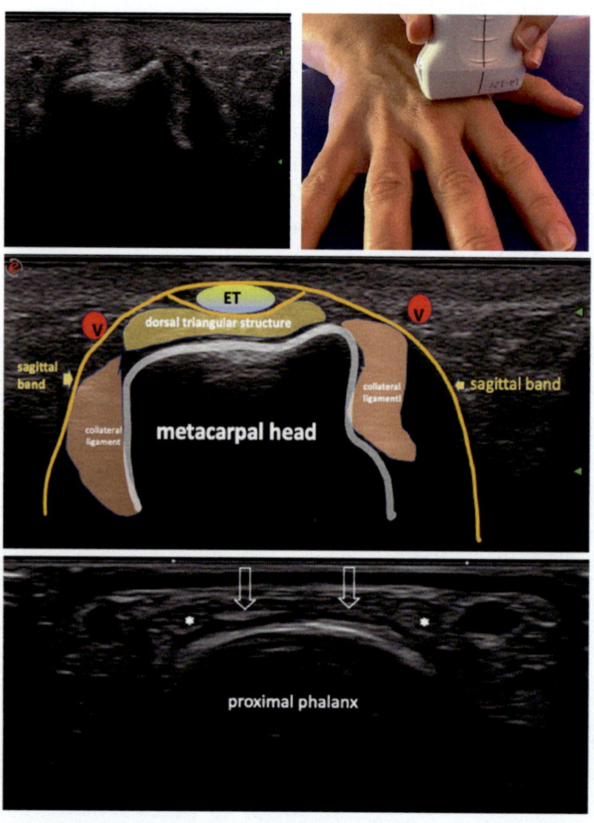

8.1.5   *Volar Longitudinal View of the PIP Joints (Standard Scan 8-5)*

The position of the hand is the same as that in Standard Scan 8-3. The probe is then moved distally to evaluate the PIP joints of digits 2–5 and the IP joint of the thumb as well as the flexor tendons. The probe can be moved around the joint in search of erosions.

Proximally to the PIP joint, the flexor superficialis tendon divides into an ulnar and radial slip, which insert along the proximal half of the middle phalanx. The PIP joint is visible, together with its cartilage, joint capsule, A3 pulley, and palmar plate.

What is normal?

Parts of the flexor tendon appear dark because of anisotropy, particularly in the areas proximal and distal to the PIP joint, where the probe is not completely perpendicular to the tendon. A certain amount of synovial material may be present in the proximal recess in healthy subjects. The mean distance between the proximal phalanx and the joint capsule is 0.8 mm (0–1.6 mm). The bone surface is regular.

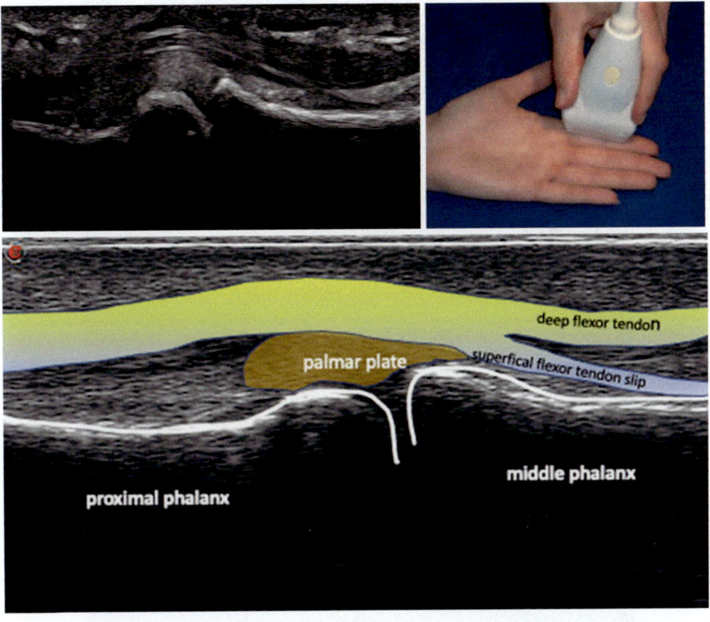

8.1.6   Volar Transverse View of the PIP Joints (Standard Scan 8-6)

The probe is turned 90° with respect to the previous scan to visualize the PIP joint, flexor tendons, and other soft tissue structures in a second plane.

On the transverse scan, at the level of the PIP joint, the deep flexor tendon can be seen in the center of the scan, just superficial to the palmar plate. The A3 pulley is also seen here in the transverse plane. On both sides of the deep flexor tendon the two slips of the superficialis flexor tendon can be distinguished before they insert at the proximal one third of the middle phalanx.

What is normal?

The flexor tendon may have a very small hypoechoic rim as described in Standard Scan 8-2, but it is smaller than it is at the MCP joint. The probe should always be parallel to the tendon to avoid anisotropy. The finger arteries may be evaluated with color Doppler ultrasound (see Chap. 13).

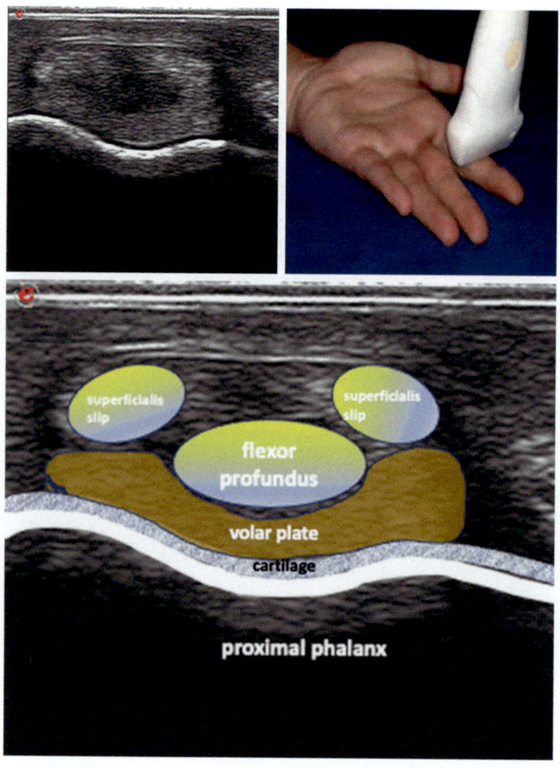

8.1.7   *Dorsal Longitudinal View of the PIP Joints (Standard Scan 8-7)*

The probe is moved directly from Standard Scan 8-3 to evaluate the PIP joint from the dorsal aspect. At the PIP joint the extensor apparatus splits into two lateral bands and one central band. The central band continues its course and inserts at the base of the middle phalanx. Both lateral bands merge at the level of the DIP joint and insert as one entity just distal of the DIP joint.

Bony spurs may be visualized more frequently than with the volar scans. The ultrasound image shows the second PIP joint, which is clearly delineated from its surroundings. The proximal phalanx is localized on the left side. The middle phalanx is localized on the right side. The hyaline cartilage covering the head of the PIP is clearly visible as a anechoic band. The triangular hyperechoic structure filling the space deep to the extensor tendon and superficial to the synovial capsule is composed of fibrocartilagenous tissue. The extensor tendon is isoechoic with hyperechoic boundaries.

What is normal?

The bone surface is regular. Osteophytes occur frequently in older patients due to osteoarthritis.

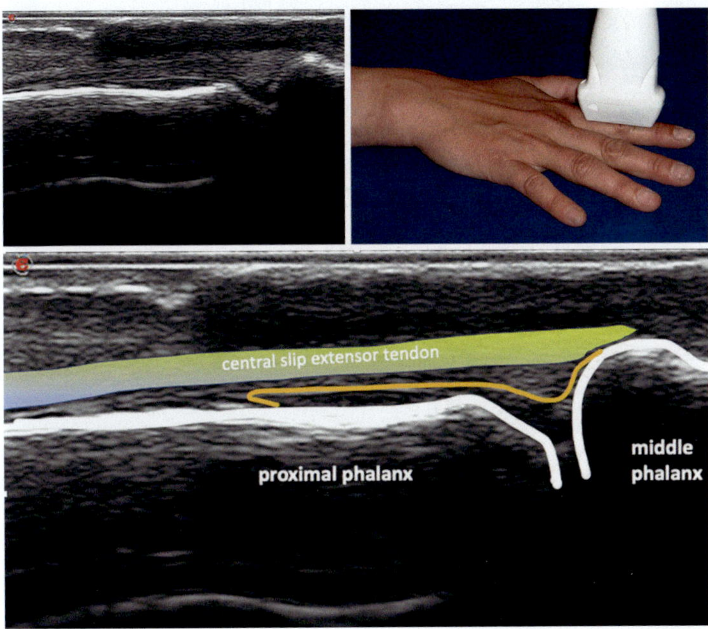

8.1.8   *Volar Longitudinal View of the DIP Joints (Standard Scan 8-8)*

For evaluating the DIP joint and the soft tissues in this region the probe is moved distally from its position in Standard Scan 8-5. The probe may be moved around the joint. Pathologies should also be examined in a transverse plane. This region is difficult to evaluate with low-frequency and low-quality probes.

The profundus flexor tendon passes between the superficialis tendon slips and inserts at the base of the distal phalanx, as this longitudinal palmar scan of the distal phalanx shows. Again, parts of the tendon are hypoechoic because of anisotropy.

In a normal DIP joint, the bone surface is regular. Osteophytes are more clearly visible in the dorsal scan of the DIP joint.

What is normal?

There are no normal values for the DIP joints.

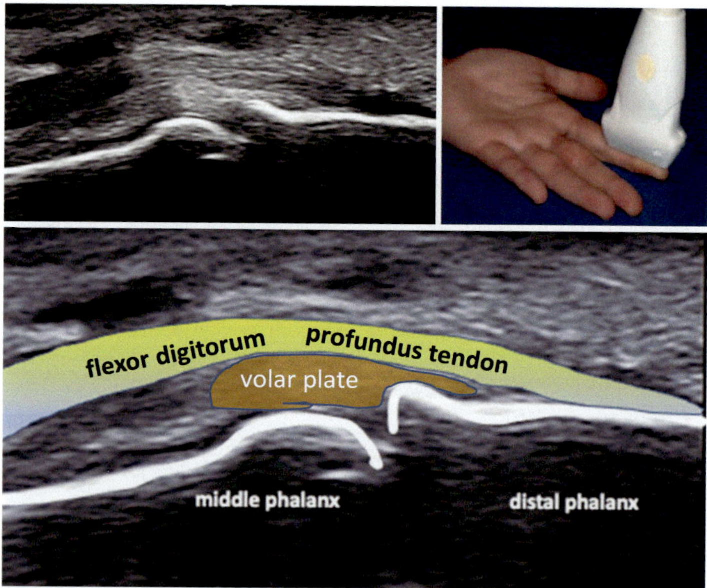

8.1.9 Dorsal Longitudinal View of the DIP Joints (Standard Scan 8-9)

The probe is moved distally from the position in Standard Scan 8-7. The probe may be moved around the joint. Abnormalities including osteophytes and nail irregularities should also be examined in a second, transverse, plane.

The dorsal longitudinal scan informs of the insertion of the extensor tendon just distal to the DIP joint. The nail bed and nail plate can be seen at the right side of the scan. Normal nails show a typical triple layer, i.e., a hyperechoic dorsal plate, a hypoechoic interplate space and a hyperechoic, more volarly localized plate. Doppler application shows the vascularity of the nail bed. Both the nail and the insertion of the extensor tendon may be involved in psoriatic arthritis. The characteristic ultrasound trilayer appearance of the nail can then become obliterated.

The extensor tendon inserts at the base of the distal phalanx close to the DIP joint and just distal to the insertion of the joint capsule.

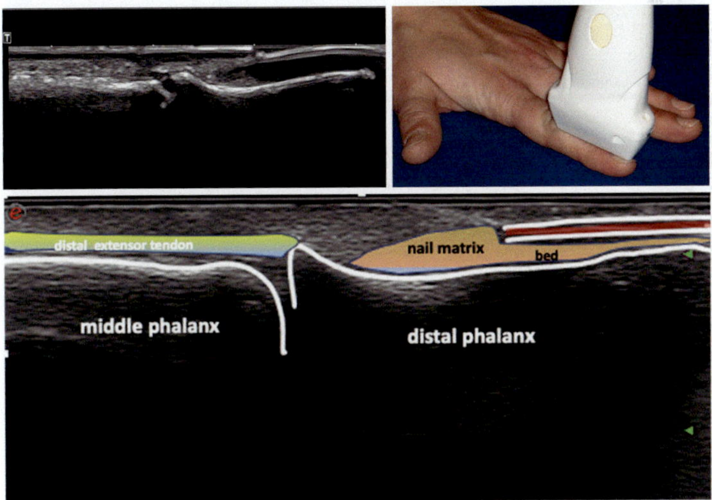

8.1.10   *Ultrasound-Guided Injection of Tendon Sheaths*

In tenosynovitis, injection of a finger flexor tendon sheath can best be done in a volar transverse plane perpendicular to the axis of the finger. It can also be done in a longitudinal plane, but then the position of the needle bevel has to be checked by means of a second transverse scan in order to exclude the possibility that the needle tip might be outside the flexor sheath. First, the site of maximum tenosynovial extension should be marked. The needle is introduced at the foot of the transducer and directed into the synovial sheath under real-time ultrasound guidance as shown in this image. The needle is maneuvered forwards parallel to the probe.

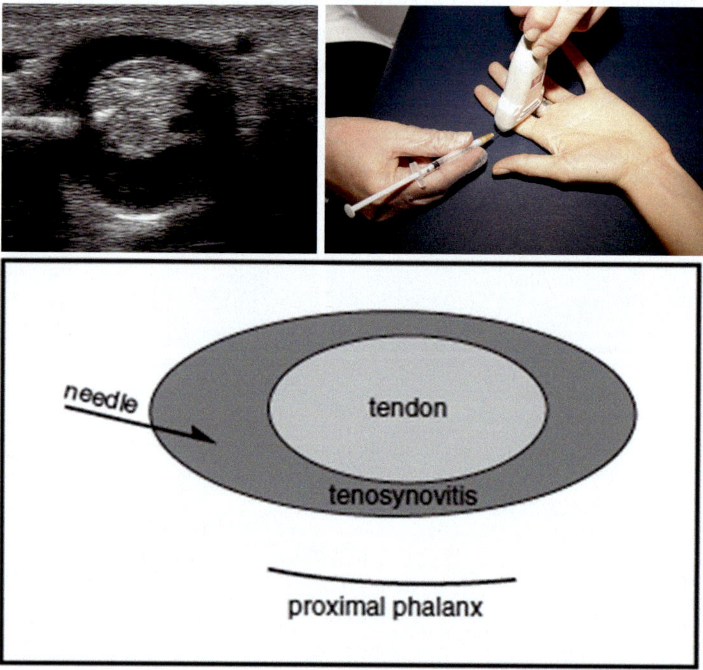

8.1.11 *Ultrasound-Guided Injection of the MCP Joint*

Injections into the small finger joints are generally done from the dorsal side. The hand of the patient is comfortably and firmly placed on a table.

Firstly, a long axis prescan is done to mark the exact site of the joint space. A small needle is inserted into the foot of the transducer proximally to the joint and directed through the capsule into the synovium under direct ultrasound guidance.

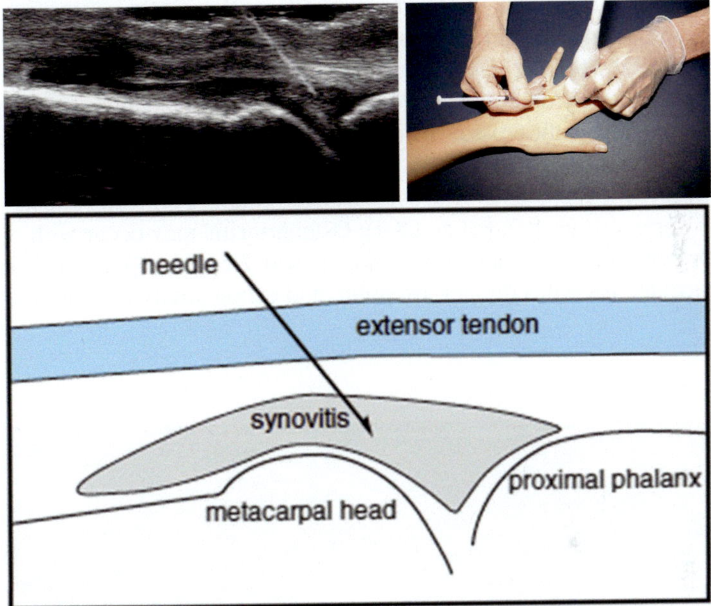

8.2   Pathology of the Fingers

8.2.1   Erosions and Osteophytes of Finger Joints

Several studies have shown that ultrasound reliably detects erosions in early RA. Erosions, such as the one in Fig. 8.1 (⇑), are defined as an intra- or extraarticular discontinuity of the bone surface that is visible in two perpendicular planes. The floor of the erosion is often irregular in RA. The majority of erosions in RA occur at the radial and ulnar sides of MCP joints adjacent to the collateral ligaments, as a result of a predilection of synovitis at these sites. Ultrasound detects erosions particularly at the radial side of the MCP 2 joints and at the ulnar side of MCP 5 joints because these areas are not hidden by other bones. Power Doppler can detect increased vascularity in active pannus within the erosion, in a similar way as dynamic gadolinium-enhanced MRI can discriminate between active and inactive RA.

In contrast to the erosions of RA, osteoarthritic changes typically appear as osteophytic bony spurs (Figs. 8.2, 8.3 and 8.4). Osteoarthritis may occur with or without effusion or synovitis that often show fewer power Doppler signals than in RA. In OA, the cartilage becomes thinner, irregular, and echogenicity increases (Fig. 8.4).

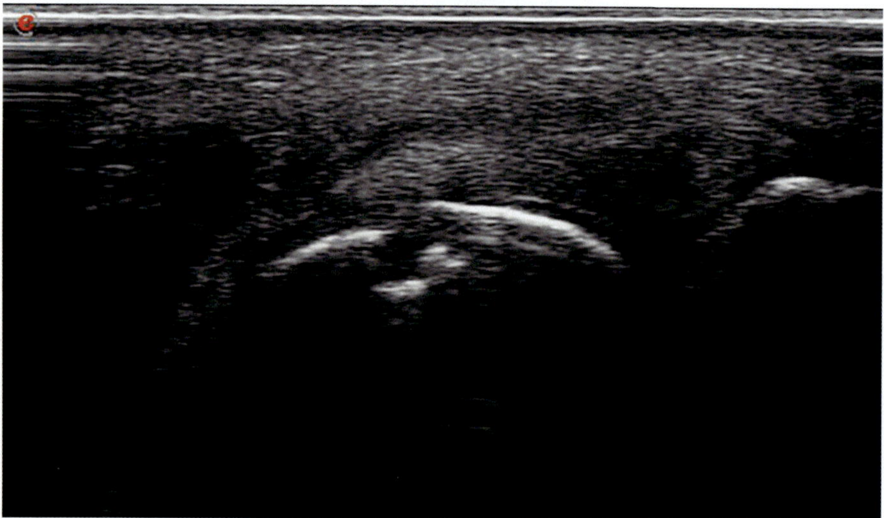

Fig. 8.1 Erosion at the radial aspect of the metacarpal bone proximal to the second MCP joint in early RA (longitudinal radial view)

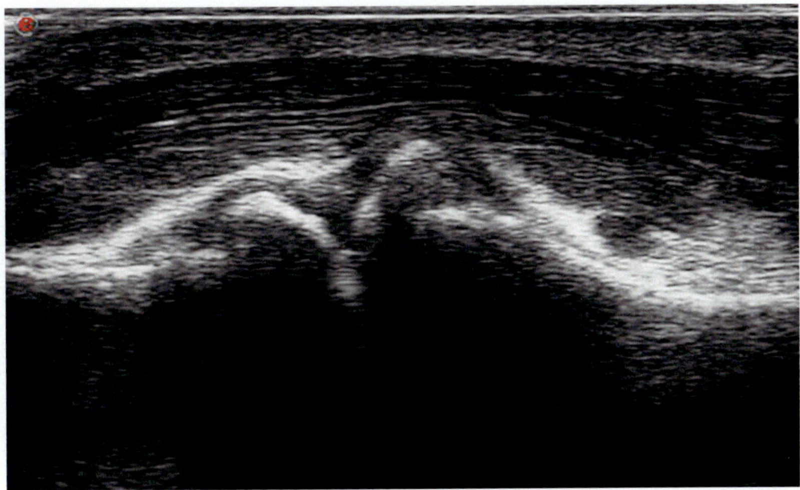

Fig. 8.2 Osteoarthritis with osteophytes of the first carpometacarpal joint (volar longitudinal view)

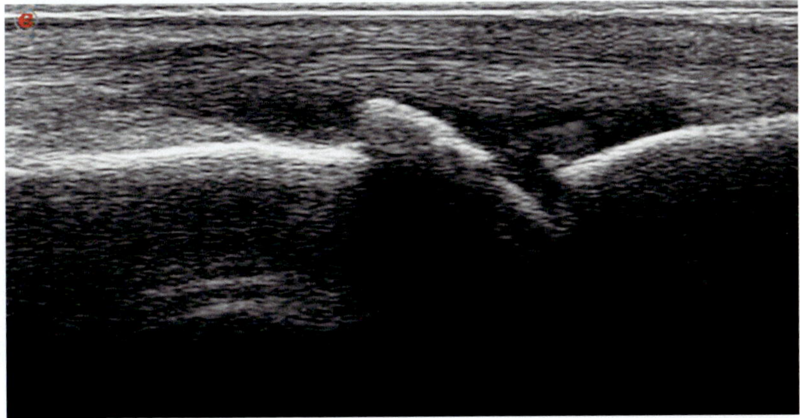

Fig. 8.3 Dorsal longitudinal scan of a second MCP joint showing osteoarthritis with mild synovitis

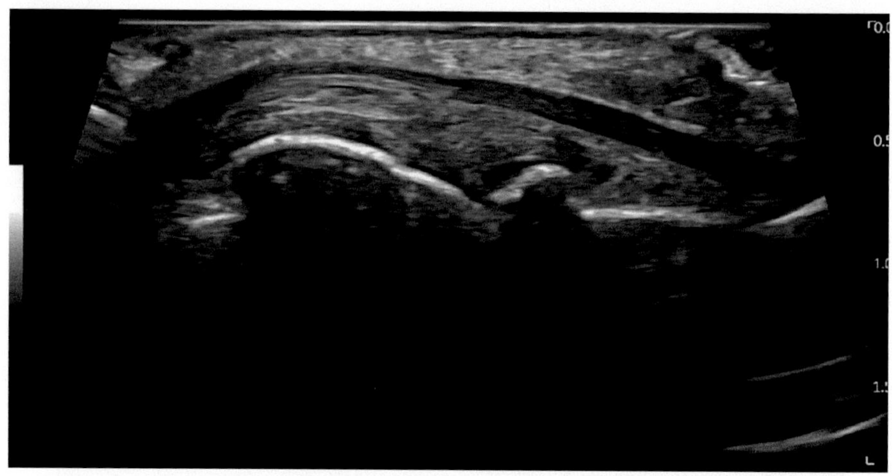

Fig. 8.4 Osteoarthritis of fourth MCP joint, showing thinned cartilage (dorsal longitudinal view)

8.2.2 *Synovitis/Effusion of the Finger Joints*

Best scans: Standard Scans 8-9, 8-11, 8-12, and 8-14

Additional scans: Standard Scans 8-10 and 8-13

Synovitis or effusion may be detected both volarly and dorsally, or only at one of these sides. Dorsally localized effusion or synovitis can be found clinically in most cases, whilst capsular distension is very difficult to palpate at the volar side because the flexor tendons are thicker.

Figure 8.5 shows anechoic material (⇓) in the volar proximal recess of a MCP joint representing effusion. It takes the shape of a tear drop. No erosions are visible in this plane. MCP joints are invariably involved in rheumatoid arthritis, and so their assessment is of utmost importance.

Figure 8.6 shows synovitis (arrowhead) with hyperperfusion (power Doppler grade 2) at the dorsal side of a MCP 1 joint in RA. One of the vessels enters a small erosion. Above the erosion is a rheumatic nodule with clear borders, similar echogenicity, and less intense vascularity. Both B-mode ultrasound and power Doppler ultrasound are reproducible tools for determining synovitis.

Figure 8.7 shows a PIP joint filled with hypoechoic material compatible with synovitis. Synovitis again extends proximally (⇓), along the shaft of the proximal phalanx. The joint capsule is not parallel to the bone.

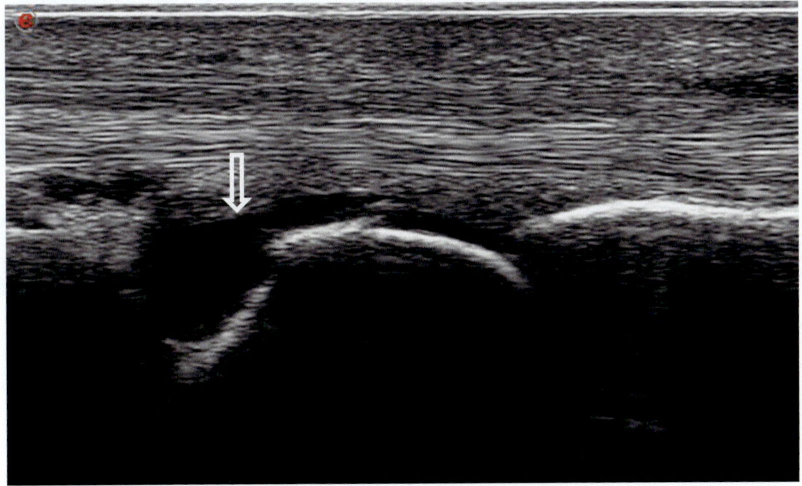

Fig. 8.5 Volar longitudinal scan showing effusion of the first MCP joint

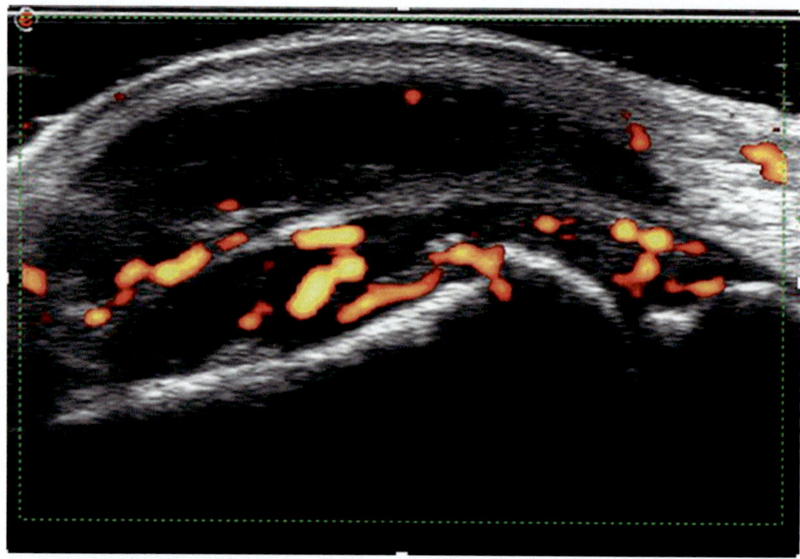

Fig. 8.6 Synovitis of an MCP joint and a rheumatic nodule (dorsal longitudinal scan)

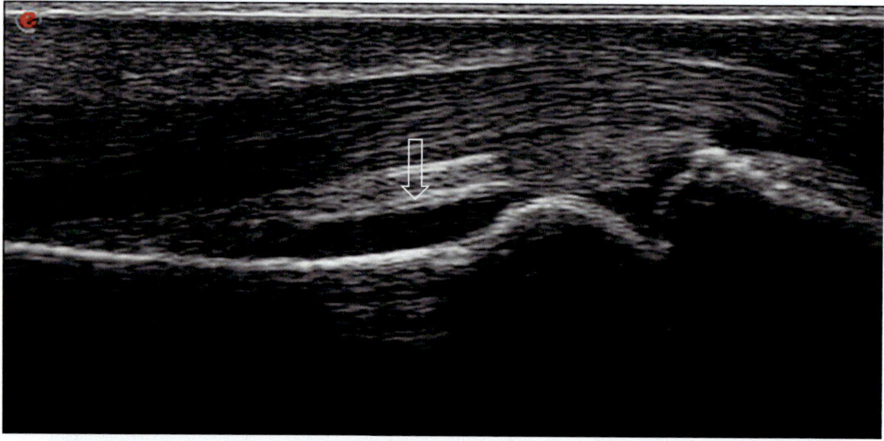

Fig. 8.7 Synovitis of a PIP joint (volar longitudinal scan)

8.2.3 *Tenosynovitis of the Finger Flexor Tendons*

Best scans: Standard Scans 8-10 and 8-13

Additional scans: Standard Scans 8-9, 8-12 and 8-15

The sensitivity of ultrasound in detecting tenosynovitis and tendon abnormalities is high. A high-frequency transducer of at least 10 MHz is required, and a frequency even higher for the extensor tendons of the fingers. It is important to shift the probe from palmar distally over the finger joints in order to detect smaller regional tenosynovitis.

Figure 8.8 depicts a superficial and a deep flexor tendon at the level of the second MCP joint, surrounded by a distended synovial sheath in a patient with SLE. The transverse plane clearly shows hypoechoic material indicating tenosynovitis. Hypoechoic material is also localized between the superficial and deep flexor tendons, enabling them to be distinguished more easily from each other than in a normal situation.

Figure 8.9 shows the longitudinal scan of the same flexor tendon. The fibrillar pattern of the tendon is normal, precluding damage to the tendon. Loss of the normal fibrillar echotexture is one of the earliest signs of tendon damage both in inflammatory and degenerative disorders.

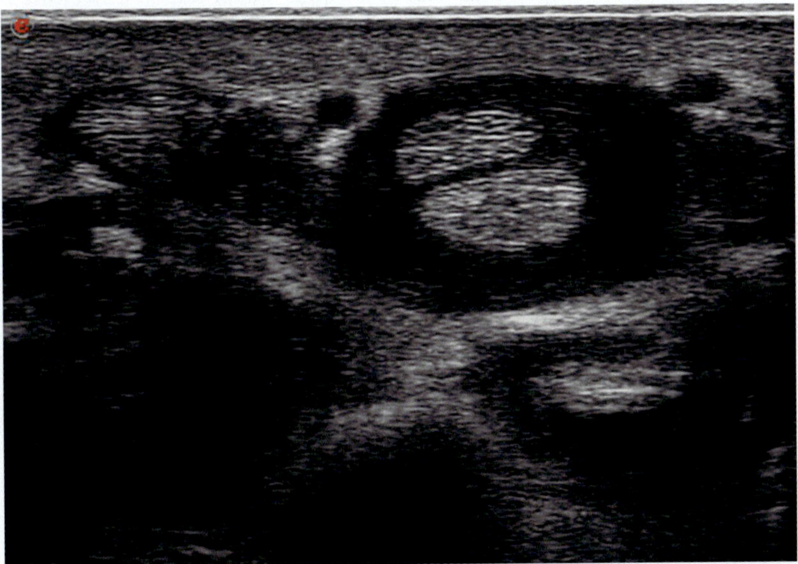

Fig. 8.8 Tenosynovitis of the fourth finger flexor tendons proximal to the MCP joint (volar transverse scan)

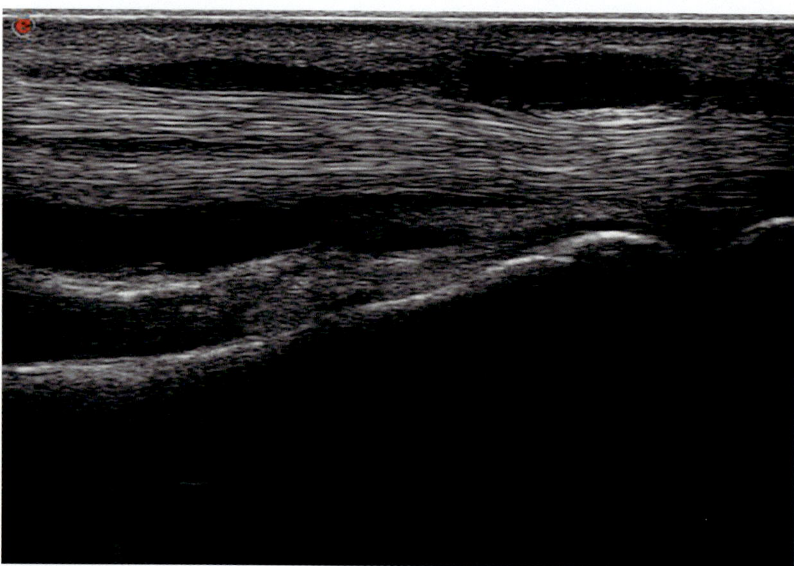

Fig. 8.9 Tenosynovitis of the fourth finger flexor tendons at the MCP Joint (volar longitudinal scan)

Figure 8.10 shows a longitudinal scan of a trigger finger due to a swelling of the A1 pulley. When flexing the finger, the flexor tendon bulges distally to the pulley instead of moving smoothly along the MCP joint.

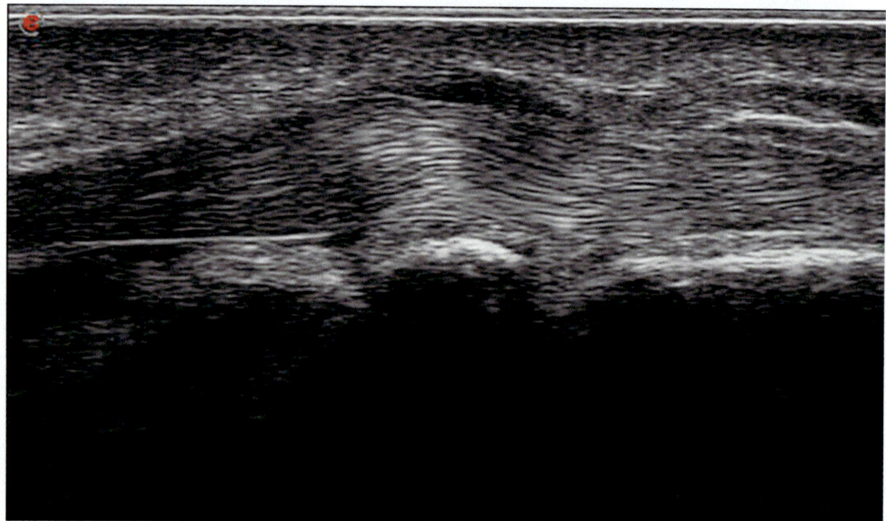

Fig. 8.10 Swelling of the A1 pulley with trigger finger (volar longitudinal scan)

Figure 8.11 shows a longitudinal volar scan of a dactylitis in psoriatic arthritis. There are small pockets of hypoechoic material at various locations around the flexor tendon visible proximally to the PIP joint (⇑), compatible with tenosynovitis. In addition, the A3 pulley seems to be thickened and hypoechoic (⇓).

Figure 8.12 depicts the same finger flexor tendon at a slightly more distal site with power Doppler. Clear signals are visible both in the subcutaneous tissue and

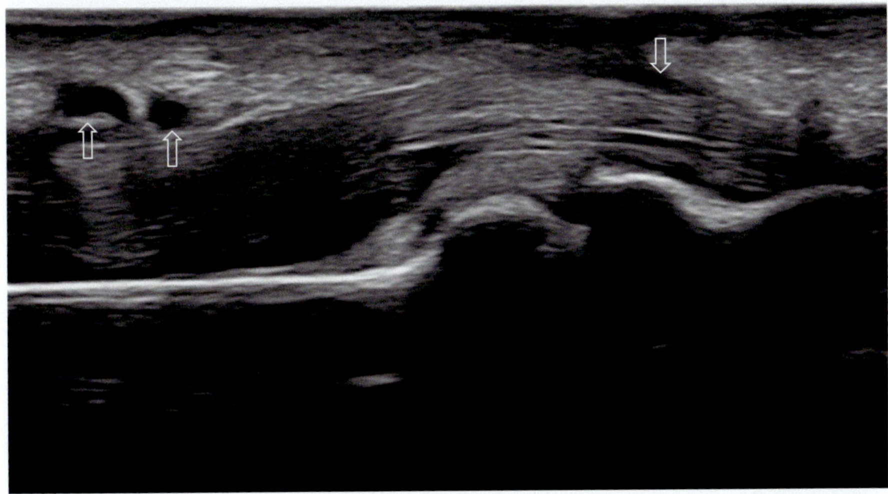

Fig. 8.11   Dactylitis in psoriatic arthritis

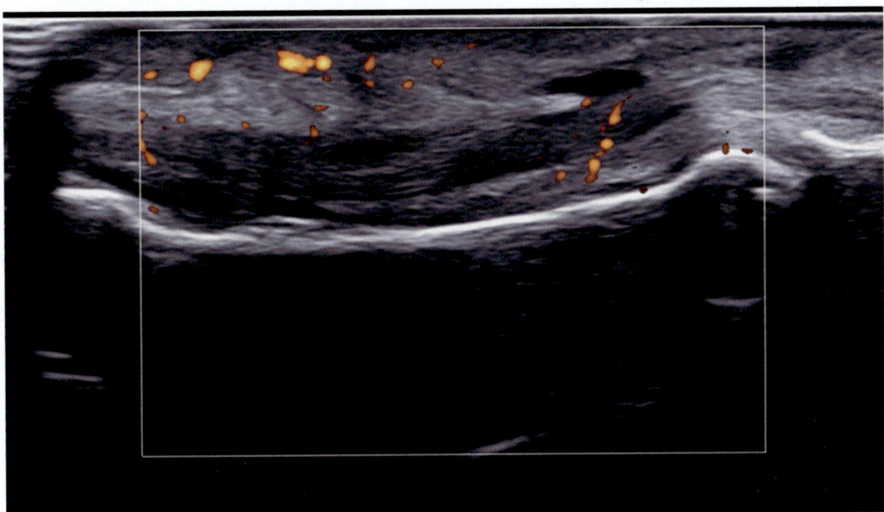

Fig. 8.12   Power Doppler scan of dactylitis in psoriatic arthritis showing inflammation of the subcutaneous tissue

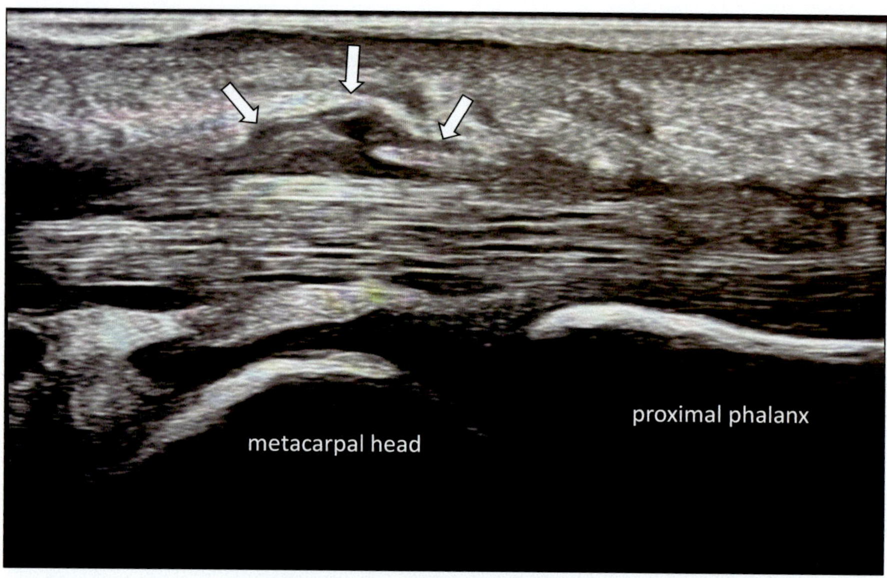

Fig. 8.13   Markedly enlarged A1 pulley in psoriatic arthritis

around the tendon. Figure 8.13 shows a significantly thickened A1 pulley (arrows) in a patient with psoriatic arthritis. Such pulleytis may be viewed as part of inflammation of the small finger entheses.

Chapter 9
The Pelvis, including the Sacroiliac Joint, the Sacral Hiatus, and the Ischial Tuberosity

9.1 The Sacroiliac Joints

Many attempts have been made to perform ultrasound of the sacroiliac joints (SI) for diagnosing sacroiliitis including the use of Doppler. There is no good literature evidence for a reliable ultrasound diagnosis. However, considering the therapeutic efficacy of image-guided intraarticular SI joint injections performed by CT, fluoroscopy, or MRI in patients with sacroiliac pain or inflammation, sonographic landmarks may be used to guide the needle to the superior entrance of the SI joint for the purpose of intraarticular SI joint injection.

Patient positioning. The patient is placed in a prone position with a bolster under the abdomen to facilitate the opening between sacrum and ilium. Either a linear or curved array probe of 5–10 MHz may be used. The SI joints are at about 3–9 cm under the skin surface, depending of the posture of the patient. In the midline, the spinal process of L5 should be identified in a transverse plane. Then the probe is shifted slightly caudally over the median sacral crest to the level of the sacral foramen 1 (S1). Between the median sacral crest and the gluteal surface of the ilium, two hypoechoic clefts are visualized, the medial one correlating to the foramen S1, the most lateral the SI joint (Fig. 9.1). Slightly more caudal is the foramen S2, which generally is a somewhat easier level to successfully inject the SI joint.

Ultrasound needle guidance. In general, the procedure is performed without local anesthesia. The needle should be advanced towards the hypoechoic cleft of the SI joint parallel to the probe, in a medial to lateral direction. Make sure that you are at the second hypoechoic cleft counted from the median crest, as the first one, more medial, relates to the S1 foramen. Once the needle tip is visualized in the hypoechoic cleft, i.e., the entrance of the SI joint, the tip of the needle should be manipulated to a more vertical position and deeper inserted (Fig. 9.2).

© The Author(s), under exclusive license to Springer Nature Switzerland AG 2023
G. A. W. Bruyn and W. A. Schmidt, *Musculoskeletal Ultrasound for the Rheumatologist*,
https://doi.org/10.1007/978-3-031-27737-5_9

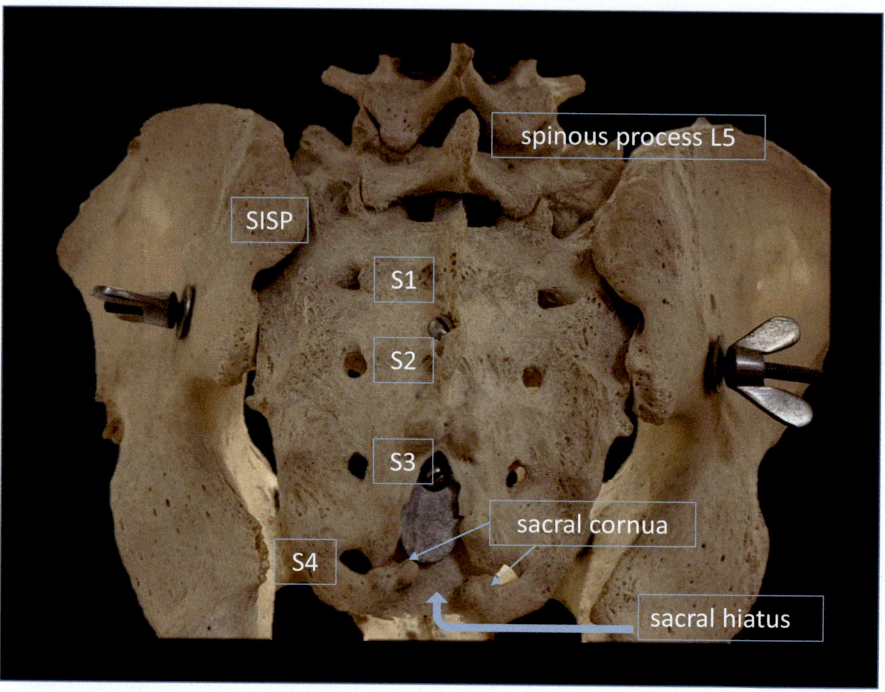

Fig. 9.1 Pelvis model showing anatomic landmarks

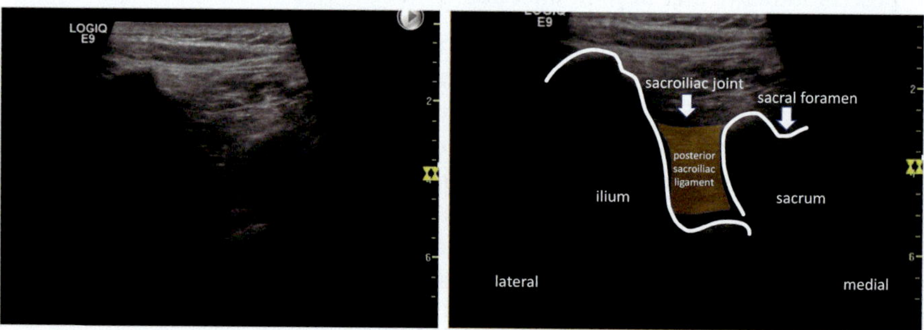

Fig. 9.2 Transverse ultrasound scan showing the bony landmarks of left sacroiliac joint (lateral) and first sacral foramen (medial)

9.2 The Sacral Hiatus

In patients with lower back pain or lumbar radicular pain, an epidural glucocorticoid injection through the sacral hiatus can be beneficial. Ultrasound-guided needle placement may be an aid to a successful outcome.

The patient is placed in prone position with a bolster under the abdomen to facilitate the opening of the sacral hernia. In general, no local anesthesia is applied to the skin or subcutaneous tissues. In a transverse plane, the bony landmarks of the two cornua are identified at the proximal end of the gluteal cleft (Fig. 9.3). The epidural needle is inserted in-plane at a 45° angle to horizontal until the hiatus entrance (Fig. 9.4). The needle has to be pushed through the strong sacrococcygeal ligament, then horizontalized and gently advanced further to the level of S4.

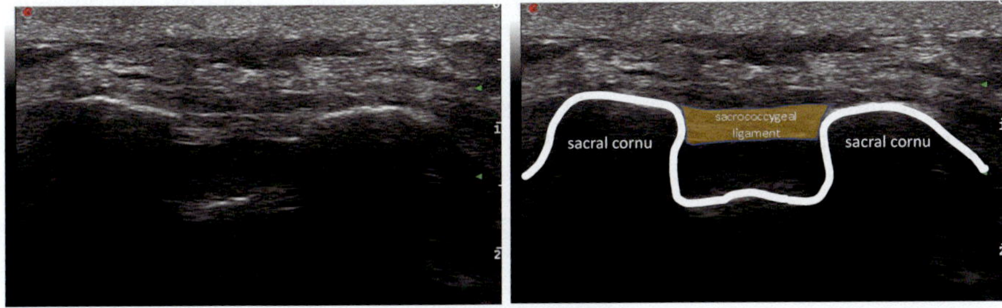

Fig. 9.3 Transverse scan of the entrance of the sacral hiatus

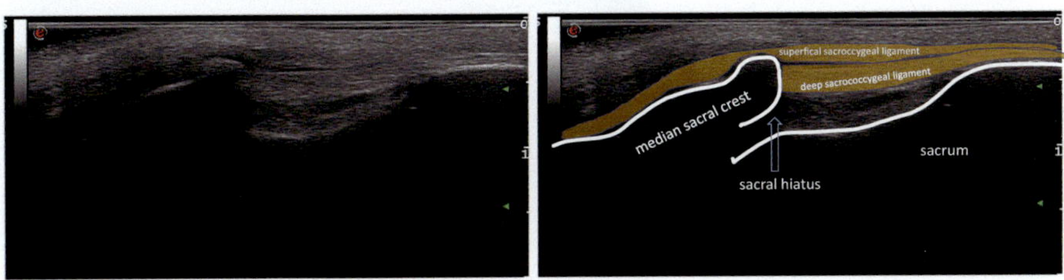

Fig. 9.4 Longitudinal scan of the sacral hiatus

9.3   The Ischial Tuberosity

The ischial tuberosity, or sitting bone, is the origin to the hamstrings, i.e., the common tendon ("conjoint") of the biceps femoris and the semitendinosus muscles, and the tendon of the semimembranosus muscle. The conjoint tendon inserts at the medial facet, whereas the semimembranosus tendon inserts at the lateral facet. In healthy athletes, a variety of disorders may occur in the gluteal-ischial region, including the saddle pressure induced hygroma in cyclists and the hamstring injury in football players. Pathology also occurs in rheumatic disorders including polymyalgia rheumatica, spondyloarthritis, and diffuse idiopathic hyperostosis. In the latter disease, a characteristic calcification of the nearby located sacrotuberous ligament may also be found. Ultrasound can be used both for diagnosis and for guidance of glucocorticoid injection.

Patient positioning. The patient is placed in a prone position, feet hanging off the table. Linear or curved array probes usually are 5–10 MHz, with lower frequencies for the region around the ischial tuberosity. Due to the massive muscle complex in this area, sonoanatomy of the proximal hamstrings region may appear difficult at first sight, and one needs to press the probe more than usually. It is easiest to start in a transverse plane on the medial site a few cm down with respect to the ischial

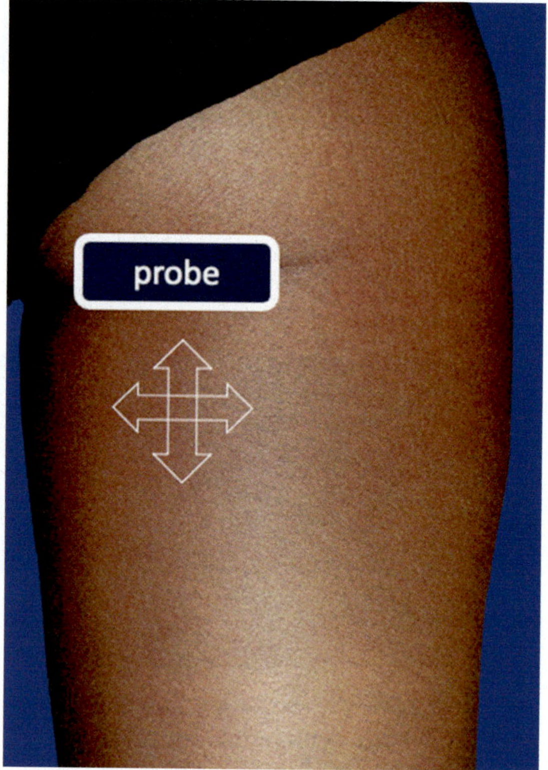

Fig. 9.5 Prone patient positioning for examination of the insertion of the hamstrings to the ischial tuberosity. Arrows indicate direction of probe shifting

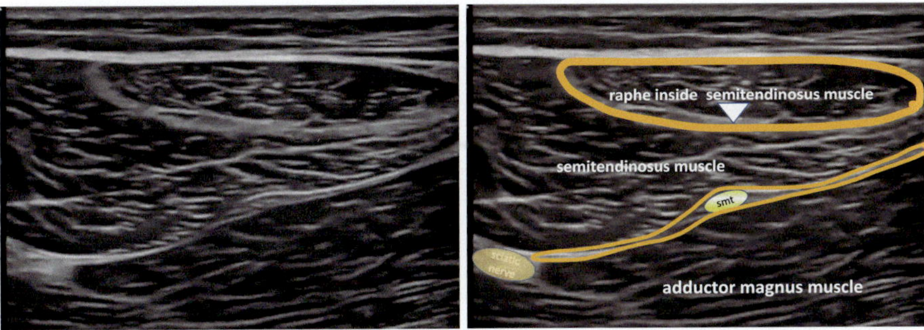

Fig. 9.6 Transverse scan medial and distal to ischial tuberosity showing the semitendinosus muscle and more posterior, the adductor magnus muscle. Smt stands for the tendon of the semimembranosus muscle

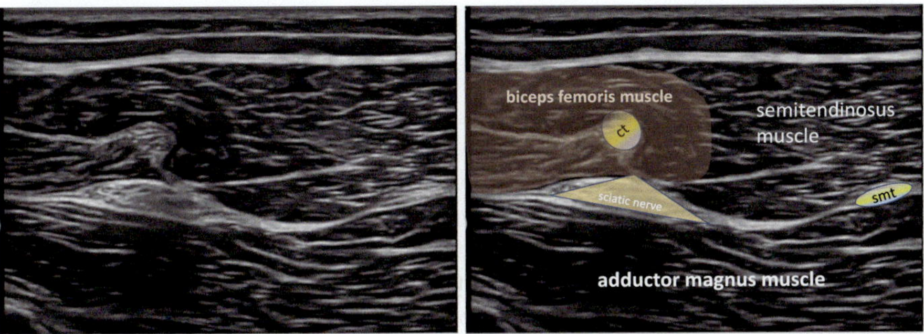

Fig. 9.7 Transverse scan distal to the ischial tuberosity showing the socalled "Mercedes" sign, consisting of the sciatic nerve and the conjoint tendon (ct) of the biceps femoris muscle and the semitendinosus muscle (smt)

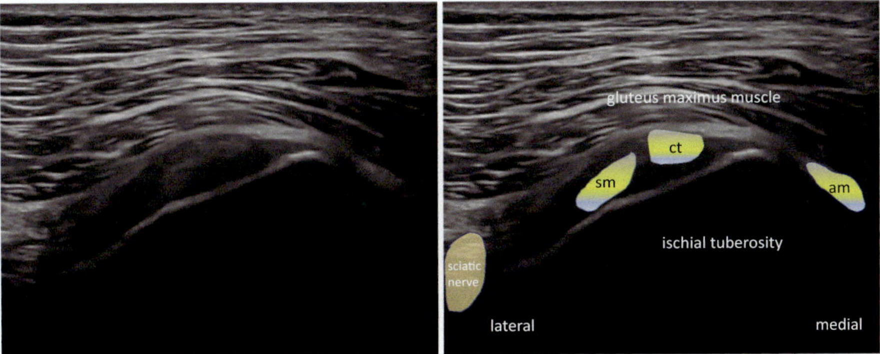

Fig. 9.8 Transverse scan showing the insertion of the hamstrings to the ischial tuberosity. Sm: semimembranosus tendon; ct: conjoint tendon; am: adductor magnus tendon

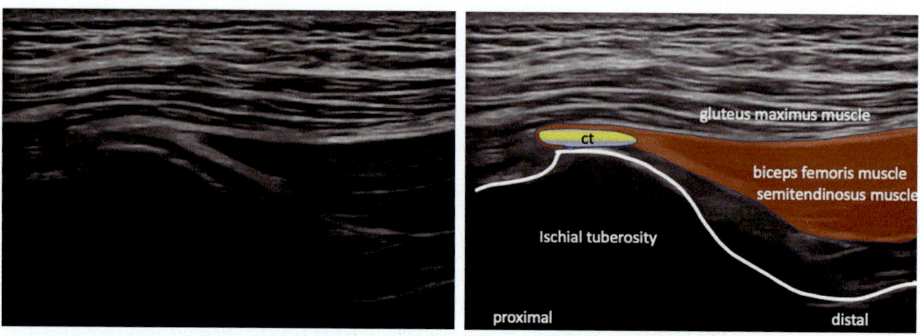

Fig. 9.9 Longitudinal scan of the insertion of the hamstrings to the ischial tuberosity

tuberosity, the latter palpated just below the gluteal fold (Fig. 9.5). First, the triangular shaped semimembranosus muscle is identified medially. Check whether this triangular structure grows quickly bigger when shifting the probe distally in a transverse plane. From the starting position, we shift the transducer laterally and identify the more rounded shape of the semitendinosus muscle. Most laterally, the biceps muscle is identified and the sciatic nerve that travels through it. Inside the semitendinosus muscle, the characteristic raphe, i.e., a fibrous reminder of the bigastric nature of this muscle, is visualized, shaped as an inverted comma (Fig. 9.6). Next, the so-called "Mercedes" sign should be identified. The two wings of this key landmark are formed by the tendon of the semimembranosus medially, the sciatic nerve laterally, and its vertical part by the conjoint tendon of the biceps muscle and the semitendinosus muscle (Fig. 9.7). The probe is then shifted proximally till the ischial tuberosity. Due to anisotropy the enthesis of the hamstrings may be difficult to clearly visualize without tilting the probe upwards or downwards. The enthesis should be assessed both in transversally and longitudinally (Figs. 9.8 and 9.9).

9.4   Pathology

The hamstrings and their insertion at the ischial tuberosity are prone to various lesions, including enthesitis, tendinitis and tendon tear. In addition, ischiogluteal bursitis is a common cause of buttock pain or pain radiating down the thighs. This bursa is an adventitial bursa located between the gluteus maximus muscle and the ischial tuberosity, medial to the insertion of the hamstrings.

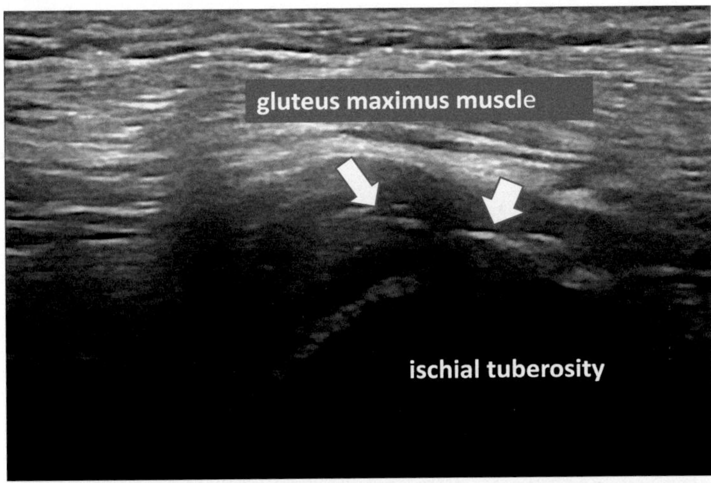

The above figure shows enthesitis of the conjoint tendon and the semimembranosus tendon enthesis at the ischial tuberosity. Enthesitis of the hamstrings origin at the ischial tuberosity in a patient with axial spondyloarthritis. Multiple calcifications in a grossly thickened insertion (arrows). Longitudinal axis scan

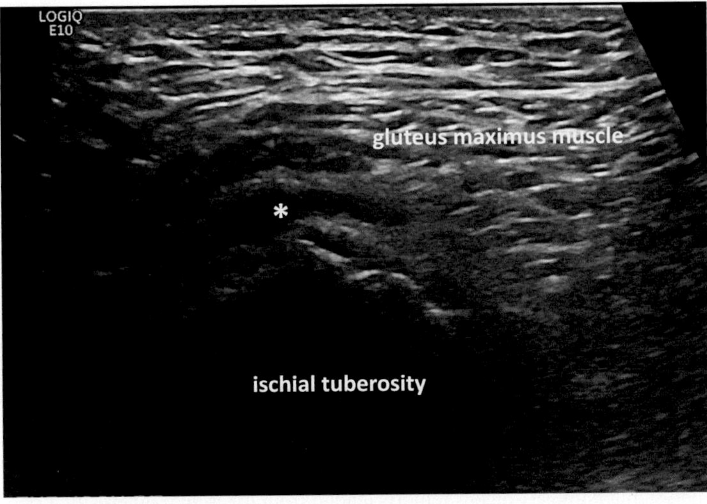

The above figure shows a bursitis (*) superficial to the ischial tuberosity. This pathology can be injected by ultrasound-guidance. Ischial bursitis. The ischial bursa (*) is visible and hypoechoic due to fluid.Short axis scan

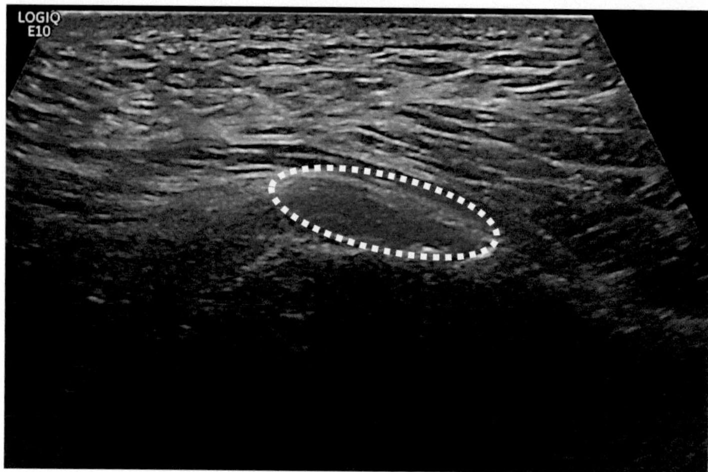

The above figure shows tendinopathy and partial thickness tear of the hamstrings near their enthesis at the ischial tuberosity. Tendinopathy and a partial thickness tear of the conjoint tendon. Cortical surface of ischial tuberosity is irregular. Short axis view

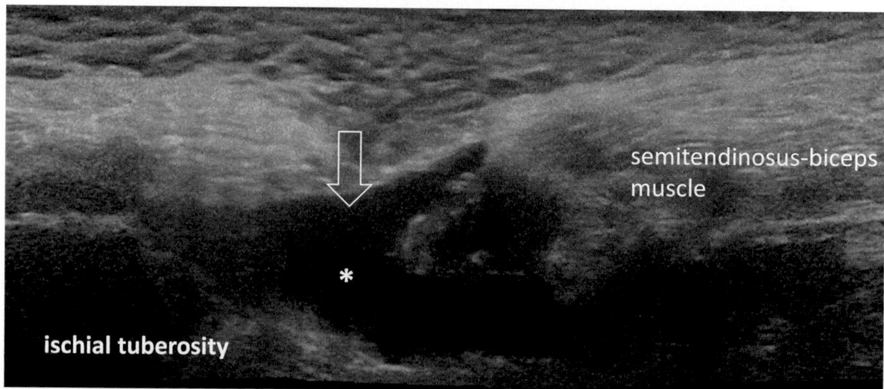

The above figure shows complete rupture of the proximal hamstrings from the ischial tuberosity. The gap is filed with fluid (*). This kind of pathology is usually seen in athletes. Complete avulsion of the common semitendinosus-biceps femoris tendon from the ischial tuberosity. Long axis view

Chapter 10
The Hip

10.1 Standard Scans of the Hip

10.1.1 Anterior Longitudinal View of the Hip (Standard Scan 10-1)

The patient lies supine with the hip in neutral position. The probe is placed parallel to the femoral neck. This scan is not completely longitudinal, but about 20° oblique with the proximal end of the probe localized medially. It is necessary to heel-toe the probe by pressing down its distal end for obtaining good ultrasound images.

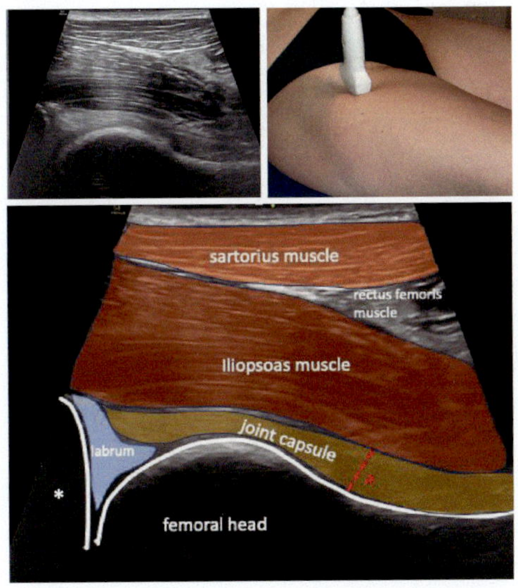

© The Author(s), under exclusive license to Springer Nature Switzerland AG 2023
G. A. W. Bruyn and W. A. Schmidt, *Musculoskeletal Ultrasound for the Rheumatologist*,
https://doi.org/10.1007/978-3-031-27737-5_10

The probe should be shifted from medial to lateral or vice versa. For dynamic examination, the hip can be rotated both externally and internally to detect smaller effusions.

Short linear probes cannot depict all structures of interest in one image. Several linear probes offer the option to provide a trapezoid view as seen in this ultrasound image. Lower frequencies between 3 and 7 MHz may be needed, particularly in obese subjects. Convex abdominal probes may be an alternative in very obese patients.

The first scan is by far the most important scan to assess the hip joint. It depicts the acetabulum (*) and the femoral head and neck together with the anterior joint capsule that extends over the femoral head and neck to its insertion at the proximal femoral shaft. The iliofemoral ligament forms the anterior joint capsule and is superficial to the recess. It may be seen anteriorly to the joint space when shifting the probe slightly laterally.

What is normal?

The mean distance between bone and the anterior rim of the joint capsule at the middle of the concavity of the femoral neck **(a)** is 5.2 mm (2.4 mm–8.0 mm). The difference between right and left neck should be <1.5 mm. The joint capsule runs parallel to the femoral head and neck.

10.1.2 Anterior Transverse View of the Hip (Standard Scan 10-2)

The patient lies supine with the hip in a neutral position. Rotate the probe 90° in relation to the first standard hip scan, Standard Scan 10-1. Again, this scan is not completely transverse but about 20° oblique. The lateral end of the probe is localized proximally. Shift the probe from the acetabulum to the femoral head and neck. The femoral vein may be compressed to exclude thrombosis.

Here it is again possible to use larger convex probes with frequencies of about 4–7 MHz or apply the trapezoid view as mentioned above.

This scan depicts the structures seen in the first plane in a second, transverse plane. The rectus femoris and iliopsoas muscles can be identified as well as the tendons of these muscles.

Abnormalities like iliopsoas bursitis and soft tissue masses may be missed when using only the longitudinal scan. The femoral artery and vein can be seen in the upper right corner of the ultrasound image. The femoral nerve localizes lateral to the artery. It is often not well visible. The joint capsule appears anechoic if the probe is held parallel to the skin surface due to anisotropy. Anisotropy may be avoided by tilting the probe in a way that it points more cranially.

What is normal?

No large amounts of fluid and no soft tissue masses are found.

The femoral vein should be compressible.

The femoral artery should be pulsating.

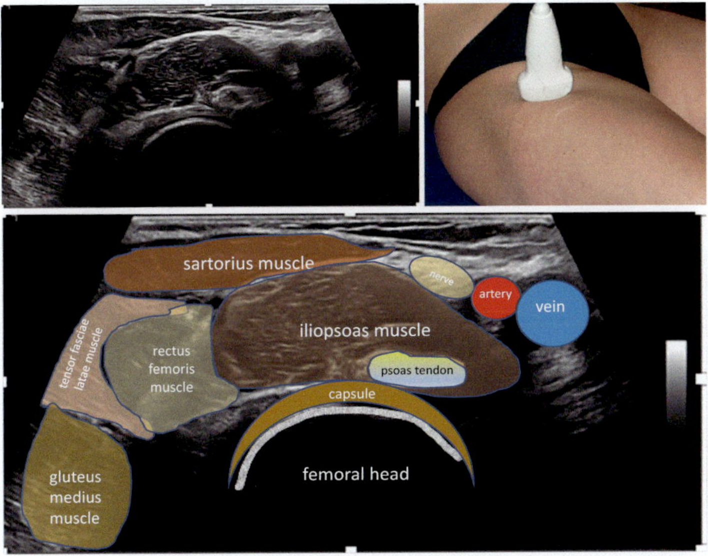

10.1.3   *Lateral Longitudinal View of the Hip (Standard Scan 10-3)*

The patient lies supine with the hip in neutral position. The probe is shifted longitudinally along the anterolateral regions of the hip joint from the position in Standard Scan 10-1 to the lateral areas of the hip joint. The probe is then shifted from anterior to posterior. It is possible to shift the probe completely to the posterior region of the hip joint, where additional information on hip joint abnormalities including effusion can be obtained. The standard scan shows the lateral slightly posterior longitudinal view of the hip joint.

Again, a low frequency linear probe with or without trapezoid view or a convex probe may be used for this scan. This image is from a linear 3–9 MHz probe that was adjusted at 6 MHz.

This scan also allows to detect synovitis and effusion of the hip joint, irregularities of the acetabulum and the femur, and soft tissue masses.

What is normal?

The joint capsule is parallel to the femoral head and neck. The normal distance between femoral neck lateral rim of the joint capsule is about 6 mm. Exact normal values in this area have not been evaluated.

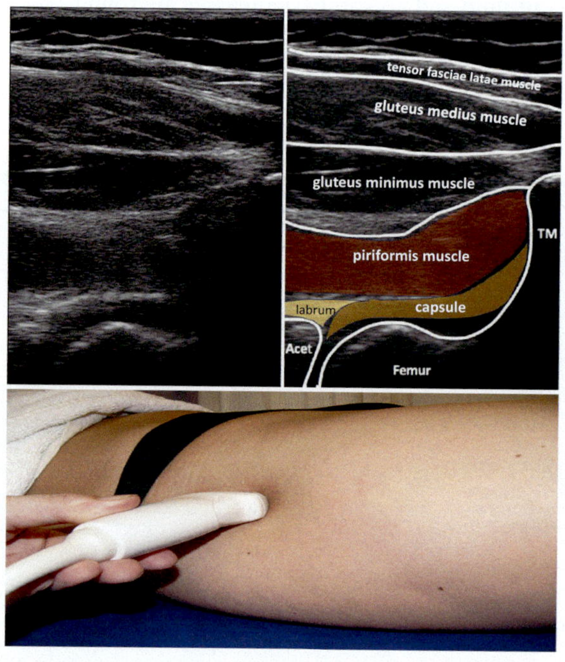

10.1.4 Longitudinal View of the Greater Trochanter (Standard Scan 10-4)

The patient is supine with the hip in neutral position. An alternative patient positioning is the lateral decubitus position with the patient lying on the contralateral side and the ipsilateral knee flexed. This scan is similar to Standard Scan 10-3 of the hip. The probe should only be positioned slightly distally and to the level of the greater trochanter. From this position, it may be swept further anteriorly and posteriorly.

Depending on the thickness of fat and soft tissue, frequencies may vary largely between 5 and 20 MHz; linear or convex probes can be used. This ultrasound image was acquired with 2–9 MHz linear probe in a rather obese person.

This scan delineates the lateral aspects of the greater trochanter including the insertions of the gluteus medius and minimus tendons. The tendon insertions may be hypoechoic due to anisotropy.

Therefore, the sonographer should change the position of the probe until it is perpendicular to the tendon fibers. The trochanteric bursae are localized above and below the tendons.

What is normal?

The trochanteric bursae are only visible when filled with fluid in case of bursitis.

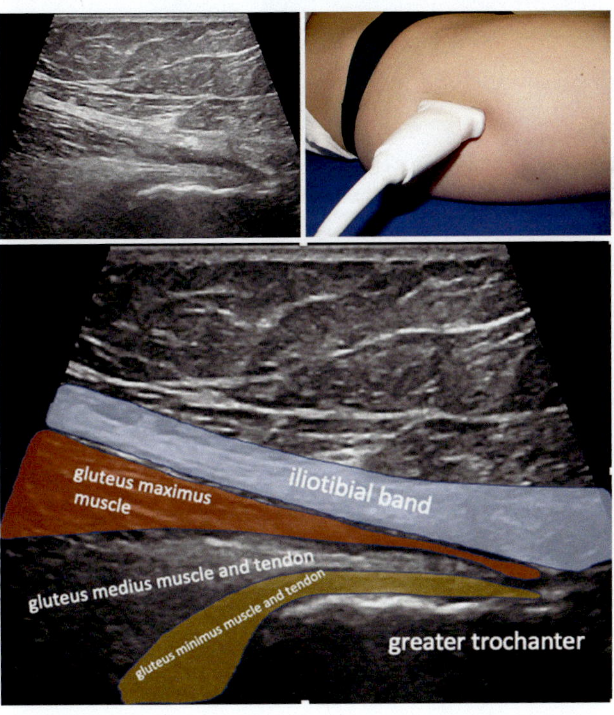

10.1.5   Transverse View of the Greater Trochanter (Standard Scan 10-5)

The patient is supine with the hip in neutral position or alternatively, in a lateral decubitus position with the ipsilateral knee flexed. More fluid may be seen in a bursa in supine position. The probe is rotated by 90° from the previous scan to depict the same structures in a second plane.

The gluteus medius tendon inserts with two tendons, one on the lateral facet and the other one on the superoposterior facet of the greater trochanter. The gluteus minimus tendon insertion localizes more anteriorly on the trochanter. It lies below the gluteus medius tendon close to the trochanter.

This scan is important to evaluate tendon structures. As with the rotator cuff, tendons may be partially anechoic due to anisotropy. It enables the delineation of a trochanteric bursa in the second plane.

Additionally, the transverse diameter of a calcification may be larger than the longitudinal diameter. Then it is easier to detect calcification on the transverse scan.

What is normal?

The posterior facet has no insertions.

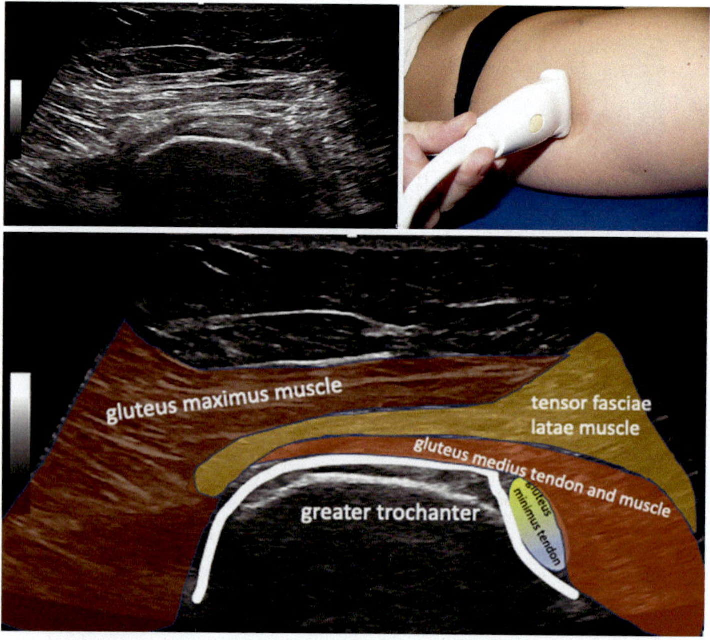

10.1.6   Ultrasound-Guided Injections of the Hip

Ultrasound-guided injection of the hip is particularly valuable, as this joint is deeply seated and hence, injections or aspirations are less accurate if done blindly.

After informed consent and the usual antisepsis, the patient is placed in a supine position with slight external rotation of the hip. The probe (either curved or linear array) is placed at the level of the femoral neck. Some probes allow the image to be angled towards the needle in order to make it more parallel to the needle which is then better visualized (as shown in ultrasound image). The prescan should show the femoral neck and the effusion. The target site, about 2 cm lateral of the neurovascular bundle, is marked. The needle is inserted distally to the foot of the probe. It is then advanced under direct vision into the anterior recess of the hip joint. A long needle is necessary, particularly in large patients. The prescan before puncture allows estimating the minimum length of the needle required.

For trochanteric bursa injection, the patient may be either supine or placed in the lateral position with the affected side facing upwards.

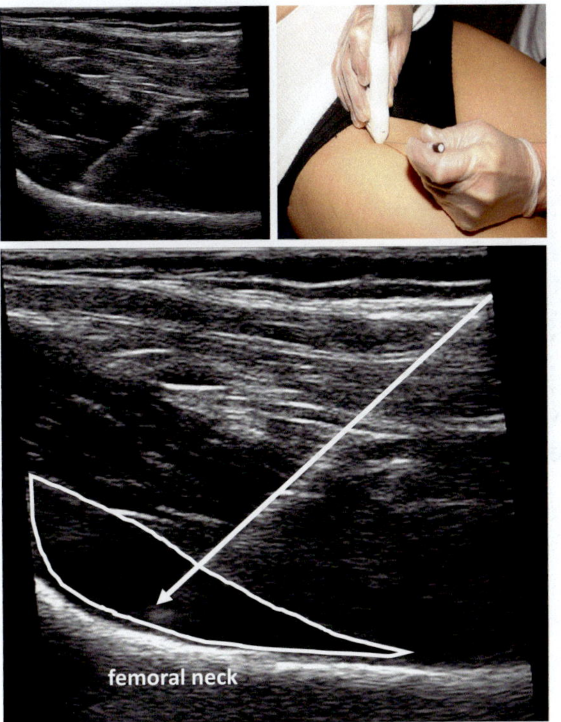

10.2   Pathology of the Hip

10.2.1   Synovitis/Effusion of the Hip I

Best Scan: Standard Scan 10-1.

Additional Scans: Standard Scans 10-2 and 10-3.

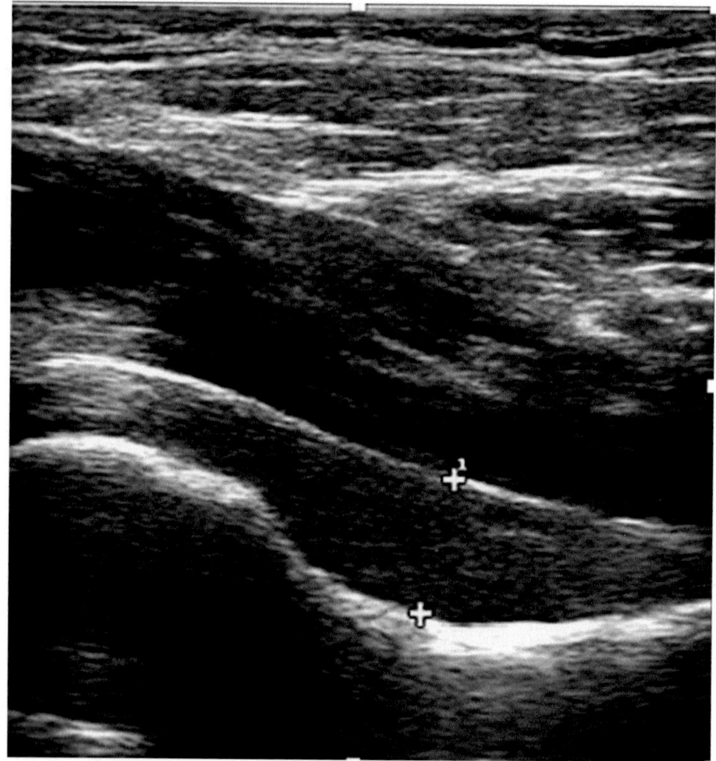

Fig. 10.1 Synovitis of the hip joint with normal bone surface (anterior longitudinal view)

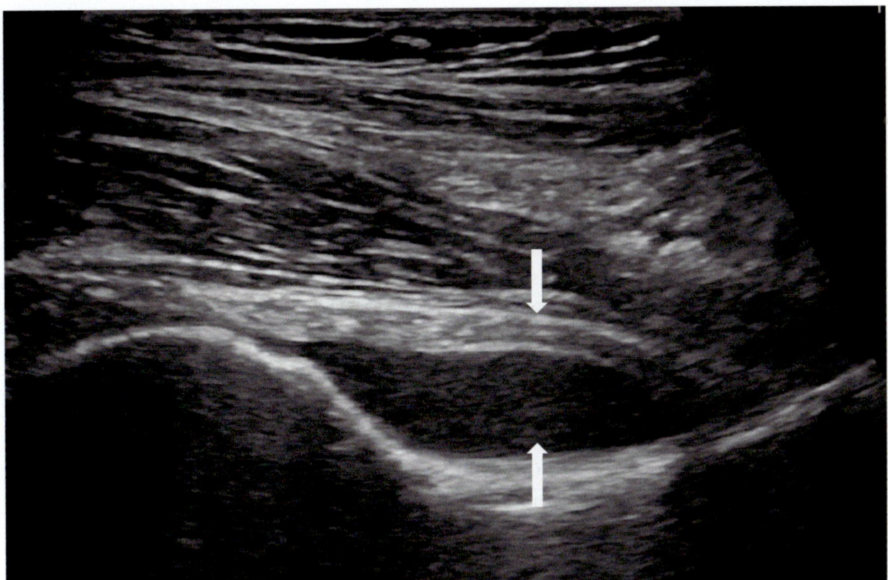

Fig. 10.2 Large effusion of the hip joint with normal bone surface (anterior longitudinal view)

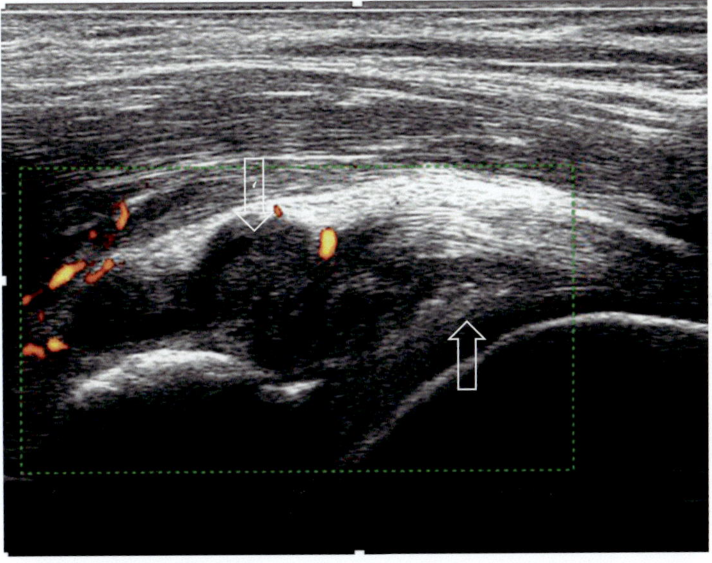

Fig. 10.3 Synovitis of hip joint with minor inflammatory activity (color) and slight bony irregularities of the acetabulum (longitudinal view)

Synovitis frequently occurs in inflamed hip joints (Fig. 10.1). The synovial material makes the joint capsule bulge anteriorly meaning it is no longer parallel to the bone surface. The distance between the bone surface and the anterior border of the joint capsule increases to more than 8 mm. As individual distances display a greater variability, the distances can be compared with the other side. Unilateral synovitis is probable if the difference between sides is >1.5 mm, and the morphology is different. The distance between the bone and the anterior border of the joint capsule in Fig. 10.1 is 10.2 mm, and it is not parallel to the bone because of synovitis. If findings are ambivalent the hip can be rotated internally and externally to detect smaller effusions.

If an effusion is present as depicted in Fig. 10.2 the finding is clearer as the anechoic (black) area which represents fluid ($\Uparrow$) contrasts with the joint capsule ($\Downarrow$) that is pushed out anteriorly.

Linear probes with higher resolution may show further details (Fig. 10.3), but they fail to provide a good overview. This image was made with a frequency of 18 MHz. The synovial proliferation extends over the acetabulum ($\Downarrow$). The cartilage of the femoral head is more homogenic ($\Uparrow \Leftarrow$).

10.2.2   Iliopsoas Bursitis

Best Scan: Standard Scan 10-2.

Additional Scan: Standard Scan 10-1.

An iliopsoas bursa is localized between the iliopsoas muscle and the hip joint. In healthy subjects it does not contain fluid visible by ultrasound.

If bursitis occurs, a hypoechoic or anechoic area can be seen below or next to the iliopsoas muscle.

Figure 10.4 shows fluid ($\Downarrow$) right anterior to the hip joint ($\Rightarrow$) and the iliofemoral ligament ($\Leftarrow$) in a longitudinal scan.

Figures 10.5 and 10.6 show iliopsoas bursitis in longitudinal and transverse scans. Figure 10-5 demonstates the bursitis close to the joint and the labrum, and below the iliospsoas muscle. Figure 10.6 depicts the communication between the right hip joint and the bursa lateral to the iliopsoas muscle ($\Leftarrow$). The fluid that is located anteriorly ($\Rightarrow$) is also part of the bursa, but the connection between these two areas is invisible on this image.

Ultrasound may fail to detect bursitis, as bursa and muscle may display similar echogenicities. In addition, bursal fluid may be localized either between an area directly anterior to the hip joint or further medially or laterally.

Just as in a Baker's cyst of the knee, iliopsoas bursitis is often a consequence of an increased amount of fluid in the adjacent joint. Bursitis can occur both with and without hip joint effusion or synovitis.

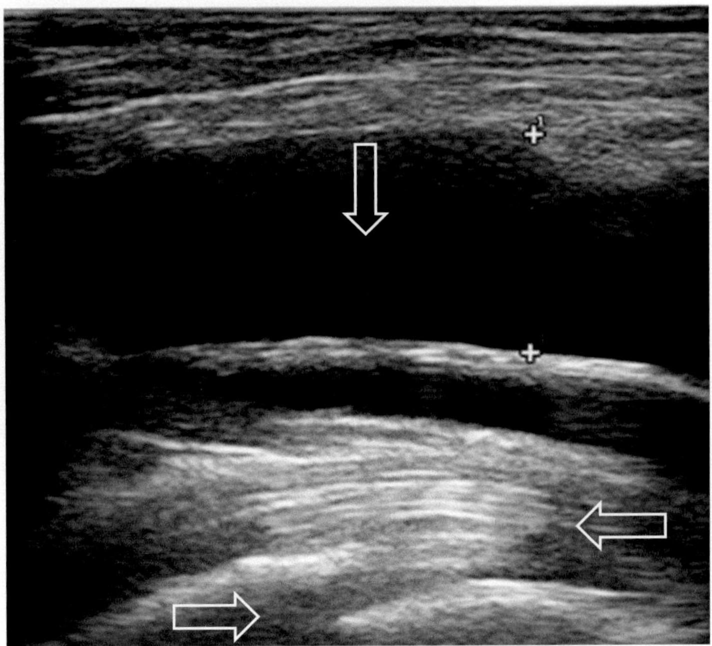

Fig. 10.4 Iliopsoas bursitis (anterior longitudinal view)

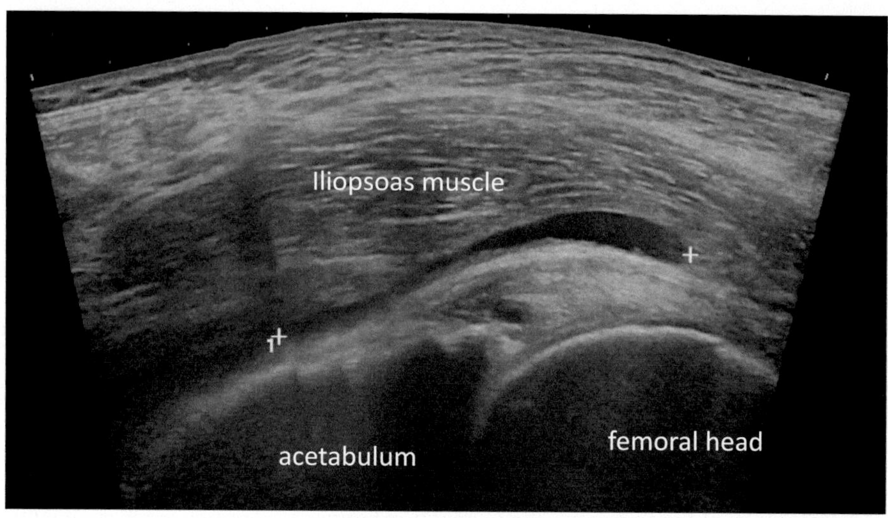

Fig. 10.5 Iliopsoas bursitis (anterior longitudinal view)

Fig. 10.6 Iliopsoas bursitis (anterior transverse view). Medial is left

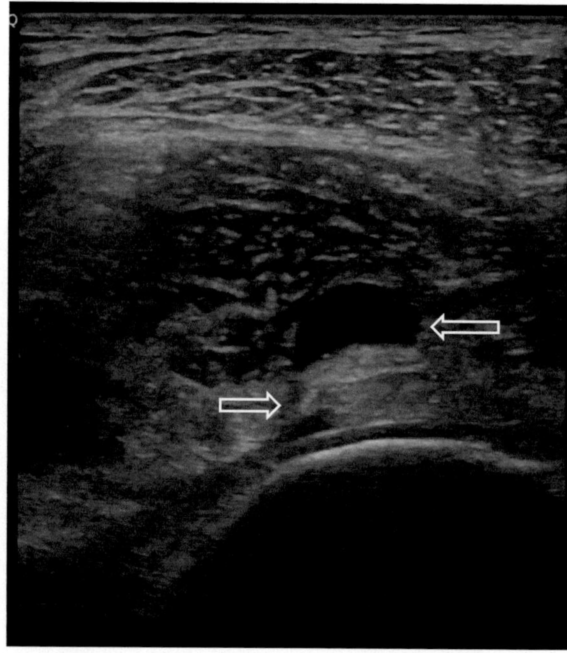

10.2.3   Osteoarthritis/Osteonecrosis of the Hip

Best scans: Standard Scan 10-1 and 10-3.

Additional Scan: Standard Scan 10-2.

Radiography is the imaging method of choice to diagnose osteoarthritis. However, ultrasound, too, can delineate typical abnormalities in osteoarthritis. It is very sensitive in detecting osteophytes that can occur at the acetabulum and/or at the femur. Ultrasound is less sensitive in detecting joint space narrowing as the joint space is not completely accessible by ultrasound.

Figure 10.7 shows osteophytes of the femoral head (⇑) but not of the acetabulum.

In addition, the ultrasound image displays a marked effusion anterior to the femoral head (⇓).

The joint capsule and the femur are not parallel to each other.

Figure 10.8 shows osteophytes only at the acetabulum (⇑). The surface of the femoral head including the cartilage is regular. There is no effusion. Both Figs. 10.7 and 10.8 show osteoarthritis.

Figure 10.9 The appearance of an erosion (⇒) is entirely different to the shape of osteophytes. Erosions may occur for instance in osteonecrosis (as in this case), in RA or in septic arthritis. Synovitis/effusion (⇐) pushing up the joint capsule (⇓) is also present.

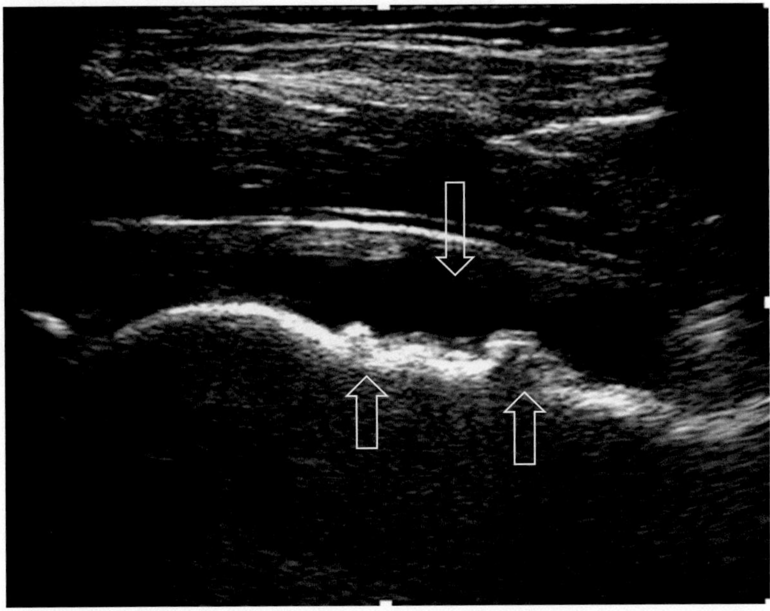

Fig. 10.7 Major irregularities of the femur in osteoarthritis (anterior longitudinal view)

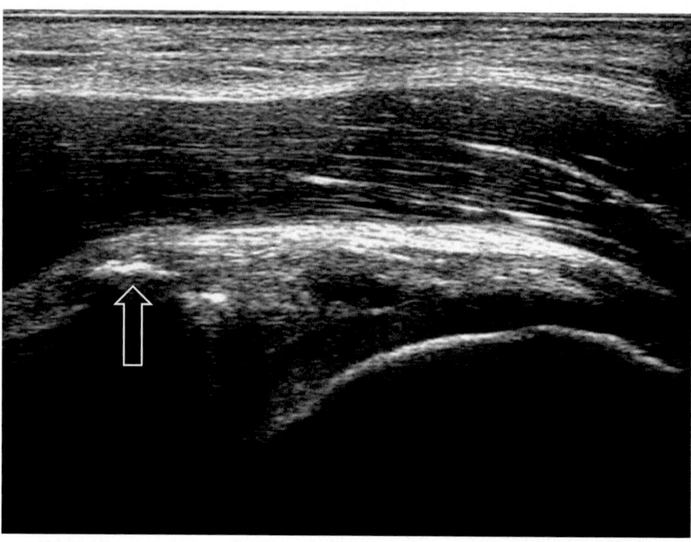

Fig. 10.8 Major irregularities of acetebulum in osteoarthritis (anterior longitudinal view)

Fig. 10.9 Large erosion of the femoral head in osteonecrosis with hip joint effusion (anterior longitudinal view)

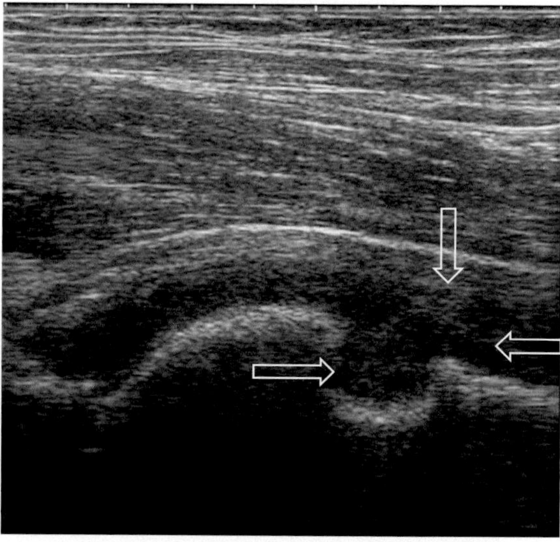

10.2.4 Crystal Arthropathy and Arthroplasty of the Hip

Best Scans: Standard Scans 10-1 to 10-3.

Chondrocalcinosis is characterized by the deposition of pyrophosphate crystals in hyaline or fibrocartilage. Ultrasound displays crystal deposits as hyperechoic areas within the cartilage as shown in the fibrocartilage of the labrum of the hip joint (Fig. 10.10; $\Rightarrow$).

Metal is as hyperechoic as bone. Ultrasound with frequencies between 5 and 15 MHz neither penetrates bone nor metal surfaces. A metal surface is more homogeneous than bone. In total hip joint arthroplasty, the surface of a prosthesis can be depicted (Fig. 10.11; ⇑). Months after surgery a pseudo-capsule develops (⇓) which is usually localized 5–6 mm anterior to the prosthesis. In this figure, the distance is 12 mm indicating that there is more material than expected. The pseudo-capsule normally does not appear as hyperechoic and as thick as the original joint capsule. As

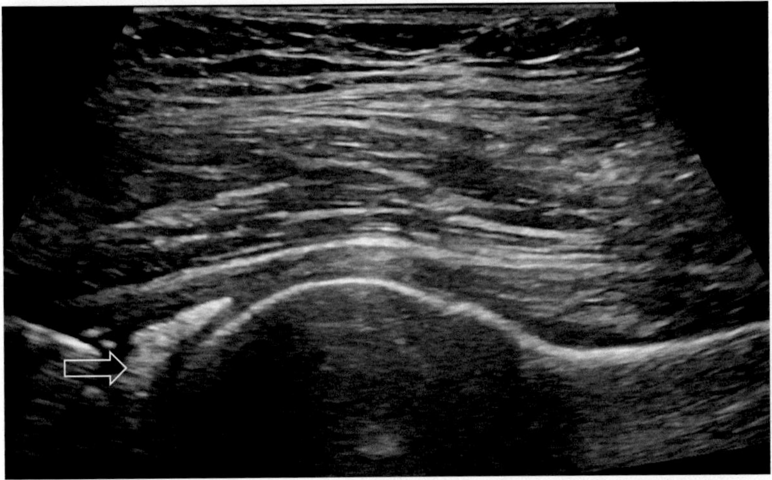

Fig. 10.10 Calcified labrum of the hip joint in chondrocalcinosis (anterior longitudinal view)

Fig. 10.11 Total hip joint
arthoplasty with elevated
pseudo-capsule (anterior
longitudinal view)

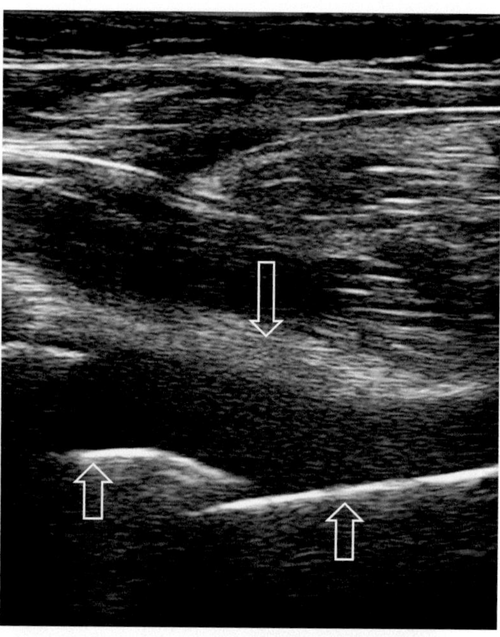

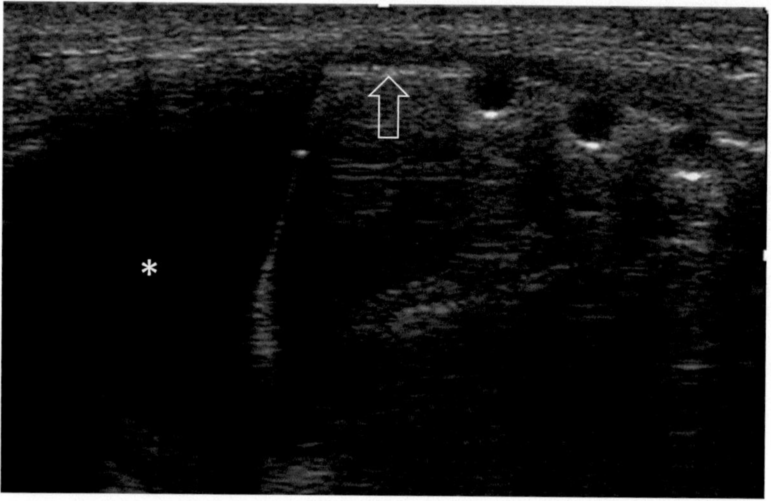

Fig. 10.12 Osteosynthesis of the femoral head and effusion (lateral longitudinal view)

in this patient it can be only assumed in the area where the hypoechoic intra-articular
material is adjacent to the more hyperechoic fibers of the iliopsoas muscle.

Figure 10.12 depicts osteosynthetic material (⇑) at the femoral head with a large
effusion proximal to it (*).

10.2.5 Greater Trochanter Abnormalities

Best Scans: Standard Scans 10-4 and 10-5.

Patients with pain in the hip region often display abnormalities around the greater trochanter. Usually, the trochanteric bursa contains very little fluid making it invisible in healthy subjects.

Bursitis may occur in inflammatory diseases such as polymyalgia rheumatica. Less commonly, bursitis may also be purulent. Ultrasound aids in detecting areas containing fluid that may be aspirated.

Trochanteric bursitis may contain midechoic material. In this case it is often difficult to differentiate the bursitis from the surrounding tissue. The tendons inserting at the trochanter may be inhomogeneous and hypoechoic because of anisotropy. Therefore, if a patient complains of pain in the lateral trochanteric region, it is necessary to look carefully in two planes for a dark, compressible structure with defined borders (Fig. 10.13; ⇒) in this region.

It is possible to differentiate between superficial trochanteric bursitis (Fig. 10.13) that is localized above (lateral to) the gluteus minimus and medius tendons and deep trochanteric bursitis that is localized below the tendons (Fig. 10.14).

Figure 10.14 additionally shows hypoechoic thickened tendons (⇓) representing tendinopathy/enthesopathy.

Chronic enthesopathy may be also characterized by calcifications as shown in Fig. 10.15 (⇑).

Fig. 10.13 Bursitis of the superficial trochanteric bursa in polymyalgia rheumatica (lateral longitudinal view)

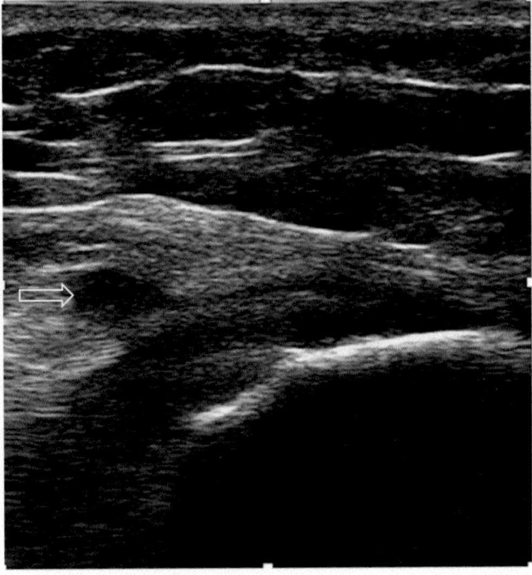

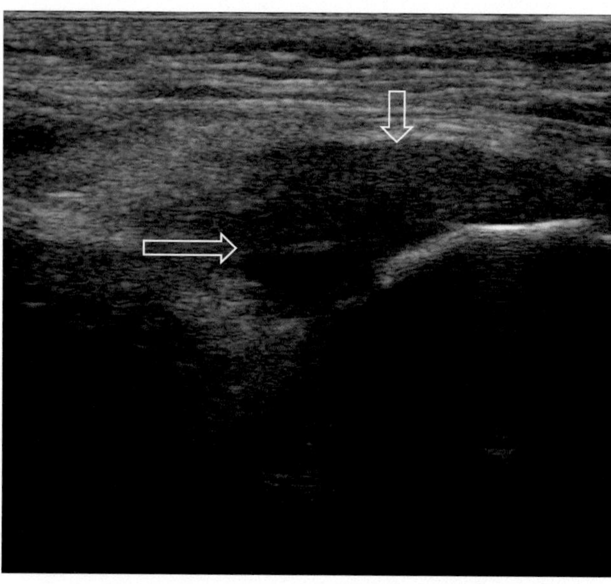

Fig. 10.14 Enthesiopathy and bursitis of the deep trochanteric bursa (lateral longitudinal view)

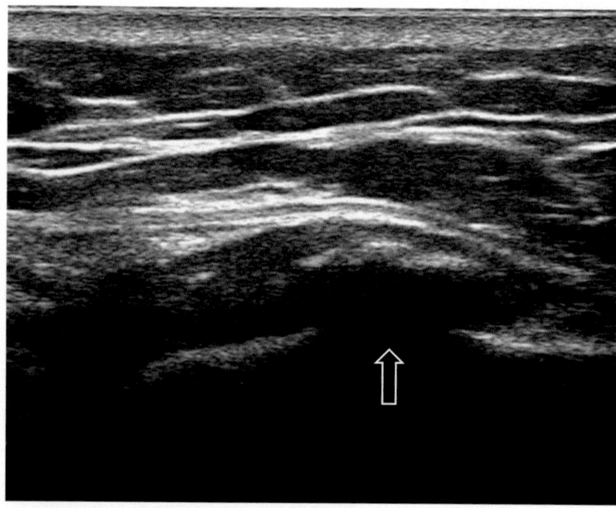

Fig. 10.15 Calcification of the gluteus medius tendon in chronic enthesopathy at the greater trochanter (lateral longitudinal view)

Chapter 11
The Knee

11.1 Standard Scans of the Knee

11.1.1 Suprapatellar Longitudinal View of the Knee (Standard Scan 11-1)

The patient lies supine with the knee in neutral position. The probe is placed parallel to the femur directly proximal to the patella. The patient tightens the quadriceps muscle for displaying small amounts of fluid in the suprapatellar recess. Alternatively, the knee may be 30° flexed by putting for instance a roll of towels under the knee. The sonographer can also press the synovial fluid from the region below the patella to the suprapatellar recess. Then the probe is shifted continuously to the lateral region and finally to the medial region.

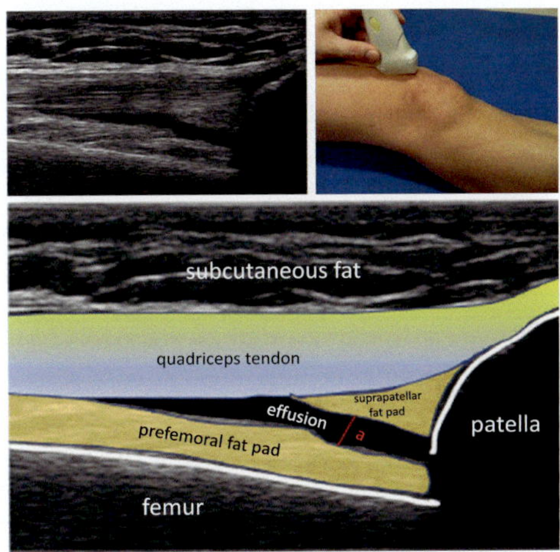

© The Author(s), under exclusive license to Springer Nature Switzerland AG 2023
G. A. W. Bruyn and W. A. Schmidt, *Musculoskeletal Ultrasound for the Rheumatologist*,
https://doi.org/10.1007/978-3-031-27737-5_11

This scan is very important when searching for knee joint effusions and synovial proliferation. It depicts the quadriceps tendon, the cranial parts of the patella and the femur.

What is normal?

Physiological fluid in the suprapatellar recess occurs in most healthy subjects. In this image the distance is 2.8 mm.

(a)   2.4 mm (0 mm–4.8 mm; midline sagittally).

2.4 mm (0 mm–4.9 mm sagitally; if the probe is positioned at the lateral aspects of the suprapatellar recess).

These measurements have been evaluated with knees in neutral position with the quadriceps muscle tightened.

The amount of fluid is pathologically increased if it can be seen all the way between midline and lateral. In most cases, synovial proliferation is abnormal.

11.1.2 Suprapatellar Transverse View of the Knee (Standard Scan 11-2)

The patient lies supine. Initially, the knee is extended, and the probe is placed transversely in the area proximal to the patella. In this position, it is possible to visualize the quadriceps tendon and the suprapatellar recess. The supraspatellar recess can also be seen if the probe is placed more medially or laterally. When the patient flexes the knee to 90° or more, it is possible to partially visualize tissue that is localized under the patella. This includes the intercondylar cartilage.

This scan is used to see knee joint effusions in a second plane, to depict synovial proliferation and, if the knee joint is flexed, to evaluate the intercondylar cartilage.

Shifting the probe medially and laterally a bit more distally visualizes the medial and lateral retinaculum that connects the patella to the femur.

What is normal?

Cartilage (**a**): 3.5 mm (1.7 mm–4.6 mm), in females 2.7 mm (1.4 mm–4.1 mm).
in males 3.5 mm (2.1 mm–4.9 mm).

Normal cartilage is anechoic or very hypoechoic. Small physiological amounts of fluid may be seen in the suprapatellar recess as described above (Standard Scan 11-1).

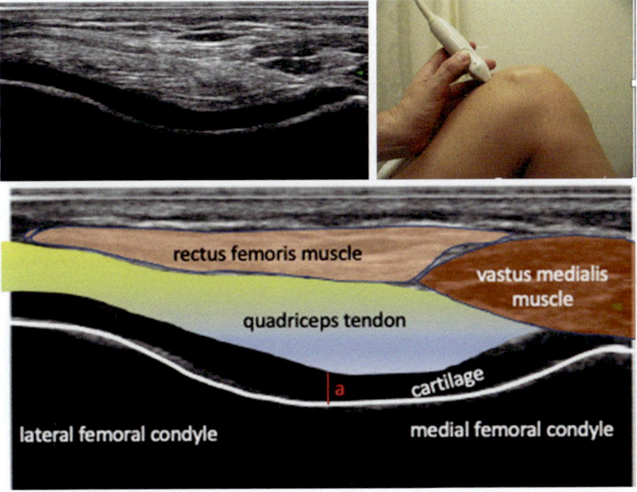

11.1.3 Lateral Longitudinal View of the Knee (Standard Scan 11-3)

The patient lies supine with the knee in neutral position. The probe is shifted continuously from the position in Standard Scan 11-1 via the anterolateral suprapatellar region to the position in Standard Scan 11-3 at the lateral joint space. In the lateral area, the insertion of the iliotibial band is visible together with the lateral meniscus. Then the probe is further shifted posteriorly, where, proximal to the joint space, the groove for the popliteal tendon can be visualized. By placing the probe more distally. i.e. distal to the joint space, and slightly further posteriorly, the fibular head can be seen.

With this scan it is possible to assess several anatomical structures and pathologies, including the presence of synovitis. Standard Scans 11-3 and 11-4 are the favorable scans for evaluating color Doppler signals.

Erosions may occur in inflammatory arthritis. Standard Scans 11-3 and 11-4 are best to show osteophytes in osteoarthritis. Ganglia or calcifications can be detected adjacent to the lateral meniscus. Larger meniscal tears can be well seen with ultrasound. Ultrasound is very sensitive to detect meniscal calcifications due to CPPD. Otherwise, it is possible to examine the lateral collateral ligament, the iliotibial band and its distal insertion to Gerdy's tubercle, biceps femoris and popliteal tendon which localize posterior to the iliotibial band. They may be torn or damaged after trauma, and they may be hypoechoic, thickened, and inhomogeneous in enthesopathy.

What is normal?

The bone surface is regular. The lateral collateral ligament is homogeneous. A little amount of intra-articular fluid is normal (see Standard Scan 11-1), particularly in the anterolateral region of the suprapatellar recess.

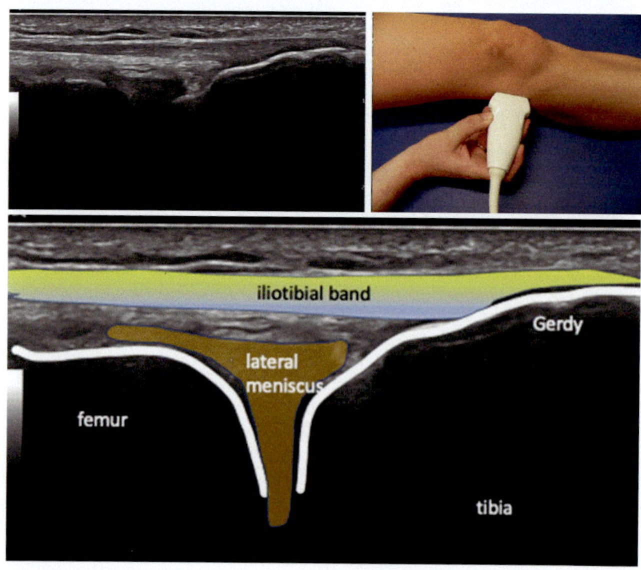

11.1.4 Medial Longitudinal View of the Knee (Standard Scan 11-4)

The patient is supine with the knee in neutral position. The probe is placed parallel to the femur at the medial joint space.

The probe can also be shifted continuously from the position in Standard Scan 11-1 via the anteromedial suprapatellar region to the position in Standard Scan 11-4 at the medial joint space. Here, the probe should be shifted from anterior to posterior or vice versa. It also can be shifted further distally to the anserine bursa. Knee pain particularly in osteoarthritis is often localized at the medial joint space, where osteophytes and protrusion of the medial meniscus may be seen. The anserine bursa area is the location where three tendons, i.e., the sartorius, the gracilis and the semitendinosus tendon, insert. However, pathology in this region is rare.

Indications are similar to Standard Scan 11-3.

What is normal?

The bone surface is regular.

The medial collateral ligament is hyperechoic and typically shows three layers, a superficial bright fibrous layer, a second hypoechoic layer consisting of connective tissue, and a deep hperechoic fibrous layer. The deep layer is the shortest band of the medial collateral ligament.

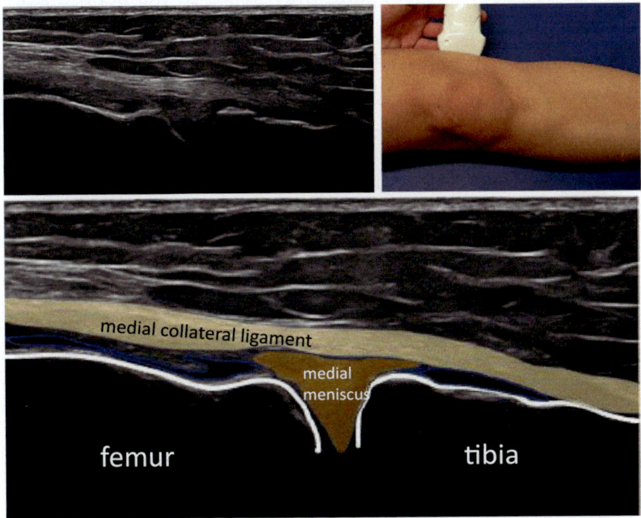

11.1.5   Infrapatellar Longitudinal View of the Knee (Standard Scan 11-5)

The patient is supine with the knee in neutral position. The probe is placed longitudinally over the midline below the patella. To examine the patellar tendon the quadriceps muscle should be tightened or the knee should be flexed, otherwise the tendon may appear irregular. Also, the probe should be shifted to the more lateral and medial infrapatellar region. Alternatively, the probe may be shifted continuously from the position in Standard Scan 11-3 or 11-4 via the lateral or medial infrapatellar region for obtaining this scan. The deep infrapatellar bursa may be filled with fluid at the medial or lateral side of the distal patellar tendon. It may often only be detected on contraction of the quadriceps muscle.

With this scan, it is possible to see anterior bursae, to evaluate the patellar tendon, to see knee joint synovitis or effusion that is sometimes localized distally to the patella. Irregularities of the femoral and tibial surface, e.g., in Osgood-Schlatter disease, can also be evaluated in this scan position. It is difficult to see the anterior cruciate ligament as it is not parallel to the probe.

What is normal?

The sagittal diameter of the patellar tendon:

(a) is 3.2 mm (1.9 mm–4.5 mm); for females: 2.9 mm (1.9 mm–3.9 mm) and for males: 3.5 mm (1.9 mm–5.1 mm).

A small amount of physiological fluid may occur in the deep infrapatellar bursa (b) in 6% of a healthy population.

Normally, no visible synovial fluid occurs in the infrapatellar region.

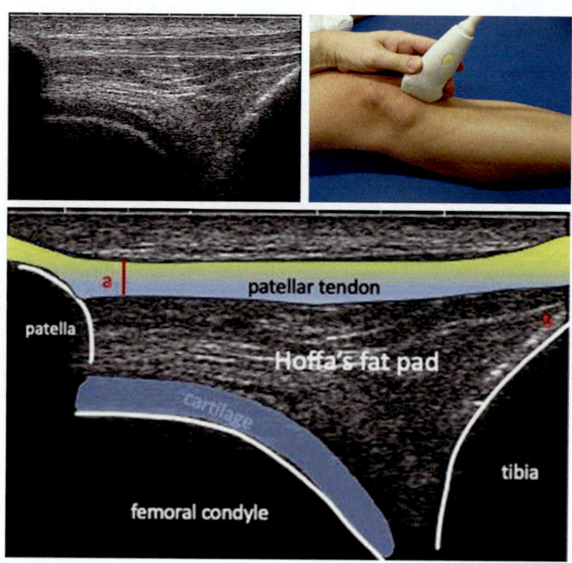

11.1.6 Infrapatellar Transverse View of the Knee (Standard Scan 11-6)

The patient is supine with the knee in neutral position. The probe is rotated by 90° in relation to the previous scan below the patella at midline. For examining the patellar tendon, the quadriceps muscle should be tightened or the knee should be flexed. The probe is shifted from proximal to distal or vice versa to see all parts of the tendon. Then it is shifted further distally to assess the infrapatellar bursa and the tibial bone surface.

Just as the previous scan, this scan enables the sonographer to assess the patellar tendon, anterior bursae, synovitis, effusion, and infrapatellar bone surfaces. Transverse scanning is also important to detect small partial patellar tendon tears, as these may be missed in the longitudinal scan.

What is normal?

See normal values for the patellar tendon on Standard Scan 11-5.

Small amounts of fluid may occur in the deep infrapatellar bursa also in healthy individuals.

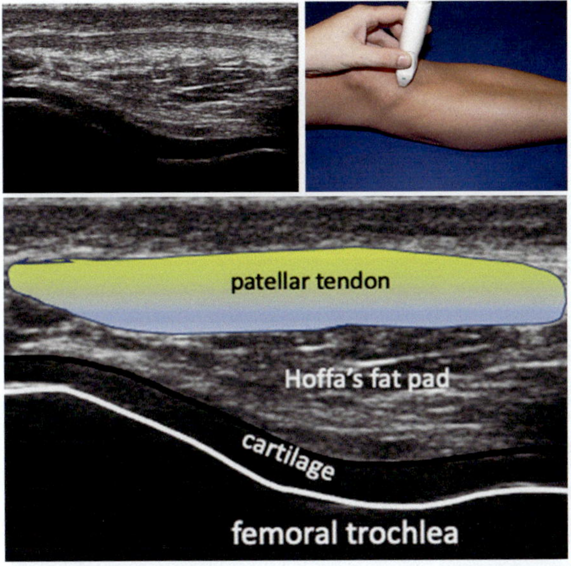

11.1.7   Posterior Transverse View of the Knee (Standard Scan 11-7)

The patient is prone with the knee in neutral position. Starting at the medial area the probe is shifted from the femoral region distal to the tibial region. This is the best area for detecting a Baker's cyst. Typically, a Baker's cyst is found between the medial head of the gastrocnemius muscle and the semimembranosus tendon. Continue this manoever towards the midline for visualizing the popliteal artery, the popliteal vein and the lateral region. It is important to look at the medial areas of the lower leg, particularly if the leg is swollen, in order to detect a ruptured Baker's cyst. A ruptured Baker's cyst may extend distally.

This scan is useful not only when looking for posterior bursitis but also for evaluating the popliteal vein. It may be compressed as seen in the ultrasound image on this page. The popliteal vein may become visible when compressing the dorsal lower leg. Further, soft tissue masses, chondrocalcinosis of the condylar cartilage, and bony irregularities can be detected with this scan.

What is normal?

A small amount of fluid in the popliteal bursa occurs in 16% of healthy individuals.
The popliteal vein is compressible.

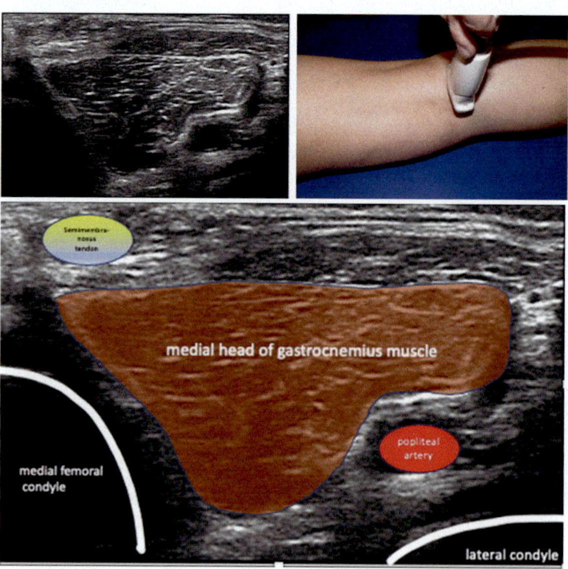

11.1.8 *Posterior Longitudinal View of the Knee (Standard Scan 11-8)*

The patient is prone. The knee is in neutral position. Beginning at the medial aspects of the dorsal knee the probe is shifted laterally or vice versa.

In the midline, the popliteal vein, the popliteal artery and the tibial nerve can be seen. Furthermore, the posterior horns of the medial and lateral meniscus can be found. In addition, the tibial insertion of the posterior cruciate ligament and the semimembranosus tendon can be visualized. This scan allows to depict the posterior structures in a second plane.

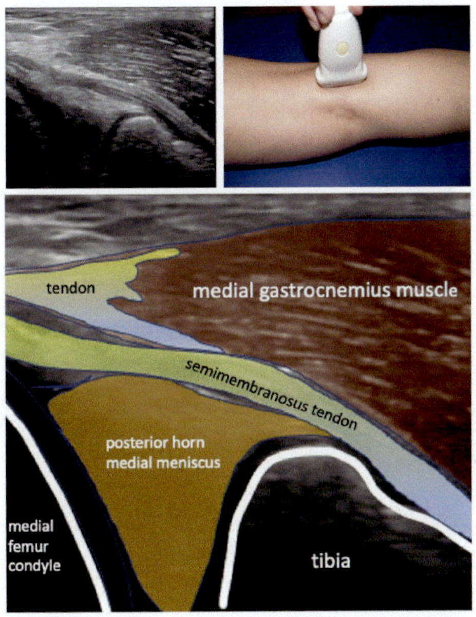

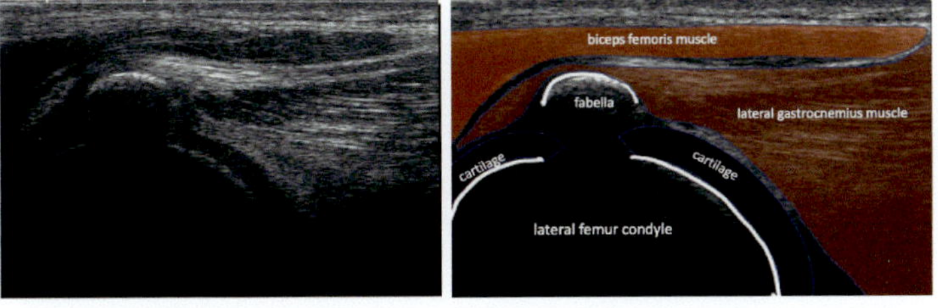

The first ultrasound image and the corresponding drawing depict the medial aspects. The second ultrasound image shows the lateral aspects with a fabella. The fabella is a sesamoid bone located in the lateral head of the gastrocnemius muscle posterior to the lateral femoral condyle. It can be found in about one third of all knees. Also in the lateral area, the common peroneal nerve can be visualized during its course towards the fibular head.

What is normal?

A small amount of fluid in the popliteal bursa may occur in healthy individuals.
   The popliteal vein is compressible.

11.1.9   Ultrasound-Guided Injections of the Knee

Ultrasound guidance may not be necessary in large effusions that can be easily aspirated.

Small effusions and synovial material that is difficult to aspirate may be punctured under ultrasound guidance. The ultrasound probe is placed transversely proximal to the patella. The needle is inserted from the lateral or medial side. The needle can be easily seen as it is parallel to the probe.

Ultrasound guidance is also possible in other structures such as small Baker's cysts or in prepatellar bursitis.

After informed consent and the usual antisepsis, the patient is placed in a supine position. The patient may be more comfortable with a small pillow under the affected knee. The knee flection increases also the amount fluid in the suprapatellar recess. The probe is placed transversely over the suprapatellar area at the level of the superior pole of the patella. To mark the effusion, a longitudinal prescan should first be performed. The prescan shows the quadriceps tendon, the suprapatellar recess effusion and the femur. The probe is then rotated by 90 degrees. Commonly, aspirations are carried out using the lateral approach, except when the effusion is more pronounced on the medial side. The needle is then inserted lateral to the foot of the transducer and advanced under direct vision into the lateral suprapatellar recess as shown here.

For Baker's cyst aspiration, the patient is placed prone and a prescan is performed to determine the target site.

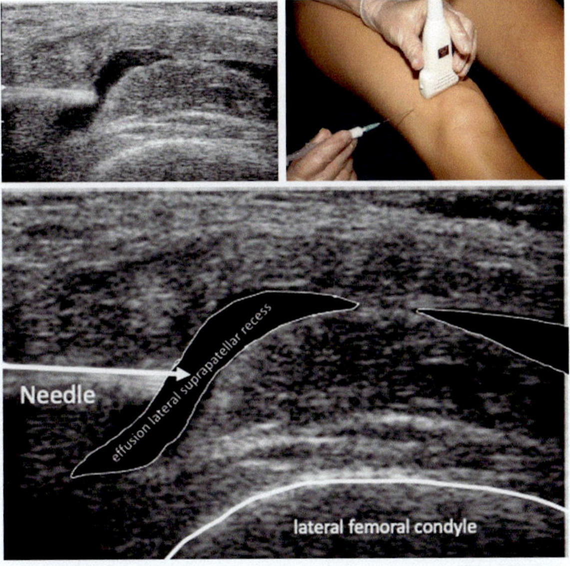

11.2   Pathology of the Knee

11.2.1   Synovitis/Effusion of the Knee I

Best Scans: Standard Scans 11-1 and 11-2.

Additional Scans: Standard Scans 11-3 to 11-8.

Effusion (anechoic, compressible and displaceable material) is found in most inflamed knees (Figs. 11.1 and 11.2; ⇐). It is impossible to determine the exact amount of synovial fluid by ultrasound. However, the longitudinal and sagittal diameters of the suprapatellar recess can be measured to compare findings in follow-up examinations.

The intra-articular material can be midechoic and heterogeneous. This may be fibrin, hematoma, cell debris, or synovial proliferation. Synovial proliferation (Fig. 11.2; ⇒) is found in most inflamed knees. It becomes thinner with a straight surface after surgical synovectomy or radiosynovectomy. It may exhibit color signals which correlate with inflammatory activity. Synovial proliferation can best be detected in the lateral area of the suprapatellar recess where it can be seen in longitudinal and transverse scans.

The best area for visualizing synovitis and its perfusion is the medial and lateral joint space (Fig. 11.3). This figure shows synovitis with inflammation (perfusion grade 2).

In addition, this figure displays slight bony irregularities, a small osteophyte (⇓) indicating mild osteoarthritis and small calcifications of the lateral meniscus (⇑).

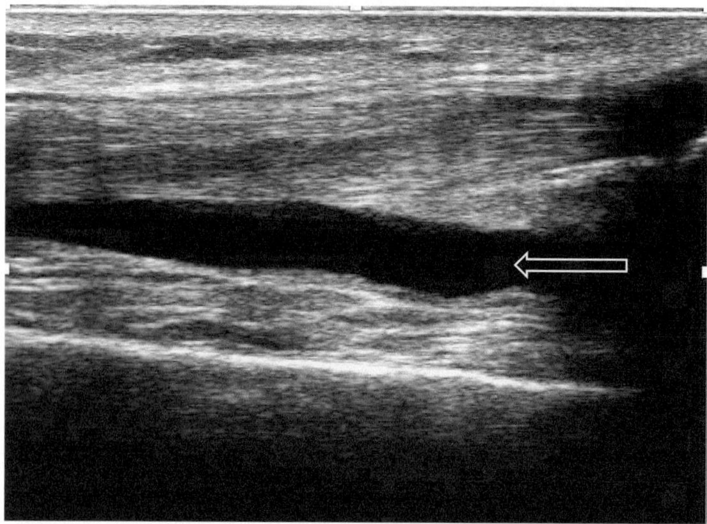

Fig. 11.1 Effusion in the suprapatellar recess (suprapatellar longitudinal view)

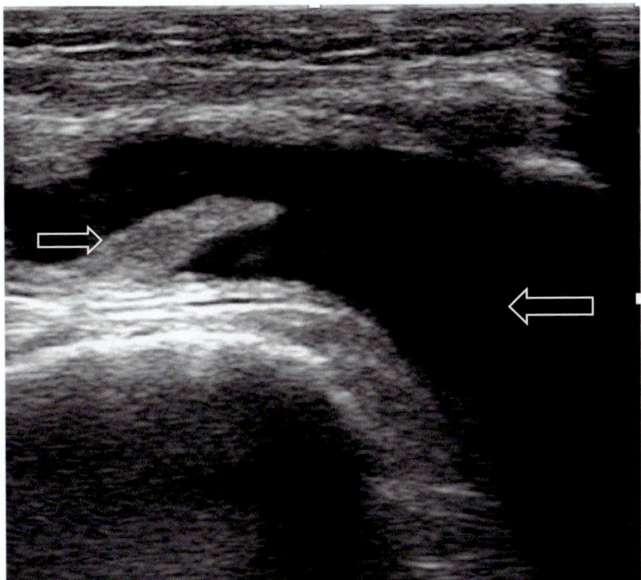

Fig. 11.2 Effusion and synovial proliferation in the suprapatellar recess (suprapatellar transverse view)

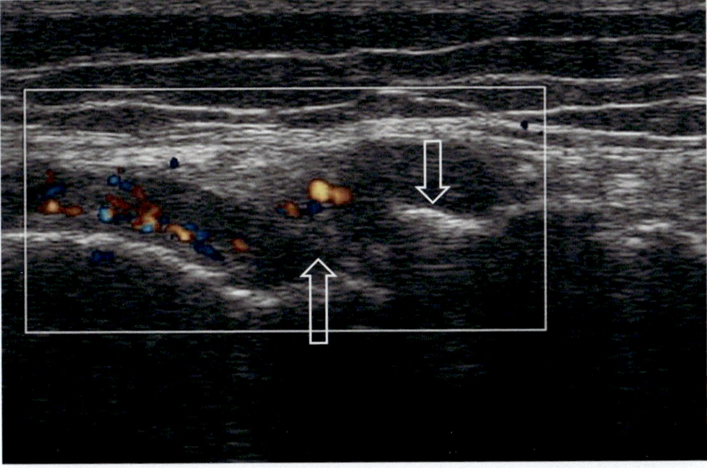

Fig. 11.3 Synovitis with hyperperfusion at the lateral joint space (lateral longitudinal view)

11.2.2 Synovitis/Effusion of the Knee II

Best Scans: Standard Scans 11-1 and 11-2.

Additional Scans: Standard Scans 11-3 to 11-8.

Although effusion is most often detected in the suprapatellar recess, it can also occur in other anatomical regions of the knee. Therefore, it is mandatory to perform a complete ultrasound examination of the whole knee in search for effusion.

In the infrapatellar region, effusion sometimes may emerge into the Hoffa's fat pad close to the tibia (Fig. 11.4; ⟸).

In patients with total knee joint arthroplasty, effusions are frequently localized in the infrapatellar region (Fig. 11.5; ⟸). In the first weeks after surgery, hypoechoic material regularly occurs close to the prosthesis. In contrast to effusions, hematomas are not completely anechoic, and they are poorly compressible. A prosthesis is depicted as a hyperechoic straight, line (⟰). In this figure, the patellar tendon is postoperatively thickened, hypoechoic and heterogeneous (⟹).

Figure 11.6 shows synovitis in the posterior compartment of the knee joint at the medial femoral condyle. Ultrasound displays hypoechoic, but no anechoic material (⟹). Thus, this material cannot be aspirated successfully. The anechoic region close to the surface of the medial femoral condyle (⟸) represents cartilage.

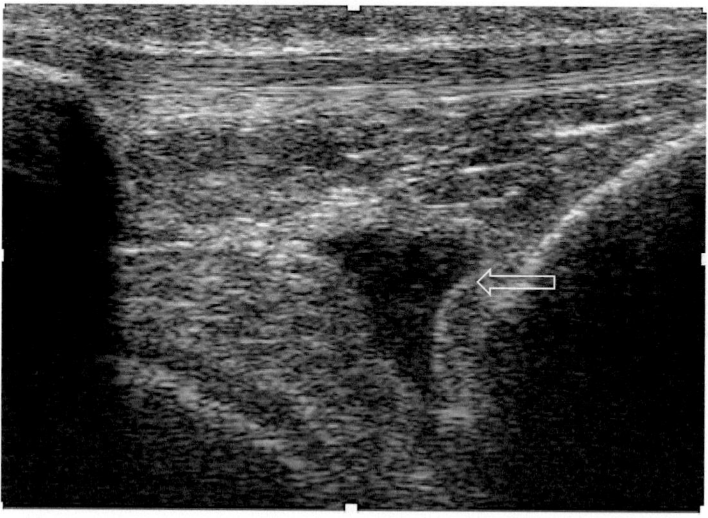

Fig. 11.4 Knee joint effusion in the infrapatellar region (infrapatellar longitudinal view)

Fig. 11.5 Knee joint effusion in the infrapatellar region, total knee joint prosthesis, and post-surgical abnormalities of the patellar tendon (infrapatellar longitudinal view)

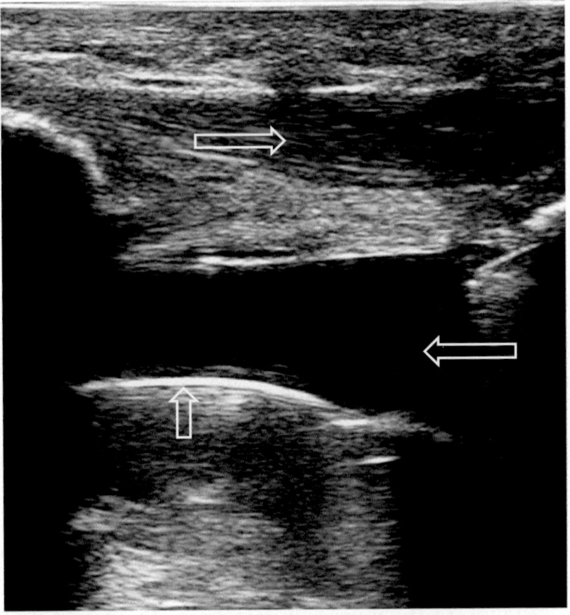

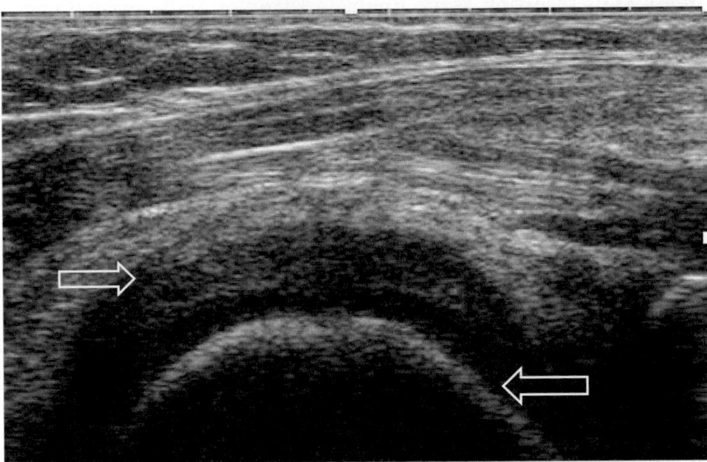

Fig. 11.6 Synovitis at the posterior region of the medial femoral condyle (posterior longitudinal view)

11.2.3   Tendon Abnormalities of the Knee I

Best Scans quadriceps tendon: Standard Scans 11-1 and 11-2.

Best Scans patellar tendon: Standard Scans 11-5 and 11-6.

Best Scans medial and lateral tendons and ligaments: Standard Scans 11-3 and 11-4.

Patients with spondyloarthrits often report pain at tendon insertions. Radiography occasionally shows calcifications or erosions. Ultrasound is particularly useful to localize these abnormalities at the insertions of tendons or ligaments together with tendon or ligament swelling. An inflamed tendon or ligament is thickened, hypoechoic and heterogeneous. In addition, power Doppler ultrasound may show increased blood flow in the tendon.

Figure 11.7 depicts the quadriceps tendon with an enthesophyte close to its insertion at the patella (⇑). This may be due either to enthesitis or enthesopathy.

Figure 11.8 shows the distal patellar tendon. It is thickened, inhomogeneous and hypoechoic when compared with the surrounding soft tissue representing tendinitis. In addition, a small partial tear (⇑ ⇓), minor color signals and some irregularities of the tibia are present. The scan also shows a small deep infrapatellar bursitis.

Figure 11.9 shows a hypoechoic, thickened and inhomogeneous distal biceps femoris tendon at its insertion at the fibula as a sign of enthesopathy (⇓). The bone surface of the femoral condyle (left), the tibia (center) and the fibula (right) is straight in this case, but it may also become irregular with erosions in chronic enthesitis (see Fig. 10.14).

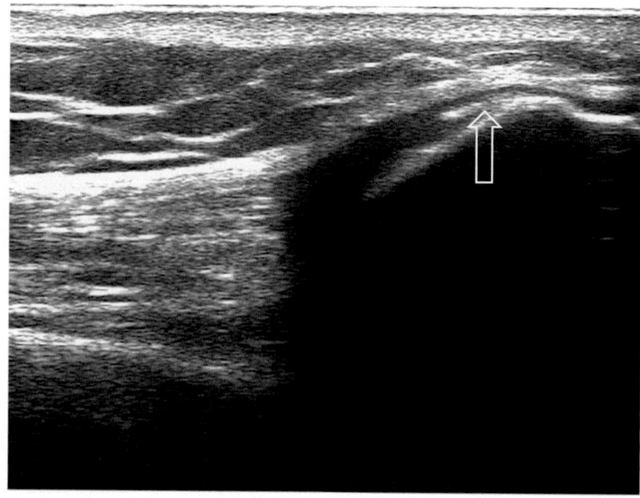

Fig. 11.7 Enthesopathy of the quadriceps tendon with an enthesophyte of the patella (suprapatellar longitudinal view)

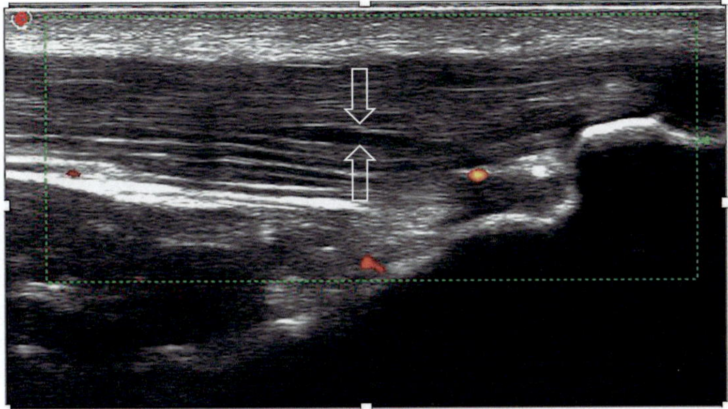

Fig. 11.8 Tendinitis of the patellar tendon (infrapatellar longitudinal view)

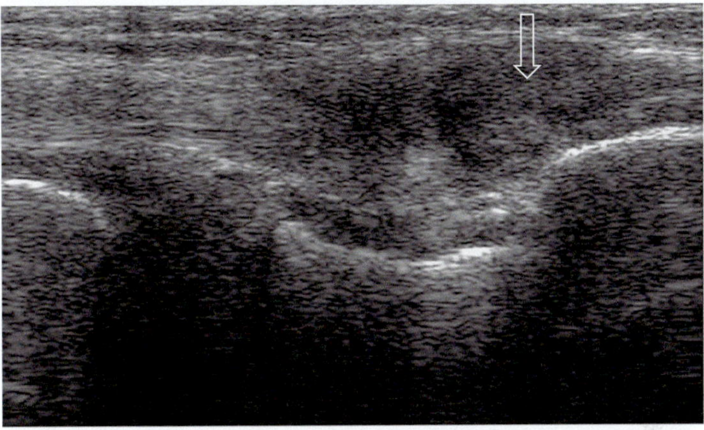

Fig. 11.9 Enthesitis of the biceps femoris tendon at its insertion at the fibula (lateral longitudinal view)

11.2.4   Tendon Abnormalities of the Knee II

Best Scans patellar tendon: Standard Scan 11-5 and 11-6.

Best Scans semitendinosus tendon: Standard Scans 11-7 and 11-8.

Figure 11.10 depicts chronic abnormalities of Osgood-Schlatter's disease. Severe irregularities of the tibia can be seen at the distal insertion of the patellar tendon (⇑). The distal end of the patellar tendon is inhomogeneous. Adolescents with acute Osgood-Schlatter's disease typically show patellar tendon tendinitis, irregularities of the epiphysial cartilage and of the bony contour of the tibia.

Figure 11.11 shows paratenonitis (⇑) of the semimembranosus tendon in a transverse view. The medial head of the gastocnemius muscle is visible medial to it (⇐). The patient presents with a painful, slightly reddened longitudinal area at the medial posterior region proximal to the knee joint. Clinically, this resembles thrombophlebitis. The ultrasound image is similar to tenosynovitis. The semimembranosus tendon has no tendon sheath and hence, this would represent paratenonitis. The tissue around the tendon is inflamed. The patient can be treated with an ultrasound-guided glucocorticoid injection.

Figure 11.12 shows a tendon tear of the quadriceps tendon (⇓). Tendon tears with or even without trauma are a common complication of rheumatic diseases. Ultrasound depicts both ends of the tendon. On dynamic examination the parts can be moved further apart from each other while flexing the knee. This patient also has a knee joint prosthesis (⇑) which is hyperechoic, straight, and horizontal.

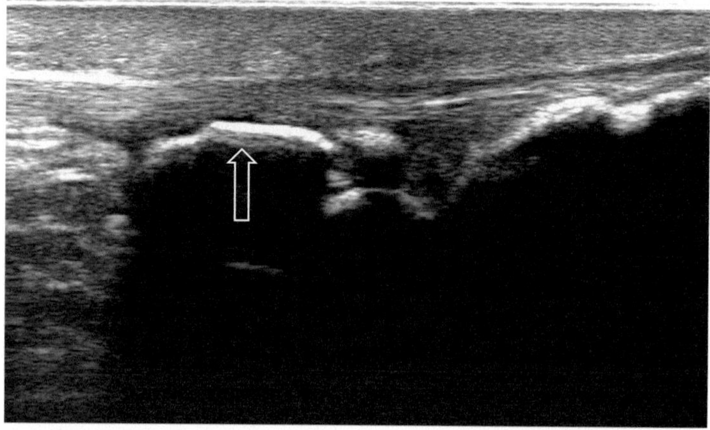

Fig. 11.10 Tibial irregularities and calcifications of the patellar tendon in Osgood-Schlatter's disease (longitudinal infrapatellar view)

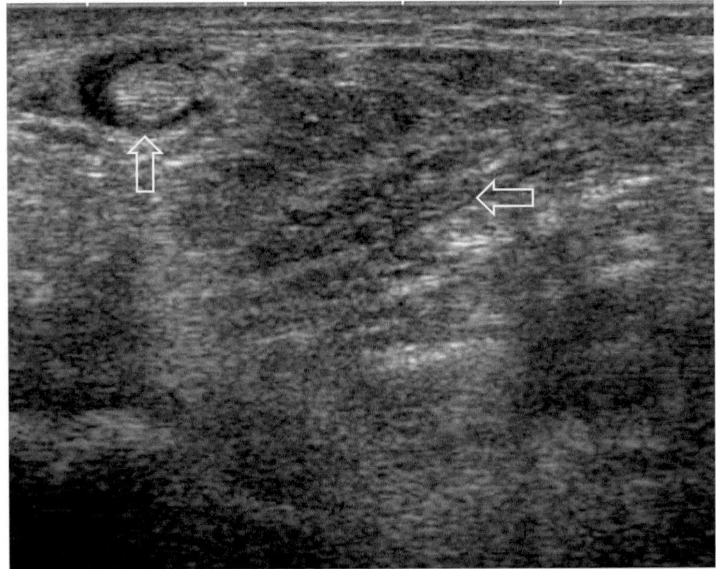

Fig. 11.11 Paratenonitis of the semitendinosus tendon (transverse posterior view)

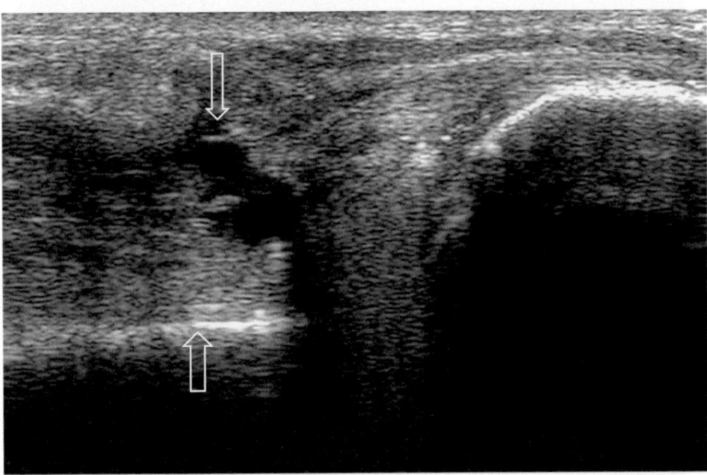

Fig. 11.12 Tear of the quadriceps tendon filled with fluid and knee joint prosthesis (suprapatellar longitudinal view)

11.2.5   *Osteophytes, Erosions and Loose Bodies of the Knee*

Best Scans: Standard Scans 11-3 and 11-4.

Additional Scans: All other Standard Scans.

Ultrasound is an excellent tool to describe the bone surface of the knee joint.

Figure 11.13a shows osteophytes (⇑) at the medial joint space in knee osteoarthritis. The medial meniscus is heterogeneous. It is pushed medially dislocating the medial collateral ligament medially (⇓). Dense hyperechoic structures within the menisicus indicate additional chondrocalcinosis (CPPD; →). Crystals are also located on the hyaline cartilage showing a double contour sign (*) which can also

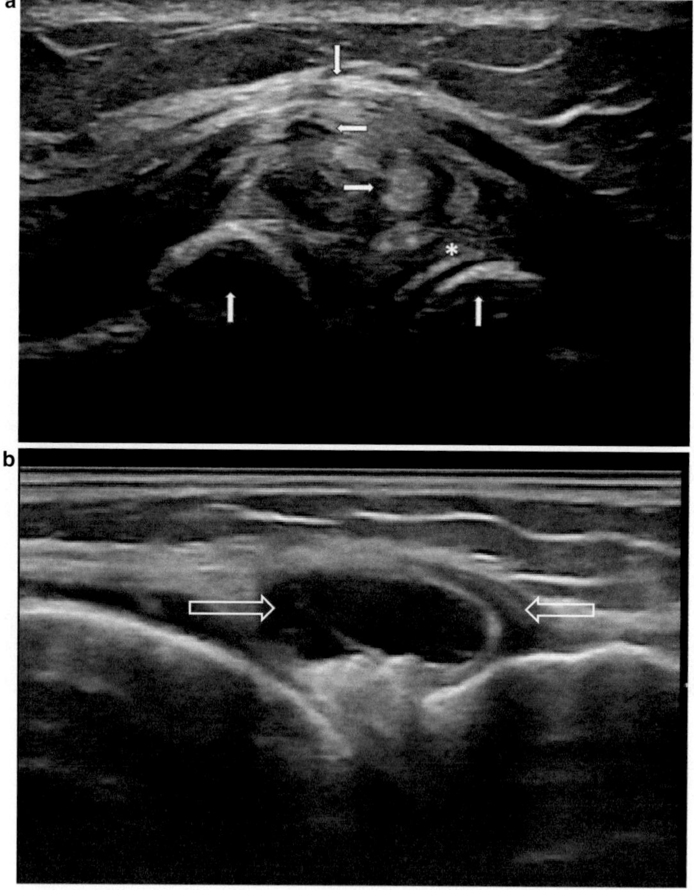

Fig. 11.13 **a** Osteophyte, chondrocalcinosis, meniscal degeneration and meniscal cyst (⇒⇐) in osteoarthritis (longitudinal medial view). **b** Meniscal cyst of the medial meniscus (longitudinal medial view)

occur in CPPD. Further, a small meniscus ganglion can be seen ($\leftarrow$). Figure 11.13b shows a well defined medial meniscal cyst ($\Rightarrow\Leftarrow$).

Figure 11.14 shows a large erosion at the lateral femoral condyle in a patient with RA ($\Rightarrow$). The detection of erosions helps to differentiate between RA and osteoarthritis as a cause of knee pain. However, erosions at the knee joint are not specific to RA. They occur also in other chronic inflammatory diseases such as chronic reactive arthritis.

Figure 11.15 shows a loose body ($\Uparrow$) that is localized next to the lateral aspect of the tibia in a patient with osteochondritis dissecans. The bone on the left is the femur. The bone on the right end is the fibula. When the probe is placed at the ends of the loose body in both a longitudinal and a transverse plane, it is impossible to delineate a connection between the loose body and the tibia.

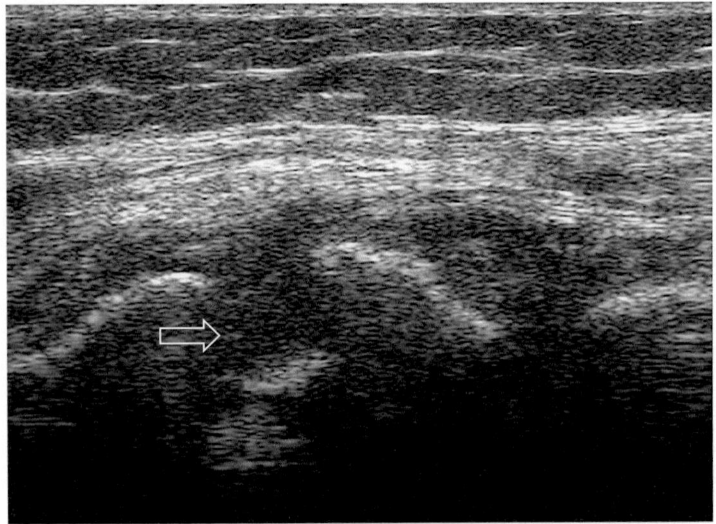

Fig. 11.14 Erosion of the lateral femoral condyle in RA (longitudinal lateral view) ($\Rightarrow$)

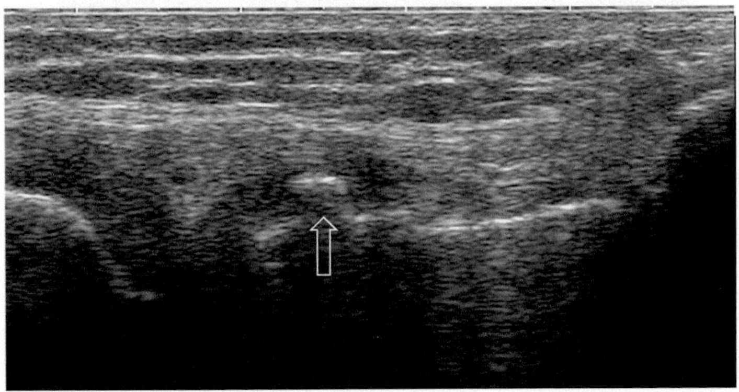

Fig. 11.15 Loose body lateral of the tibia in osteochondrosis dissecans (longitudinal lateral view) ($\Uparrow$)

11.2.6   Prepatellar and Infrapatellar Bursitis

Best Scans: Standard Scans 11-5 and 11-6.

Three types of bursitis occur in the prepatellar and infrapatellar region. Both prepatellar bursitis (Fig. 11.16) and deep infrapatellar bursitis (Figs. 11.17 and 11.18) are common. Superficial infrapatellar bursitis is a rare condition. It is localized anteriorly to the distal part of the patellar tendon. This alteration is not depicted. In bursitis the bursae should be visualized and measured in all three directions (longitudinal, transverse, and sagittal).

Prepatellar bursitis can be diagnosed clinically. Usually, it is important to know the underlying pathology of prepatellar bursitis. Ultrasound aids in differentiating the cause of bursitis. Often non-fluid material is found which cannot be aspirated successfully. Ultrasound can find areas of fluid that can be aspirated for confirming the diagnosis of gout or septic arthritis. In gout, specific hyperechoic structures with or without posterior shadowing may be found. In Fig. 11.16 the soft tissue around the bursitis is thickened and homogeneous due to generalized amyloidosis in a patient with multiple myeloma.

Infrapatellar bursitis as depicted in Fig. 11.17 (longitudinal scan) and in Fig. 11.18 (transverse scan) occurs often in conjunction with a knee joint effusion. Sometimes, infrapatellar bursitis is the only sign of inflammation in the knee region. It can be seen better when the quadriceps muscle is tightened. It is often localized at the distal lateral or medial edges of the patellar tendon.

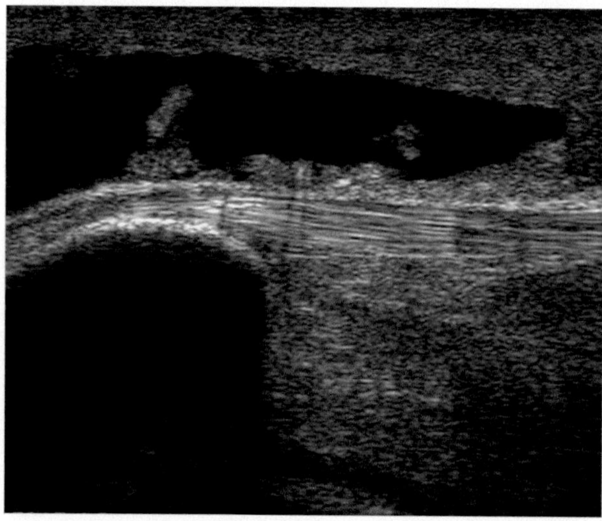

Fig. 11.16 Prepatellar bursitis and amyloidosis of subcutaneous tissue (pre- and infrapatellar longitudinal view)

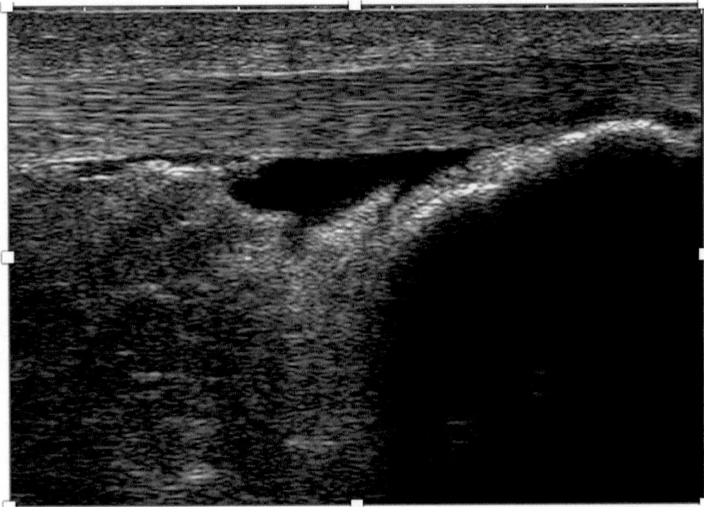

Fig. 11.17 Deep infrapatellar bursitis (infrapatellar longitudinal view)

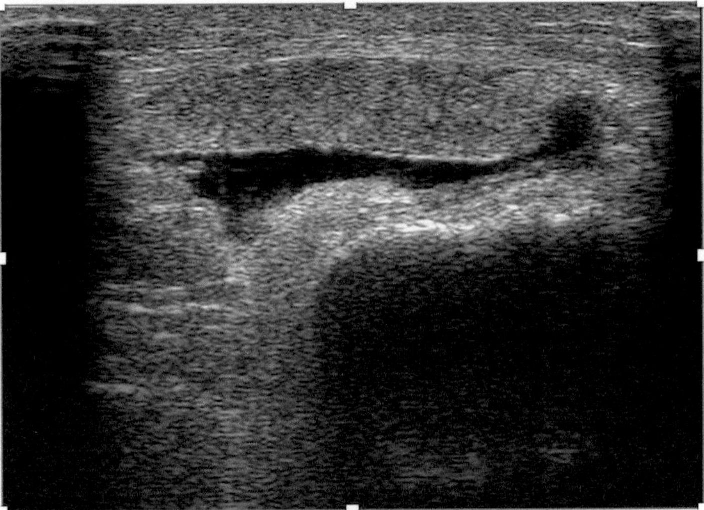

Fig. 11.18 Deep infrapatellar bursitis (infrapatellar transverse view)

11.2.7 Baker's Cyst

Best Scans: Standard Scans 11-7 and 11-8.

In the 1970s, the first indication for musculoskeletal ultrasound was the detection of popliteal Baker's cysts. A ruptured Baker's cyst is a frequent cause of a swollen leg in patients with rheumatic diseases. Ultrasound can easily differentiate between Baker's cysts and deep vein thrombosis. Baker's cysts may contain fluid, midechoic or hyperechoic material, and even calcifications.

The best way to start searching for a Baker's cyst, is to apply the transverse scan at the medial posterior side slightly distal to the knee, where more than 80% of the Baker's cysts are found, and to continue distally to the posterior and medial areas of the lower leg.

A Baker's cyst is typically localized between the medial head of the gastrocnemius muscle and the semimembranosus tendon. It may consist of three compartments that communicate with each other and with the knee joint (Fig. 11.19). The popliteal bursa ($\Downarrow$) and the medial gastrocnemius bursa ($\Leftarrow$) are most commonly involved. The semimembranosus bursa ($\Rightarrow$) that is localized posterior to the medial femoral condyle (*) is less frequently involved. Anisotropy of the semimembranosus tendon may be misinterpreted as semimembranosus bursitis.

A Baker's cyst should be displayed and measured in transverse and longitudinal views.

Figure 11.20 shows an intact popliteal cyst in a longitudinal view.

A Baker's cyst may rupture or may extend distally for more than 20 cm. The distal end of a ruptured Baker's cyst ($\Rightarrow$) becomes pointed with fluid in the adjacent tissue ($\Downarrow$) (Fig. 11.21).

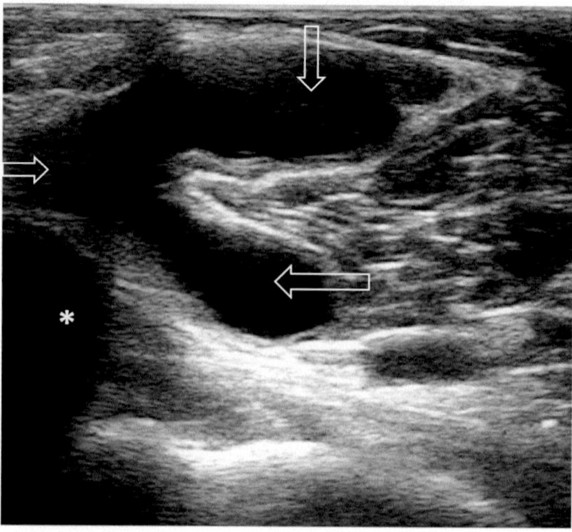

Fig. 11.19 Baker's cyst (posterior transverse view)

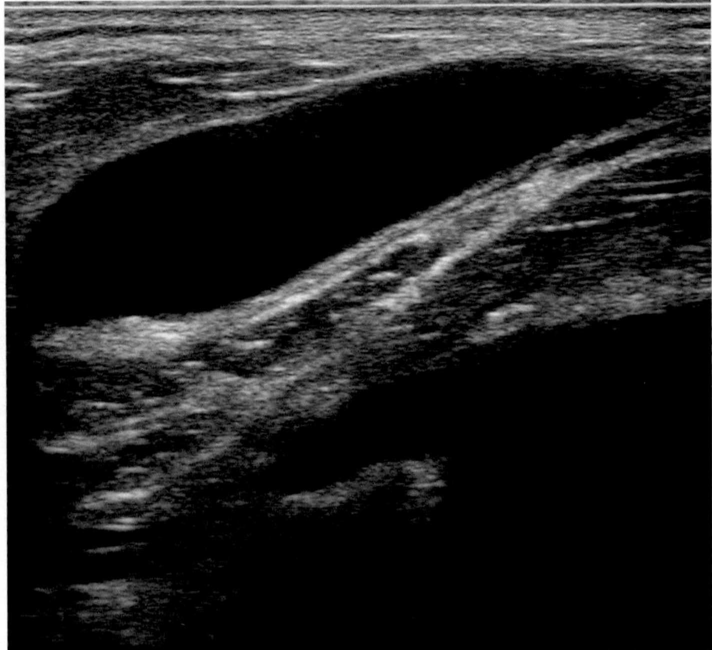

Fig. 11.20 Baker's cyst (posterior longitudinal view)

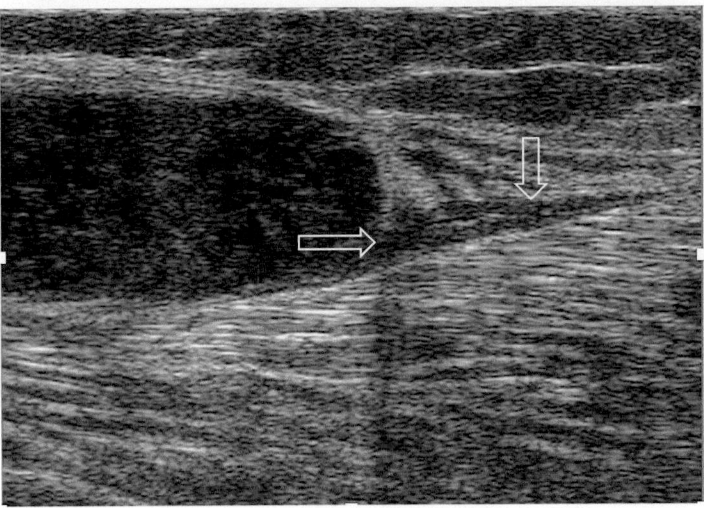

Fig. 11.21 Ruptured Baker's cyst (posterior longitudinal view)

11.2.8   Cartilage and Crystal Disease

Best Scans hyaline cartilage: Standard Scans 11-2 and 11-8.

Best Scans fibrocartilage: Standard Scans 11-3 and 11-4.

Hyaline cartilage is best seen on a suprapatellar transverse scan with 110° flexion of the knee (Standard Scan 11-2) depicting the intercondylar cartilage, and on medial and lateral dorsal longitudinal scans (Standard Scan 11-8) showing the dorsal aspects of the epicondyles.

Figure 11.22 shows thinned, slightly hypoechoic and irregular cartilage of the left knee in osteoarthritis in the suprapatellar transverse scan. The cartilage has completely disappeared in the lateral region of the intercondylar area (⇑).

Chondrocalcinosis hyaline (CPPD) is characterized by specific hyperechoic dots and lines (⇑) within the cartilage (Fig. 11.23). Further, calcifications can be seen in the menisci which consist of fibrocartilage (Fig. 11.13a). Ultrasound has a higher diagnostic accouracy than conventional radiography for CPPD.

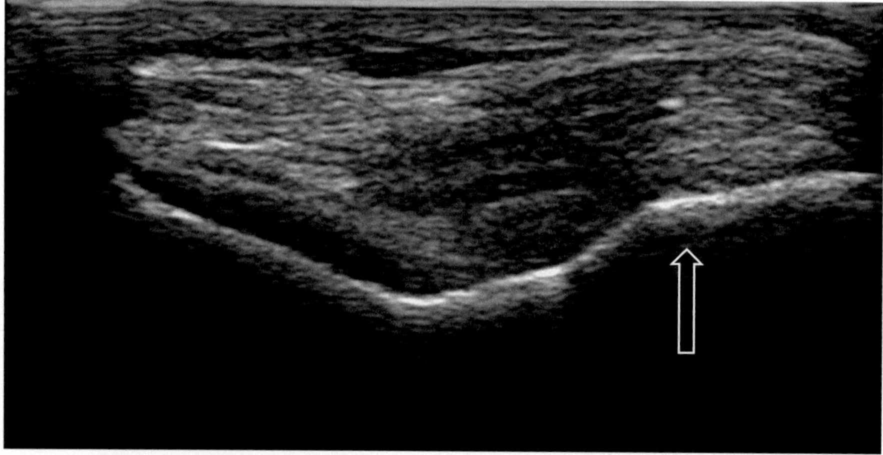

Fig. 11.22 Thinned intercondylar cartilage in osteoarthritis (suprapatellar transverse view)

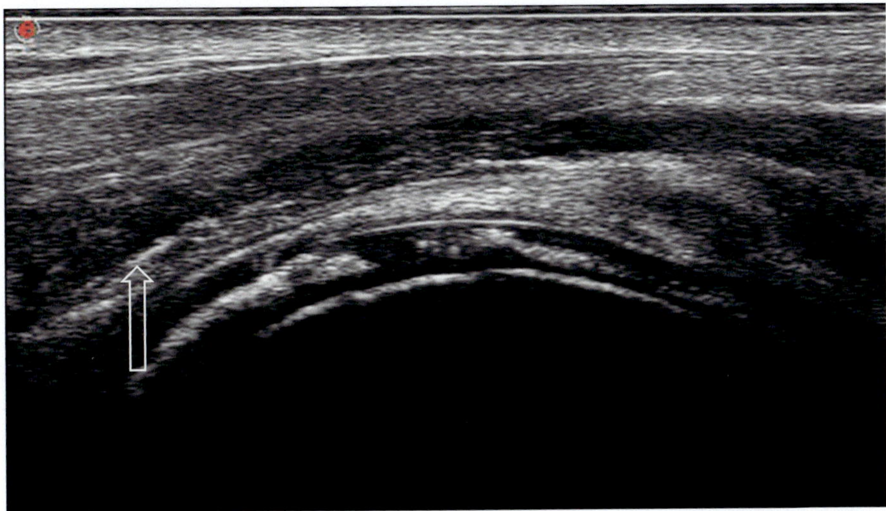

Fig. 11.23 Chondrocalcinosis of the cartilage of the dorsal femoral condyle (dorsal longitudinal view)

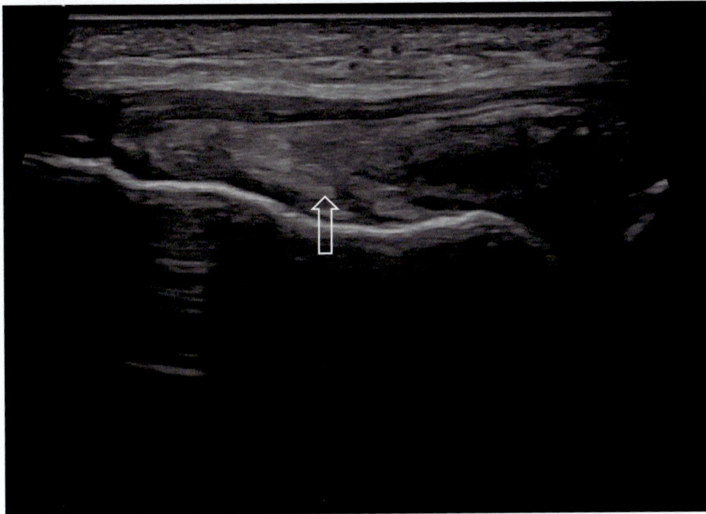

Fig. 11.24 Soft-tissue gout tophus close to the medial femoral condyle (medial longitudinal view) (⇑)

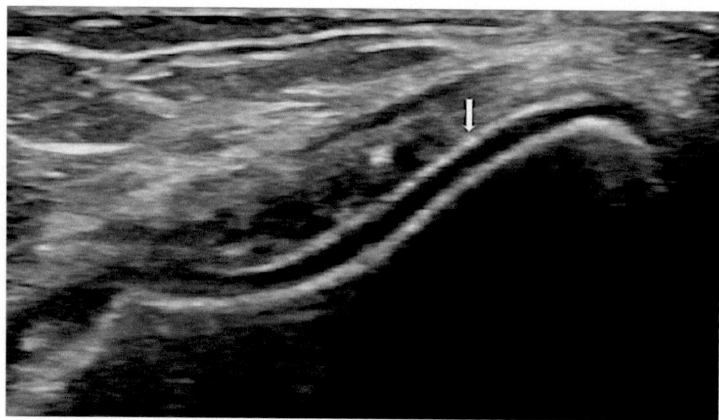

Fig. 11.25   Double contour sign in gout (suprapatellar transverse scan) (⇓)

Ultrasound provides typical images of gout tophi as shown in Figure 11.24 (⇑). A gout tophus has a hyperechoic, snowstorm-like appearance with a hypoechoic rim. If tophi are dense there will be posterior shadowing. Dense calcifications completely extinguish the signal of the bone surface. This soft tissue tophus is localized close to the medial condyle. Tophi can also appear within joints. In addition, a double contour sign is often found representing gout crystal depositions on the intercondylar cartilage (Fig. 11.25, ⇓).

Chapter 12
The Ankle, Foot and Toes

12.1 Standard Scans of the Ankle

12.1.1 Dorsal Longitudinal View of the Ankle (Standard Scan 12-1)

The patient is supine. There are two ways for positioning the leg. Either the knee is extended with the ankle in a neutral position, or the knee is 45° flexed with the foot resting on the bed as shown here.

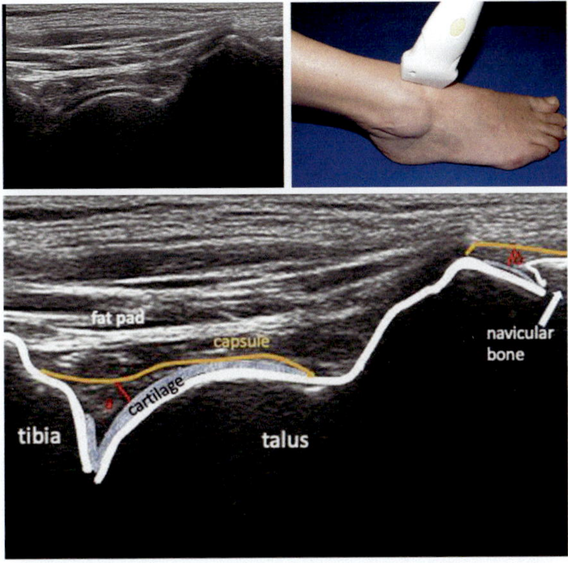

© The Author(s), under exclusive license to Springer Nature Switzerland AG 2023

G. A. W. Bruyn and W. A. Schmidt, *Musculoskeletal Ultrasound for the Rheumatologist*,

https://doi.org/10.1007/978-3-031-27737-5_12

Place the probe longitudinally at midline in the area of the ankle. Then shift the probe to the medial and lateral areas.

Short probes (<4.5 cm) delineate either the ankle joint or the talonavicular joint. Make sure that both joints are examined. For dynamic examination have the patient flex and extend the ankle to detect minor amounts of fluid. Note that the talonavicular joint is localized not at the deepest point of the talus but more distally.

This scan is useful for evaluating the ankle and the talonavicular joint as well as for detecting tenosynovitis of the extensor tendons.

What is normal?

The distance including the cartilage between talus and joint capsule 1 cm distal of the ankle joint midline sagittal (**a**) is 1.1 mm (0.1–2.1 mm).

The maximum sagittal distance including the cartilage between bone and joint capsule at the talonavicular joint (**b**) is 1.4 mm (0.2–2.6 mm).

12.1.2 Dorsal Transverse View of the Ankle (Standard Scan 12-2)

The patient's position is identical to that in Standard Scan 12-1. Place the probe transversely over the ankle joint and shift it from tibia to talus and navicular or vice versa. This scan is important for examining the structures seen in Standard Scan 12-1 in a second plane. This scan is also well suited to assess the various extensor tendons. In healthy subjects it may be difficult to differentiate the anatomical structures, in particular the tendons, unless there is a certain amount of fluid in the tendon sheaths. Moving the big toe and the other toes may be useful to differentiate their extensor tendons from the tibialis anterior tendon.

What is normal?

The normal sagittal diameter of the tibialis anterior tendon (a) at the level of the ankle joint is 2.5 mm (1.2 mm–3.8 mm). The normal transverse diameter (b) is 8.2 mm (4.7 mm –11.7 mm). The physiologic hypoechoic rim (c) is 0.8 mm (0–1.7 mm).

The maximum diameter of the tendon sheath or any extensor tendon at any location should be ≤3 mm.

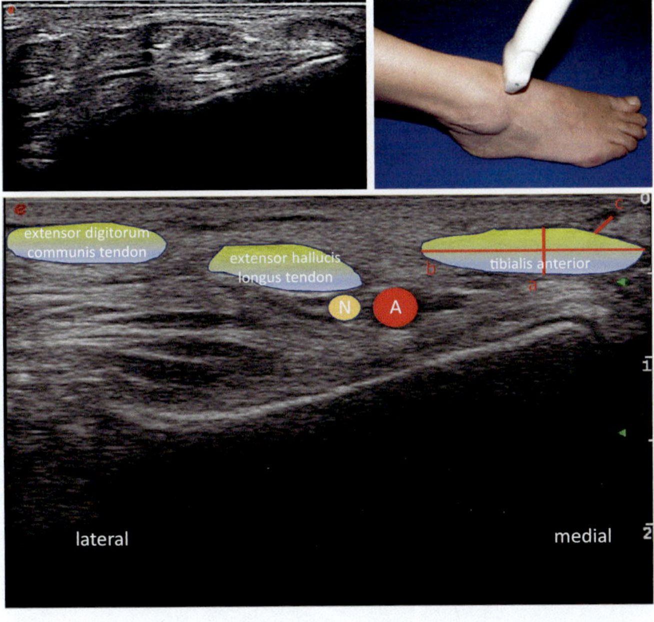

12.1.3   Medial Transverse View of the Ankle (Standard Scan 12-3)

The patient's position is identical to that in Standard scans 12-1 and 12-2. The patient only exorotates the leg. In this way it is easier to assess this region. After having started directly distal to the medial malleolus, the probe is shifted distally along the three flexor tendons. It is then shifted along the malleolus up to an area about 10 cm cranial of the malleolus as the tendon sheaths extend that far proximally.

The aim of this scan is to look for tenosynovitis of the flexor tendons. The tibialis posterior tendon is localized most anteriorly followed by the flexor digitorum longus tendon and the flexor hallucis longus tendon. The tibialis posterior tendon is markedly thicker than the flexor digitorum longus tendon. The flexor hallucis longus tendon can be only seen distally from the malleolus. The neurovascular bundle includes the tibial posterior artery (A) and the two tibial posterior veins (V) that are normally compressible. The tibial nerve localizes between the posterior tibialis vein and the flexor hallucis longus tendon (N). The neurovascular bundle passes below the flexor retinaculum of the ankle. Slightly tilting the probe under the malleolus brings the medial aspect of the subtalar joint into focus. It can be also examined from the lateral (see Sect. 12.1.5) and the posterior aspect (see Sect. 12.1.7).

What is normal?

The normal sagittal diameter of the tibialis posterior tendon directly distal to the malleolus (a) is 2.8 mm (1.0–4.6 mm), the transverse diameter (b) is 8.4 mm (4.2–12.6 mm). The normal diameter of the physiological hypoechoic rim (c) is 1.2 mm (0–2.8 mm). The maximum diameter of the tendon sheath of any flexor tendon at any location should be ≤3.5 mm.

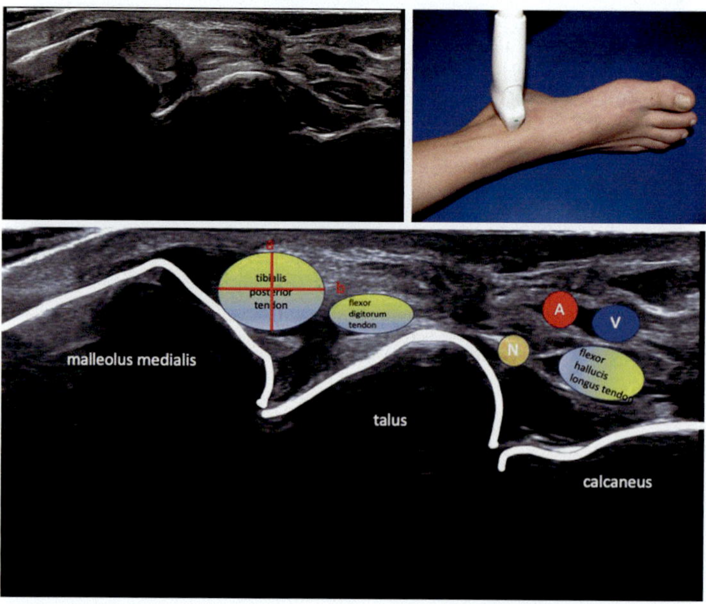

12.1.4 Medial Longitudinal Scan of the Ankle (Standard Scan 12-4)

The patient's position is identical to Standard Scans 12-1 to 12-3. The patient only exorotates the leg as shown in Standard Scan 12-3 to improve the assessment of this region. Again, after starting in the region distal to the medial malleolus the probe is shifted distally.

To completely visualize the area in which the tendons are surrounded by a tendon sheath the probe should also be shifted proximally behind the malleolus up to an area about 10 cm cranial of the malleolus.

The scan displays a panoramic view of the tibialis posterior tendon, from the level of the medial malleolus towards its main insertion on the navicular bone and a smaller portion on the medial cuneiform bone. Shifting the probe a bit more posteriorly creates a window for the other structures including the flexor tendons, the posterior tibial artery and veins, and the tibial nerve.

What is normal?

The tendons are slightly hyperechoic or isoechoic and homogeneous. They may be hypoechoic (dark) because of anisotropy in the region of their insertions. Sometimes it is difficult to visualize the tibialis posterior tendon near its insertion into the navicular bone.

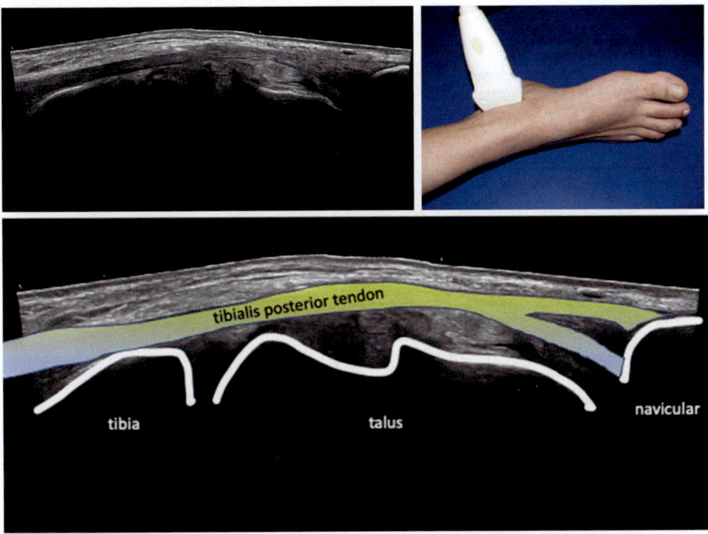

12.1.5   Lateral Transverse View of the Ankle (Standard Scan 12-5)

The patient's position is identical to that in Standard Scans 12-1 to 12-4. The patient's leg should only be rotated for assessing this region more easily. Again, starting in the area directly distal to the malleolus, the probe is shifted distally towards the insertion of the peroneus brevis tendons on the head of 5th metatarsal and proximally up to an area about 10 cm cranial of the malleolus as the tendon sheath extends that far.

This scan helps to find tenosynovitis of the paired peroneal tendons. On the transverse scan the peroneus brevis tendon is localized medially and closer to the bone than the peroneus longus tendon.

The figure shows the peroneus tendons at the level of the subtalar joint.

When tilting the probe slightly under the malleolus the lateral aspect of the subtalar joint appears. Ultrasound can detect effusions and osteophytes. Usually the ankle joint, the subtalar joint and the talonavicular joint do not communicate with each other. However, this may be the case in some individuals, particularly in patients with inflammatory diseases involving the ankle.

What is normal?

The normal sagittal diameter of the peroneus longus tendon directly distal of the malleolus (a) is 3.0 mm (1.4–4.6 mm). The transverse diameter (b) is 6.0 mm (2.3–9.7 mm). The normal diameter of the physiological, hypoechoic rim is 1.1 mm (0–2.3 mm).

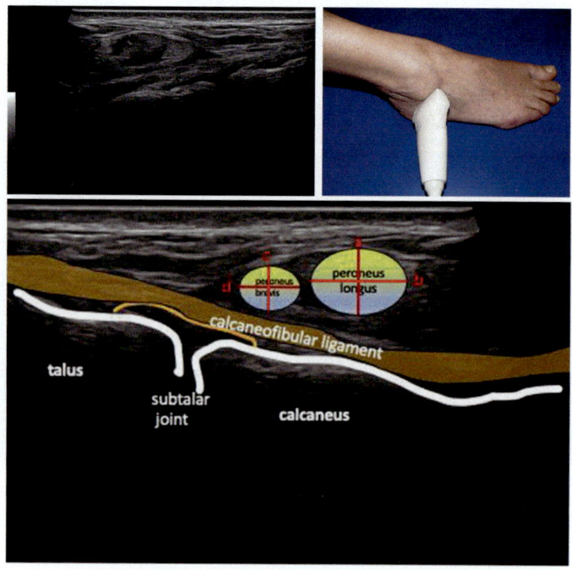

The normal sagittal diameter of the peroneus brevis tendon directly distal of the malleolus (c) is 2.5 mm (1.2–3.8 mm).

The transverse diameter (d) is 4.3 mm (1.3–7.3 mm).

The normal diameter of the physiologic hypoechoic rim is 0.9 mm (0.1–1.7 mm).

The maximum diameter of the common tendon sheath of the peroneal tendons should be ≤3 mm.

12.1.6   Lateral Longitudinal View of the Ankle (Standard Scan 12-6)

The patient's position is identical to Standard Scans 12-1 to 12-5. The patient only rotates the leg as in Standard Scan 12-5 to improve the assessment of this region. Starting at the region distal to the lateral malleolus the probe is shifted distally towards the insertions of the peroneal tendons. To completely visualize the area in which the tendons are surrounded by a tendon sheath the probe should also be shifted proximally behind the malleolus up to an area about 10 cm cranial of the malleolus.

This scan displays the paired peroneal tendons in the second plane.

The anterior talofibular ligament (↓) is the most commonly torn ligament of the foot. It becomes visible when placing the proximal end of the probe directly on the lateral malleolus and orientating the probe strictly parallel to the sole of the foot, preferably with inversion if this should not be too painful for the patient. Small amounts of fluid in the ankle below the ligament may be physiological.

What is normal?

Both the tendons and the ligament appear as hyperechoic structures with a typical fibrillar appearance as found in other tendons and ligaments.

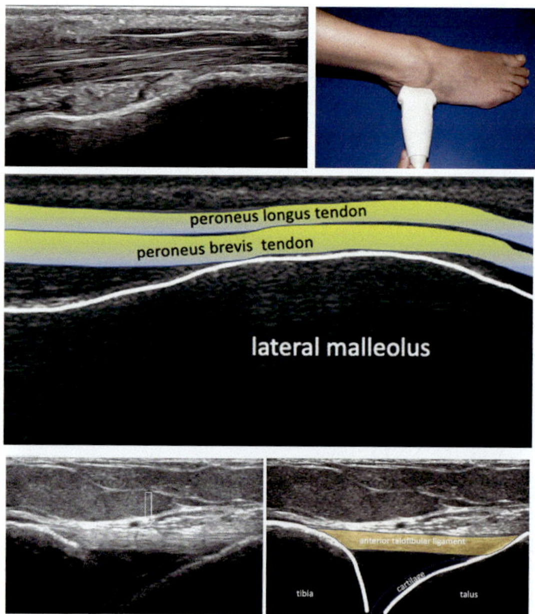

12.1.7   Posterior Longitudinal View of the Ankle (Standard Scan 12-7)

The patient is in prone position with the feet hanging over the end of the examination table. Alternatively, the patient can rest the toes on the bed with the ankle extended. For dynamic assessment, the sonographer can hold the foot and flex and extend the ankle.

First, the superficial structures including the Achilles tendon, the retrocalcaneal bursa, and the posterior area of the calcaneus are examined. Then the probe is shifted towards the proximal areas of the Achilles tendon until the gastrocnemius and soleus muscles can be seen. The Kager's triangle consists of hypo- to isoechoic fat tissue.

This scan should also be used for examining deeper structures, particularly for the assessment of the posterior recesses of the tibio-talar (ankle) and subtalar joints. Sometimes effusion or synovitis of these joints occur only in the posterior aspect. Small effusions can be detected with extending and flexing the ankle joint while ultrasound is being performed.

What is normal?

The sagittal diameter of the Achilles tendon, 2 cm proximal of the calcaneus is 4.3 mm (2.7–5.9 mm) (a). In females this is 4.1 mm (2.7–5.5 mm), and in males this is 4.6 mm (3.0–6.2 mm). A small amount of fluid occurs in 24% of retrocalcaneal bursae (b). The sagittal diameter should be ≤2.7 mm. The posterior recess of the tibiotalar joint is 1.2 mm (0.1–2.3 mm) (c).

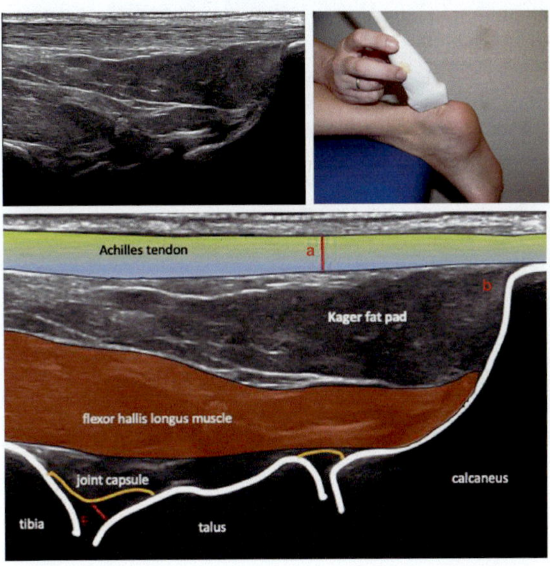

12.1.8   *Posterior Transverse View of the Achilles Tendon and the Ankle (Standard Scan 12-8)*

The patient's position is identical to that in Standard Scan 12-7. Again, all sections of the Achilles tendon should be examined starting at the posterior aspect of the calcaneus and shifting the probe about 15 cm proximally. This scan displays the anatomical structures in the second plane in the search for Achilles tendinitis, paratenonitis, enthesitis, calcaneal spurs, and effusions of the posterior recess of the ankle joint. Here, only the superficial structures are shown.

What is normal?

The echogenicity of the Achilles tendon should be identical or higher compared to the surrounding tissue. It takes the form of an ellipse with multiple hyperechoic dots corresponding to collagen bundles. Two cm proximal of its insertion in the calcaneus, the tendon has a transverse diameter (a) of 14.3 mm (10.2–18.4 mm). In females this is 13.3 mm (9.9–16.7 mm) and in males 15.4 mm (11.5–19.3 mm).

A hypoechoic rim around the Achilles tendon occurs in 13% of healthy persons. The diameter should be ≤3.3 mm. This corresponds with the paratenon. A small amount of physiological fluid may be found in the retrocalcaneal bursa (anechoic area below the Achilles tendon in the ultrasound image).

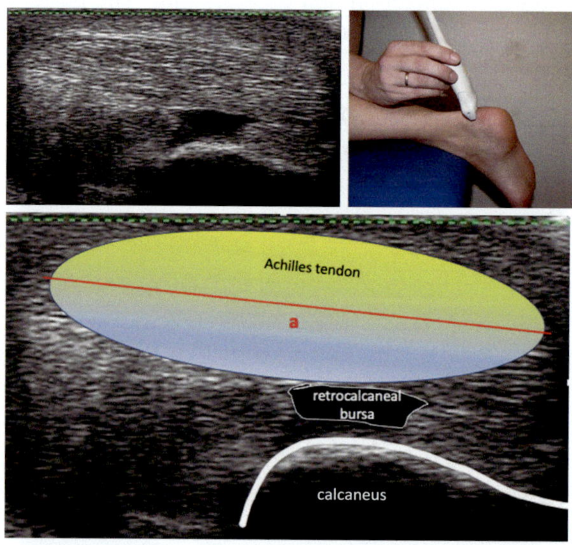

12.1.9   Plantar Proximal Longitudinal View of the Foot (Standard Scan 12-9)

The patient's position is identical to that in Standard Scans 12-7 and 12-8.

The patient lies prone with the feet hanging over the end of the examination table.

The probe is placed over the midline or slightly medially to the midline at the plantar area of the calcaneus. The distal end of the probe is directed towards the first toe. This means that the scan is not completely longitudinal but about 10% oblique with the distal end of the probe pointing medially. The probe should be shifted medially and laterally in order to scan all regions of the plantar fascia and to assess the calcaneus for spurs.

As the skin is thicker in this region, it is necessary to apply more pressure with the probe. Furthermore, the gain needs to be increased in most cases as structures often appear too hypoechoic.

What is normal?

Like most tendons the plantar fascia is hyperechoic and homogeneous.

The sagittal diameter of the plantar fascia at the distal plantar end of the calcaneus (a) is 3.4 mm (2.1–4.7 mm).

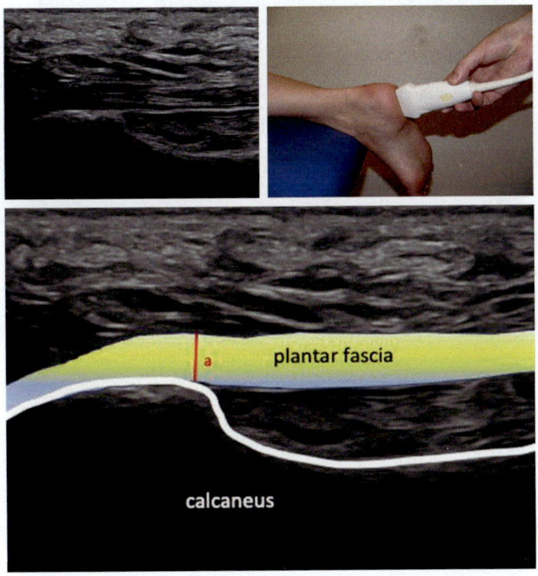

12.1.10   Dorsal Longitudinal View of the Midfoot (Standard Scan 12-10)

The patient's position is identical to that in Standard Scans 12-1 and 12-2.

Starting at the midline distal to the ankle and talonavicular joints, the naviculo-cuneiform and the third tarsometatarsal joints are shown. The probe is then shifted medially to assess the medial aspects of the naviculocuneiform joint and the first and second tarsometatarsal joints. The probe is shifted laterally to assess the lateral aspects of the naviculocuneiform joint and the fourth and fifth tarsometatarsal joints. When shifting the probe further laterally in region distal and lateral to the lateral malleolus the calcaneo-cubital joint can be seen.

The scans for the midfoot are important for detecting effusion, synovitis and bony irregularities (e.g., in osteoarthritis) of the midfoot.

What is normal?

The distance between bone and joint capsule is minimal in these joints.
Normal values have not yet been determined.

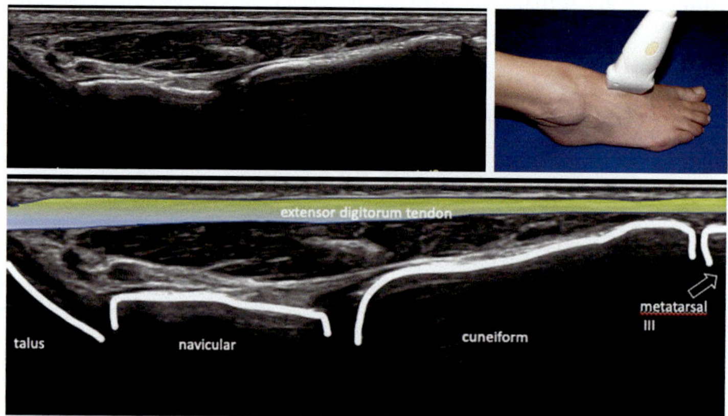

12.1.11 Dorsal Longitudinal View of the Toes (Standard Scan 12-11)

The patient's position is identical to that in Standard Scans 12-1 and 12-2 of the foot. For dynamic examination the patient should flex and extend the toes. Place the probe at the midline of the dorsal aspect of each MTP joint. This scan offers the fastest way for detecting effusions or synovitis of the toes. As synovitis may occur more medially or laterally the probe should be shifted in these directions as far as possible. The MTP I and the MTP V joints can also be assessed at their medial or lateral aspects, particularly to detect erosions or tophi and the double contour sign in gout. The probe is then shifted semi-circumferentially around these joints. All joints can also be assessed from the plantar side. Findings should be re-evaluated in a transverse plane.

The examination may be extended to the PIP, DIP, and IP joints of the toes from posterior, lateral, medial und plantar in longitudinal and transverse scans.

What is normal?

The sagittal dorsal distance between bone and joint capsule including the cartilage for an MTP I joint (a) is 1.7 mm (0–3.5 mm). For an MTP II joint it is 1.6 mm (0.1–3.1 mm).

The ultrasound figure displays physiological synovial material and cartilage in an MTP joint.

Replace ultrasound image.

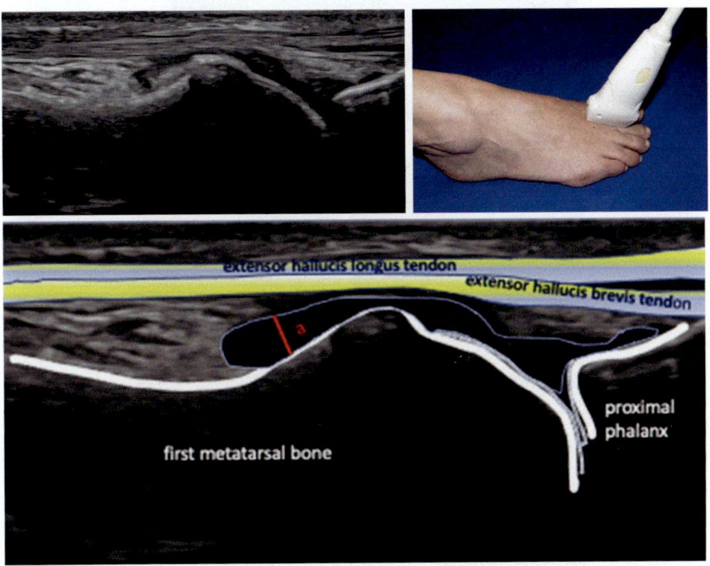

12.1.12   Ultrasound-Guided Injections of the Ankle

After informed consent and the usual antisepsis, the patient lies supine. The patient should flex the knee, and the foot should be flat on the table. The probe is placed in longitudinal orientation on the supratalar region to mark the target area where injection should take place. The prescan shows the anterior recess of the ankle joint. Then, the needle is inserted at the foot of the probe and advanced under real-time ultrasound guidance into the anterior recess of the tibiotalar joint. Alternatively, ultrasound guided injections can be performed from the lateral or medial sides with transverse ultrasound scans. With the needle and probe parallel in a transverse plane it is easier to avoid the artery compared to the longitudinal plane.

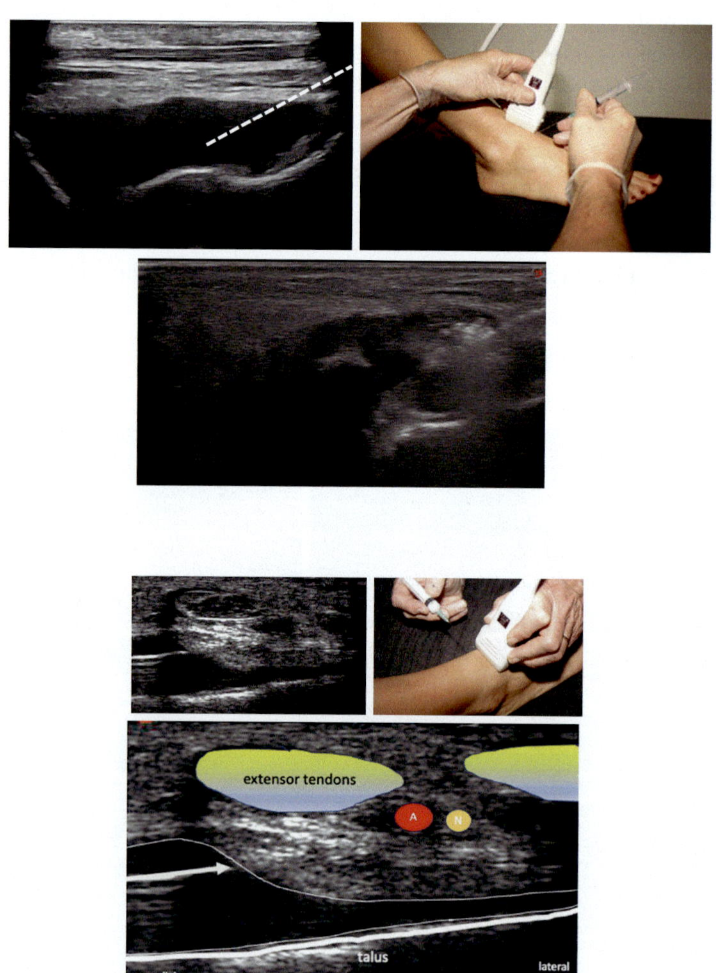

12.1.13 Injection of the Peroneal Tendon Sheath

Typical features of flexor tenosynovitis or, as in this case, peroneal tenosynovitis are swelling of the tendon, decreased echogenicity, effusion and synovial thickening of the tendon sheath. A prescan of the target area is done showing the lateral malleolus and the two peroneal tendons. A small mark is then made on the skin, to indicate the center point of the effusion. At this point, the needle is introduced and under ultrasound guidance and directed into the tendon sheath. The injection of glucocorticoids should result in a distension of the tendon sheath.

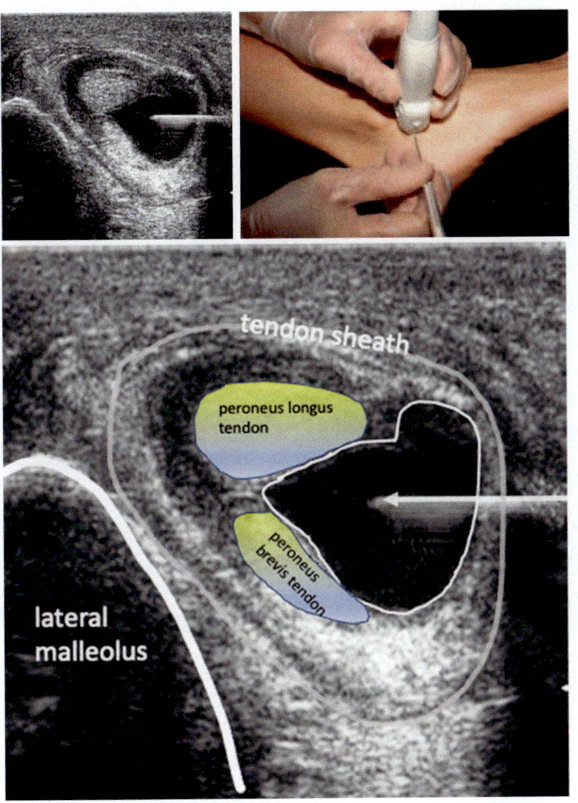

12.1.14   Injection of MTP Joints

Since the joint space can be easily accessed from the dorsal aspect, injections of the small toe joints are generally done dorsally. The foot of the patient is comfortably and firmly placed on a table.

Firstly, a long axis scan is done to mark the exact site of the joint space. A small needle is inserted at the foot of the probe and pushed forward to the joint space between the metatarsal head and the proximal phalanx of the toe under direct ultrasound guidance.

Alternatively, injections can be done on the dorsal aspect from lateral or medial with the needle out of plane.

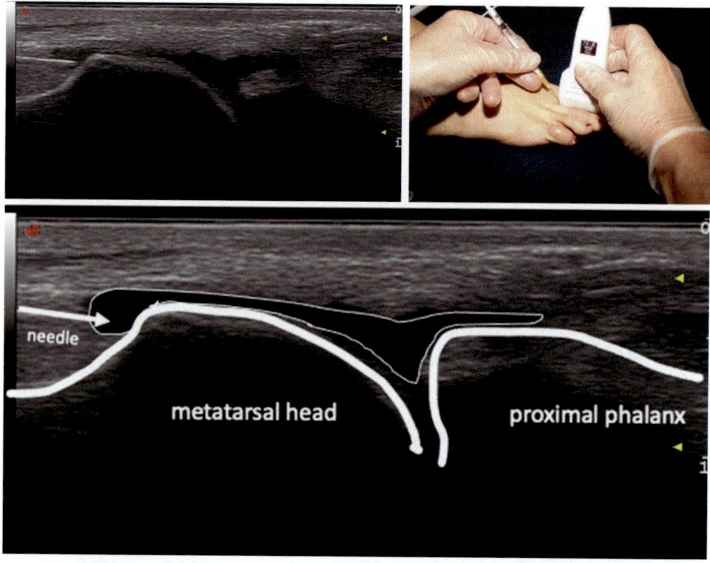

12.2 Pathology of the Ankle, Foot and Toes

12.2.1 *Synovitis/Effusion of the Ankle and Talonavicular Joint*

Best Scans: Standard Scans 12-1, 12-2, 12-7, 12-8

The capsule of the tibiotalar joint extends distally and inserts at the talus.

The capsule of the talonavicular joint follows distally. The insertions of both joint capsules are near to each other. In effusion or synovitis of the tibiotalar joint, anechoic or hypoechoic material accumulates between talus and joint capsule. Thus, the joint capsule will no longer be parallel to the bone.

Figure 12.1 depicts an effusion of the ankle joint (⇑) and an effusion with synovial proliferatons of the talonavicular joint (⇓) in a longitudinal view. The tibia is slightly irregular (⇐).

Figure 12.2 shows an effusion of the tibiotalar joint in a transverse plane at the level of talus (⇑). The extensor tendons are visible more superficially.

Figure 12.3 shows synovitis of the talonavicular joint (⇑). The intra-articular material is hypoechoic and poorly compressible. Dorsal to the joint capsule runs the dorsal pedal artery (⇒) which should not be confused with tenosynovitis of extensor tendons.

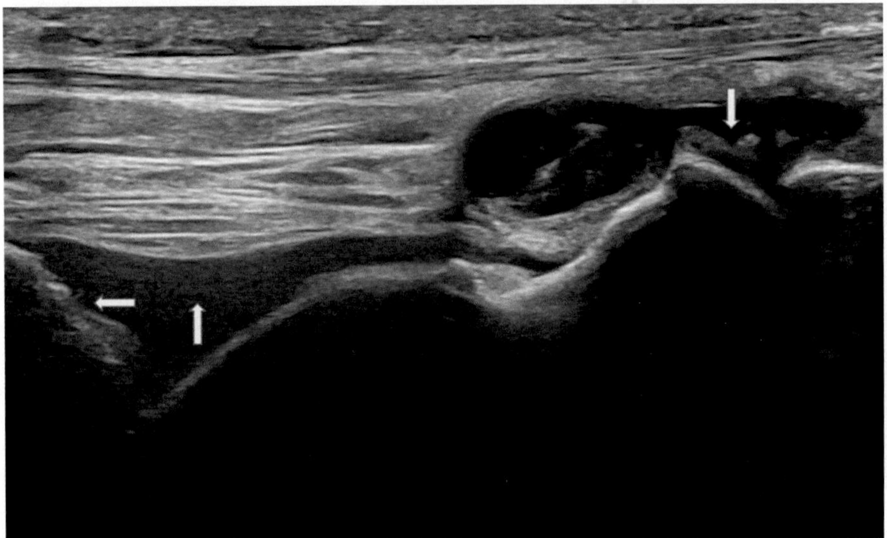

Fig. 12.1 Effusion in the tibiotalar joint and the talonavicular joint (dorsal longitudinal view)

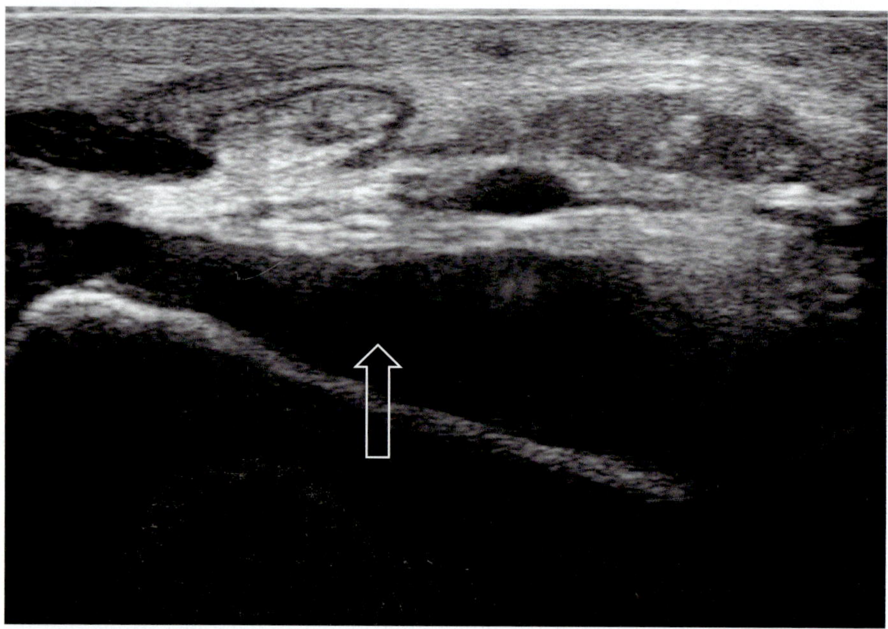

Fig. 12.2 Effusion of the tibiotalar joint (dorsal transverse view)

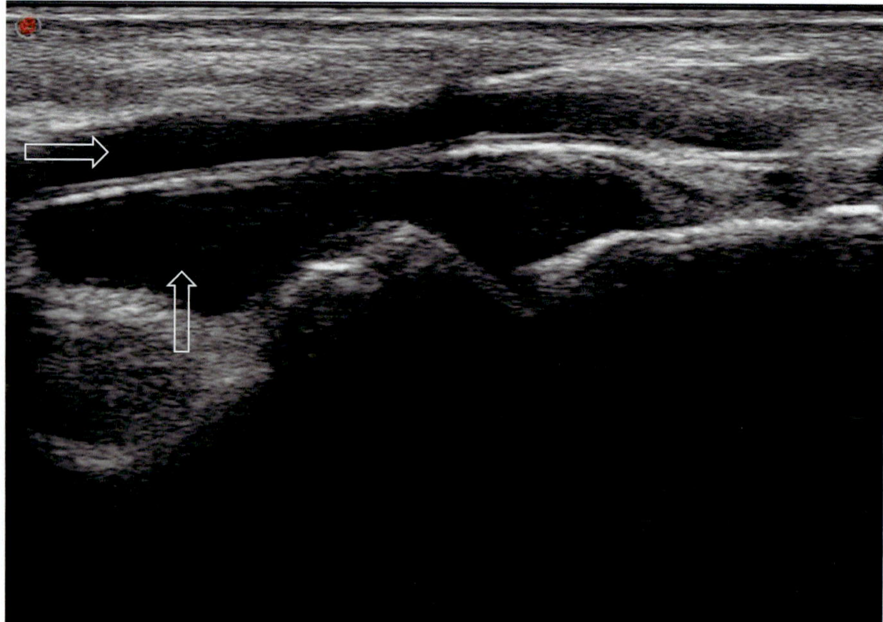

Fig. 12.3 Synovitis of the talononavicular joint (dorsal longitudinal view)

12.2.2 Tenosynovitis of the Foot and Ankle

Best Scans: 12-1 to 12-6

Tenosynovitis of flexor and peroneus tendons can occur in any segment, either at the level of the malleolus or further proximal or distal. Therefore, it is important to shift the probe along the whole area of the tendon sheath. The same applies to the extensor tendons. It is easier to detect tenosynovitis in transverse scans as the fluid or inflammatory material often extends laterally or medially. You should begin with a transverse view when looking primarily for tenosynovitis. It is easier to visualize a tendon with tenosynovitis than a normal tendon.

Figures 12.4 and 12.5 show tenosynovitis of the tibialis posterior tendon in transverse and longitudinal views (⇐). The flexor digitorum tendon shown in Fig. 12.4 is unaffected (⇑).

Figure 12.6 a and b show tenosynovitis (⇐) of the extensor digitorum tendons at the level of the talus and the navicular bone. The talonavicular and naviculocuneiform joints are normal.

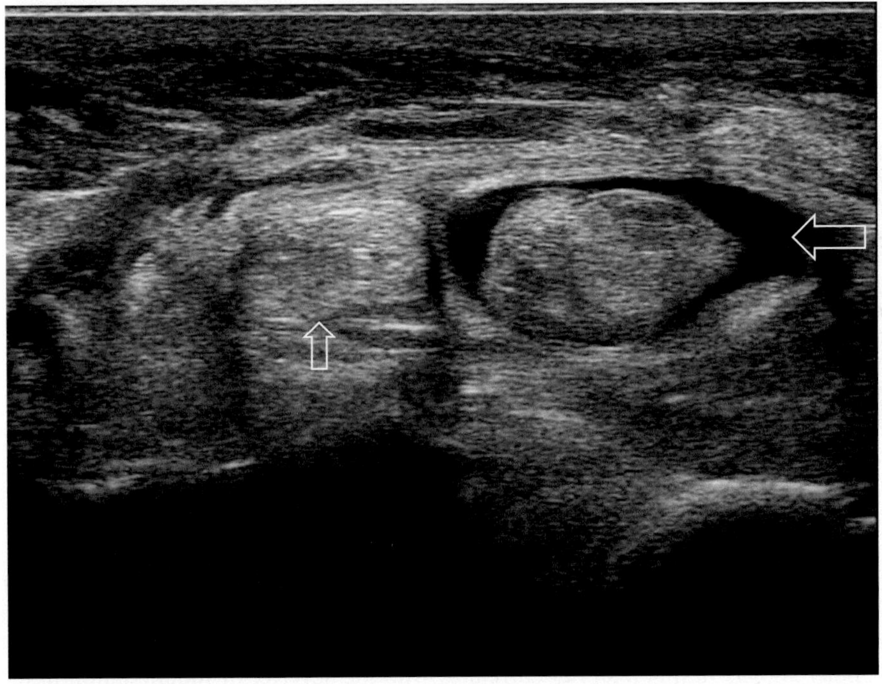

Fig. 12.4 Tenosynovitis of the tibialis posterior tendon (medial transverse view)

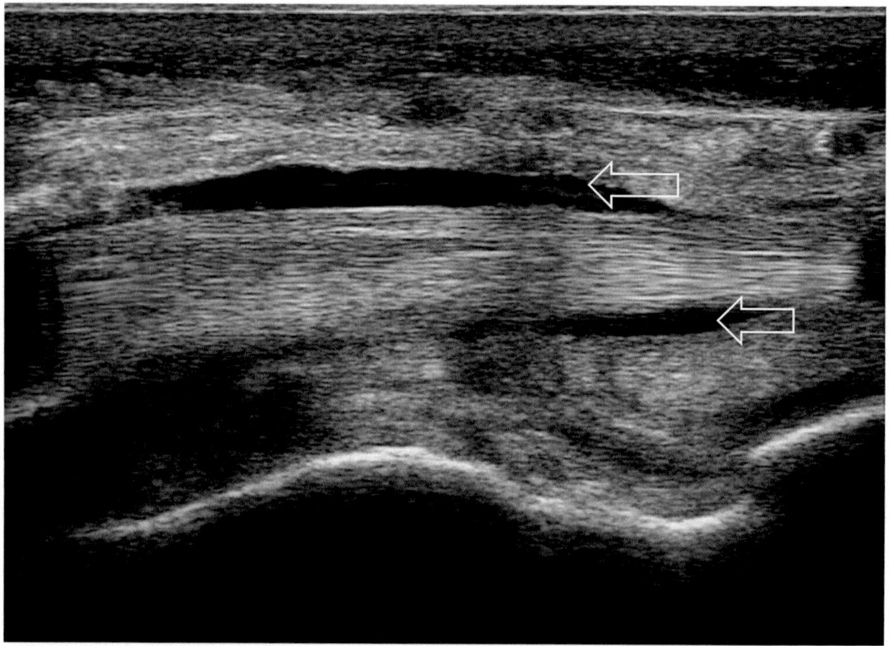

Fig. 12.5 Tenosynovitis of the tibialis posterior tendon (medial longitudinal view)

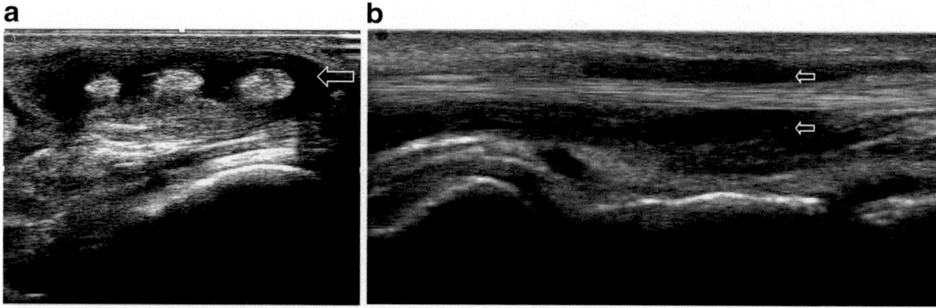

Fig. 12.6 a Tenosynovitis of the extensor digitorum tendons (dorsal transverse view). **b** Tenosynovitis of the extensor digitorum tendons (dorsal longitudinal view)

Tenosynovitis may either contain fluid as shown in Figs. 12.4 and 12.5, or hypoechoic, non-compressible material representing inflammatory tisue as shown in Fig. 12.6 a and b. In RA, this material is usually pannus. The grade of power Doppler signals in this material correlates with the severity of inflammation in the tenosynovium.

12.2.3   Pathology of the Achilles Tendon I

Best Scans: Standard Scans 12-7, 12-8

In tendinitis, the Achilles tendon is thickened and hypoechoic, i.e., the tendon is darker than the surrounding soft tissue. It may also be inhomogeneous with an increasing sagittal diameter.

Figure 12.7 shows a longitudinal scan of a patient with Achilles tendinitis. The tendon is hypoechoic when compared with the surrounding soft tissue. The sagittal diameter is 12.5 mm. Some areas are particularly inhomogeneous representing small tears ($\Downarrow$).

Figure 12.8 displays Achilles tendinitis in a transverse plane. The tendon is more spheroidal than a normal tendon because the sagittal diameter is increased to 13 mm. The anechoic areas within the tendon represent partial tears.

Figure 12.9 shows another case of Achilles tendinitis. Although the sagittal diameter of the tendon is only 6 mm, and its echotexture is rather homogeneous and only slightly hypoechoic, it displays marked hyperperfusion when applying the power Doppler mode. This represents clinically relevant inflammation of the tendon.

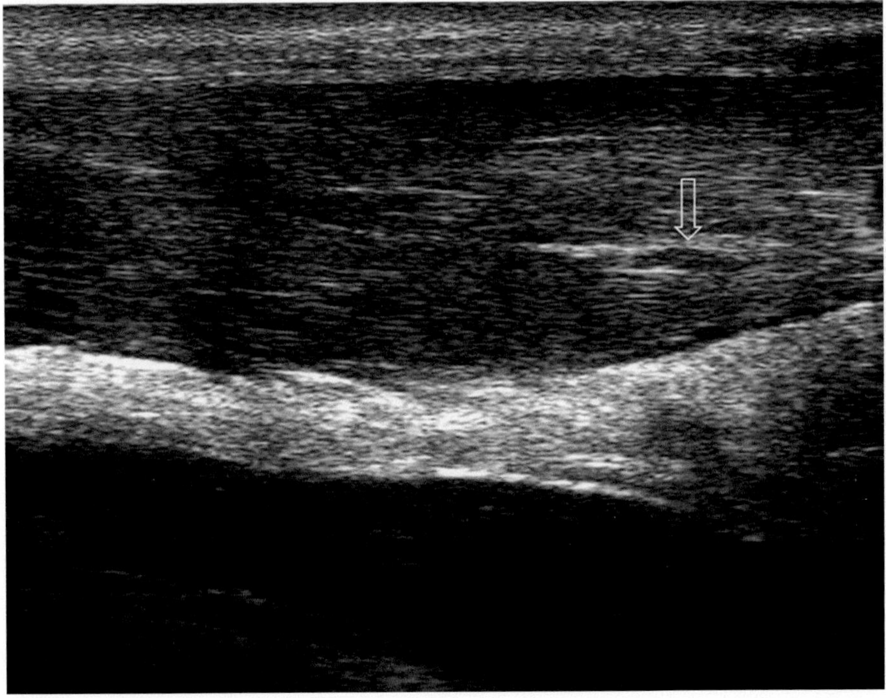

Fig. 12.7   Tendinitis of the Achilles tendon (posterior longitudinal view)

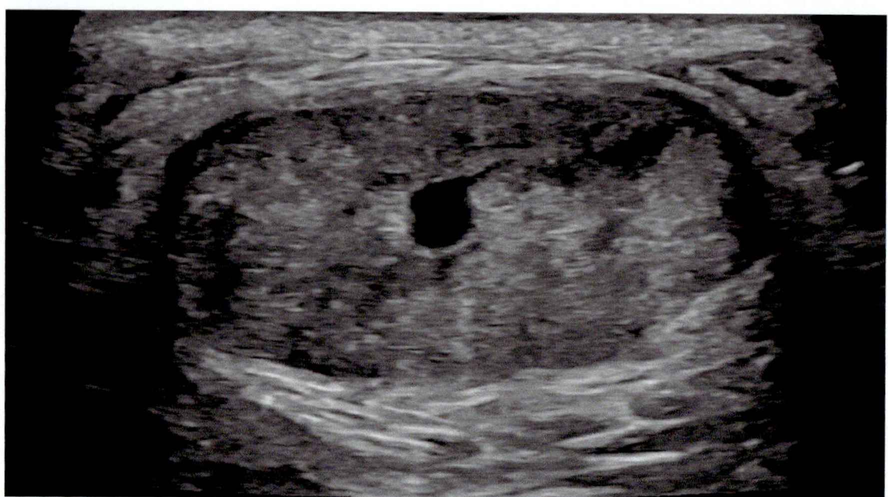

Fig. 12.8 Tendinitis of the Achilles tendon (posterior transverse view)

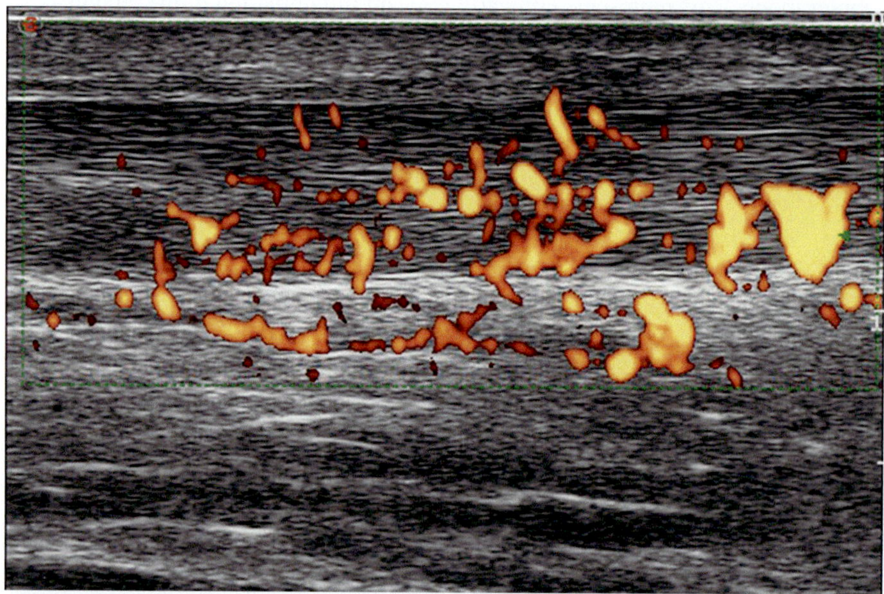

Fig. 12.9 Tendinitis of the Achilles tendon with hyperperfusion (posterior longitudinal view)

12.2.4   Pathology of the Achilles Tendon II

Best Scans: Standard Scans 12-7, 12-8

Pain and swelling of the Achilles tendon region may not only involve the body of the Achilles tendon, but also the loose connective tissue surrounding it. Figure 12.10 shows a homogeneous Achilles tendon with normal echotexture and normal echogenicity. Inside the body of the Achilles tendon, there is extensive hypervascularity. The tissue next to the Achilles tendon appears hypoechoic with hypervascularity representing paratenonitis.

Retrocalcaneal bursitis can also occur without Achilles tendinitis as shown in Fig. 12.11. It localizes below the Achilles tendon close to where it approaches the calcaneus.

Both in Achilles paratenonitis and in retrocalcaneal bursitis, ultrasound guided glucocorticoid injections or aspirations can be easily performed.

Ultrasound is an excellent technique for displaying Achilles tendon tears as it allows both static and dynamic examination.

Figure 12.12 shows an Achilles tendon tear with a discontinuity of the fibers of the Achilles tendon. The anechoic region represents hematoma ($\Uparrow$). The arrows pointing downwards ($\Downarrow$) show the ends of the remaining tendon. These deviate from each other when extending the ankle joint.

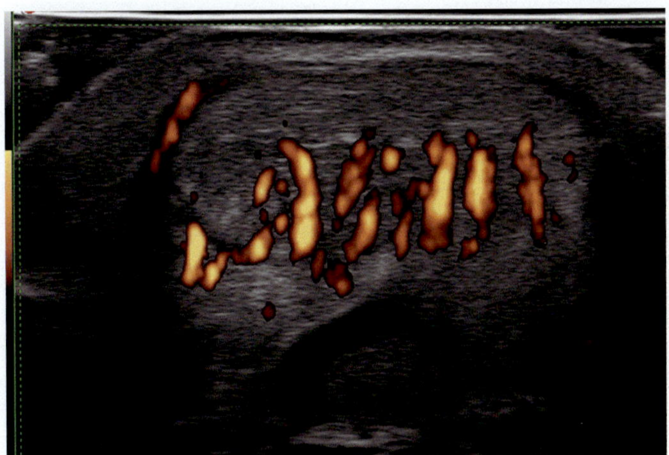

Fig. 12.10 Paratenonitis with tendinitis of the Achilles tendon (posterior transverse view)

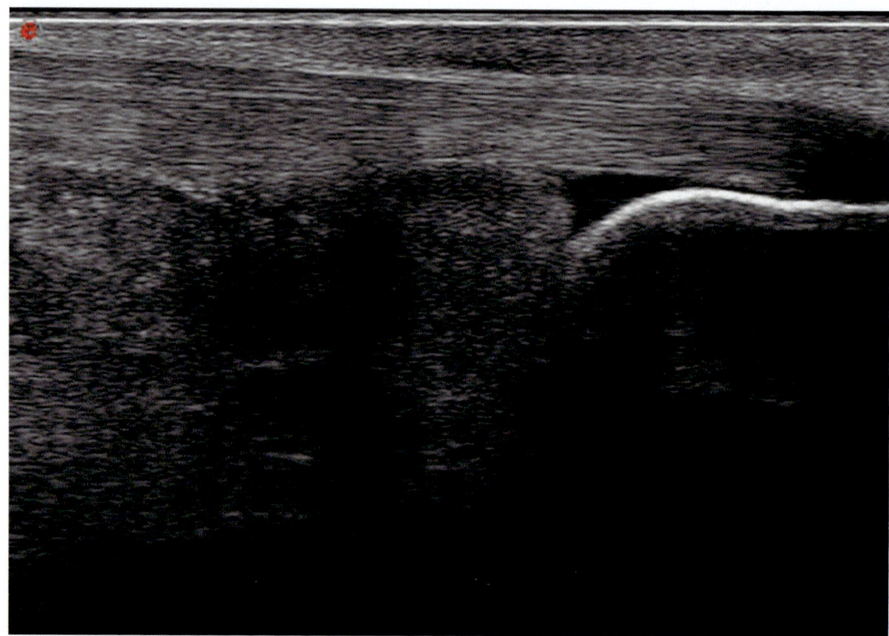

Fig. 12.11 Retrocalcaneal bursitis without Achilles tendinitis (posterior longitudinal view)

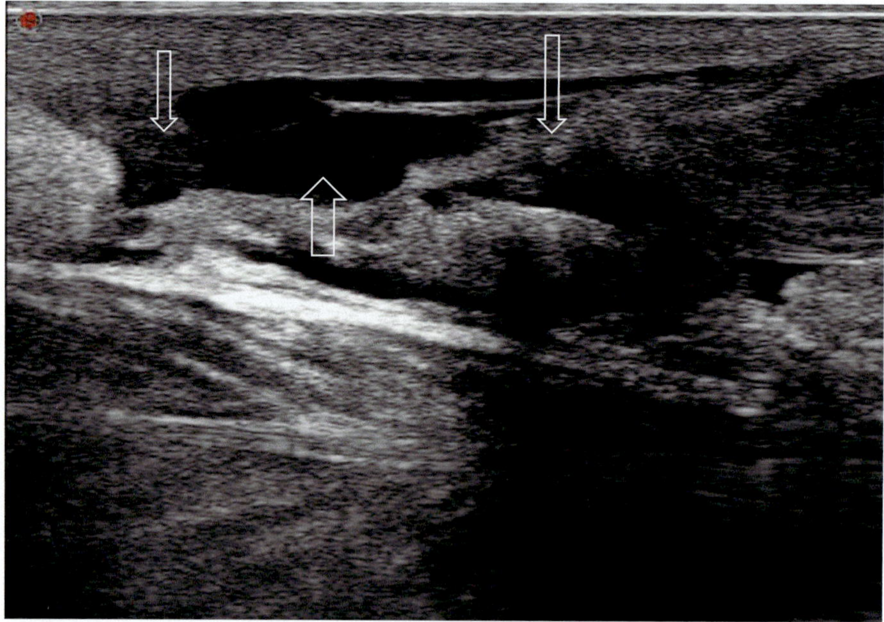

Fig. 12.12 Achilles tendon tear (posterior longitudinal view)

12.2.5   Heel Pain: Enthesopathy, Calcaneal Spurs and Effusion

Best Scans: Standard Scans 12-7 and 12-8

Enthesitis describes the inflammation of the attachment of a tendon to the bone.

This typically includes an inflammation of both the bone, characterized by bone marrow edema, that can be seen on MRI, and by inflammation of the overlying tendon, which is easily visible on ultrasound. The tendon above the enthesis is thickened, inhomogeneous and hypoechoic as in tendinitis. Power Doppler ultrasound shows hyperperfusion of the tendon close to the enthesis. In chronic enthesitis (enthesopathy) the bone surface may become irregular with erosions and enthesophytes.

Figure 12.13 shows enthesitis and tendinitis of the Achilles tendon. The Achilles tendon is thickened, inhomogeneous and hypoechoic. Hyperperfusion can be seen both close to the bone and in the Achilles tendon itself. The bone surface is irregular with small erosions (⇑) and enthesophytes (⇓).

Figure 12.14 shows chronic enthesopathy. The Achilles tendon is homogeneous. It does not show any Doppler signals. However, the bone surface of the calcaneus shows irregularities including several erosions (⇑).

In patients with heel pain, it is important not only to focus on the superficial structures such as the Achilles tendon, retrocalcaneal bursa and posterior bone surface of the calcaneus, but also to visualize the posterior recess of the ankle joint.

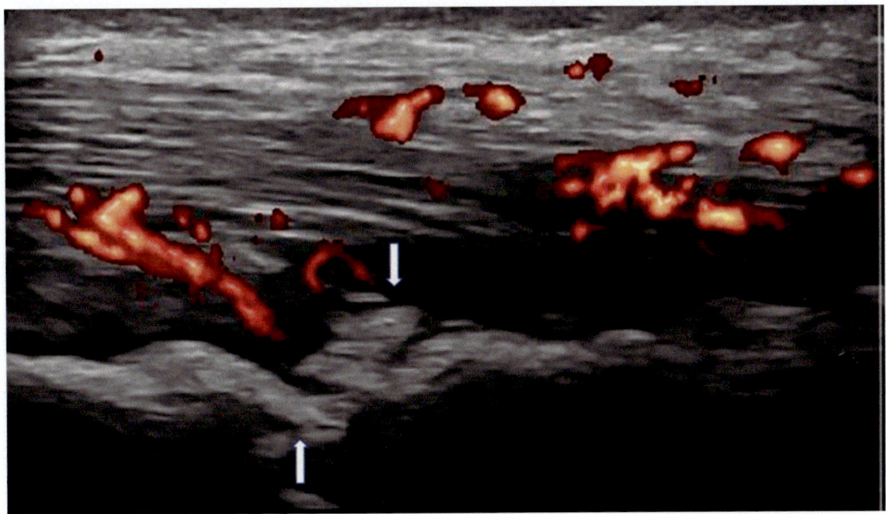

Fig. 12.13 Achilles tendinitis and enthesitis with erosions and enthesophytes (posterior longitudinal view)

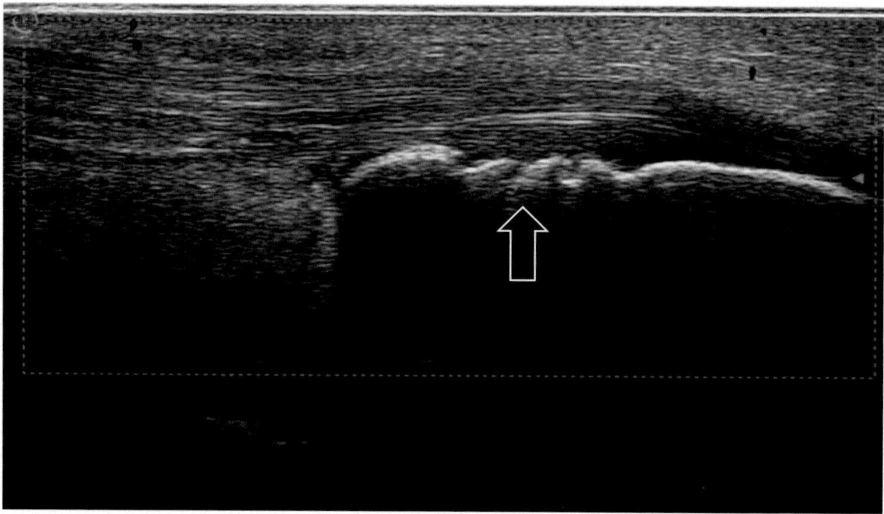

Fig. 12.14 Chronic enthesopathy with calcaneal erosions (posterior longitudinal view)

Figure 12.15 shows a large effusion in the posterior area of the ankle joint ($\Downarrow$) with a connection to the subtalar joint. Effusions or synovitis sometimes occur only on the posterior side of the ankle joint. Arthritis of the ankle may be missed if only dorsal scans are performed.

Fig. 12.15 Large effusion in the posterior recess of the ankle and subtalar joint (posterior longitudinal view)

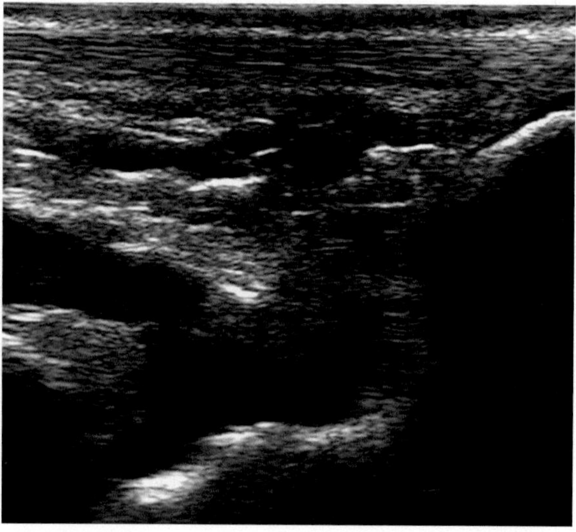

12.2.6 Plantar Fasciitis and Pathologies of the Midfoot

Best Scan plantar fascia: Standard Scan 12-9

Best Scan midfoot: Standard Scan 12-12

The plantar fascia becomes hypoechoic, inhomogeneous, and thickened in case of plantar fasciitis. The image is similar to that of tendinitis and enthesitis, but power Doppler rarely shows hypervascularity.

Figure 12.16 shows plantar fasciitis. The plantar fascia is hypoechoic and inhomogeneous (⇓). The sagittal diameter is increased to 6.5 mm. In addition, there is a plantar calcaneal spur (⇑). Its appearance is like a step on the bone surface. Spurs without abnormalities of the plantar fascia usually do not cause relevant symptoms.

Less commonly, more distal aspects of the plantar fascia present with a painful swelling at the plantar region of the midfoot, called Ledderhose's disease. This is comparable with Dupuytren's disease of the palmar aspects of the hand. The affected area of the plantar fascia is thickened and hypoechoic (⇑) as seen in Fig. 12.17.

Figure 12.18 shows major synovitis of the naviculocuneiform joint (⇓) and less severe synovitis of the third tarsometatarsal joint (⇐) in a patient with osteoarthritis of the midfoot. The bony surface is irregular with osteophytes and narrowed joint spaces. Similar findings can be seen in psoriatic arthritis or diabetes mellitus.

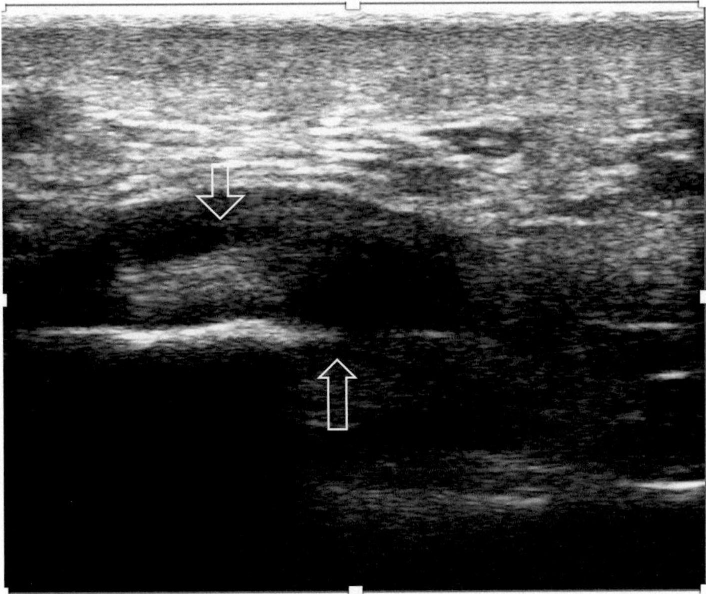

Fig. 12.16 Plantar fasciitis with plantar calcaneal spur (plantar longitudinal view)

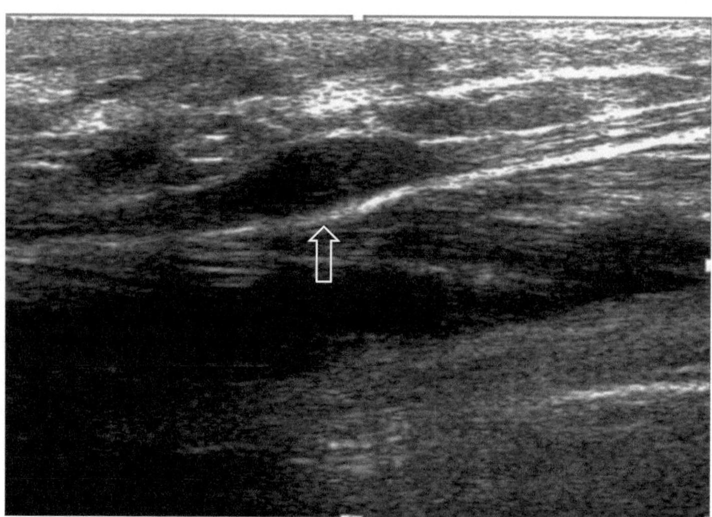

Fig. 12.17 Ledderhose's disease (plantar fibromatosis) (plantar longitudinal view)

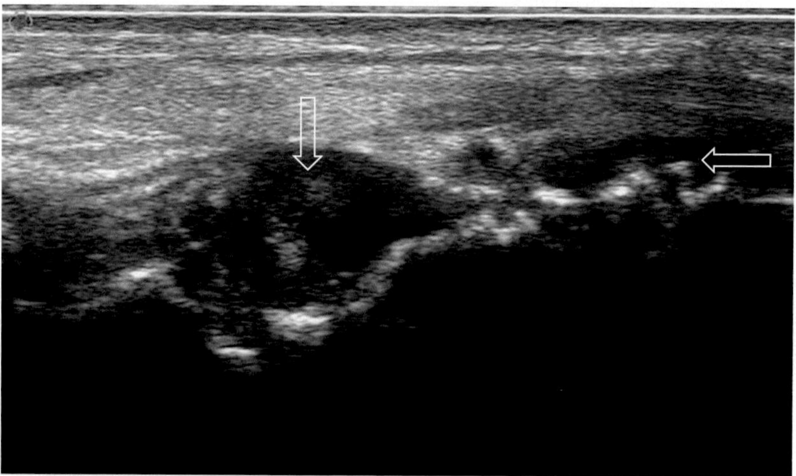

Fig. 12.18 Synovitis of the naviculocuneiform and the third tarsometatarsal joints in osteoarthritis (dorsal longitudinal view)

12.2.7 MTP Joints

Best Scan: Standard Scan 12-11

It is often difficult to decide clinically whether synovitis of the MTP joints is present or absent. The easiest sonographical access is the dorsal approach. The patient should flex and extend the toes to detect minor amounts of fluid or synovitis. If synovitis is present the joint capsule is not parallel to the bone surface.

Figure 12.19 shows both effusion (anechoic region; ⇓) and synovitis (hypoechoic region; ⇑) of the MTP joint in a patient with early RA.

Figure 12.20 shows an erosion at the lateral aspect of the 5th MTP joint that is typical for RA (⇑). All diameters of the erosion are well over 1.0 mm. The floor of the erosion is irregular, and it is localized proximal to the joint space (⇐).

Ultrasound has become an important diagnostic tool for gout. Findings that are depicted in Fig. 12.21 are pathognomonic for gout. Intraarticular tophi are hyperechoic with snowstorm appearance and often a dark rim (⇒). They may exhibit posterior shadowing if dense (⇑), i.e., the hyperechoic line of the bone is interrupted. In addition, the image shows the typical double contour sign (⇓). This is caused by deposits of urate crystals on the intra-articular cartilage. Thus, the line between synovium and cartilage appears as hyperechoic and as thick as the underlying bone surface. Aggregates (⇐) are small, dense crystal deposits. These are not as specific for the diagnosis of gout as the other parameters.

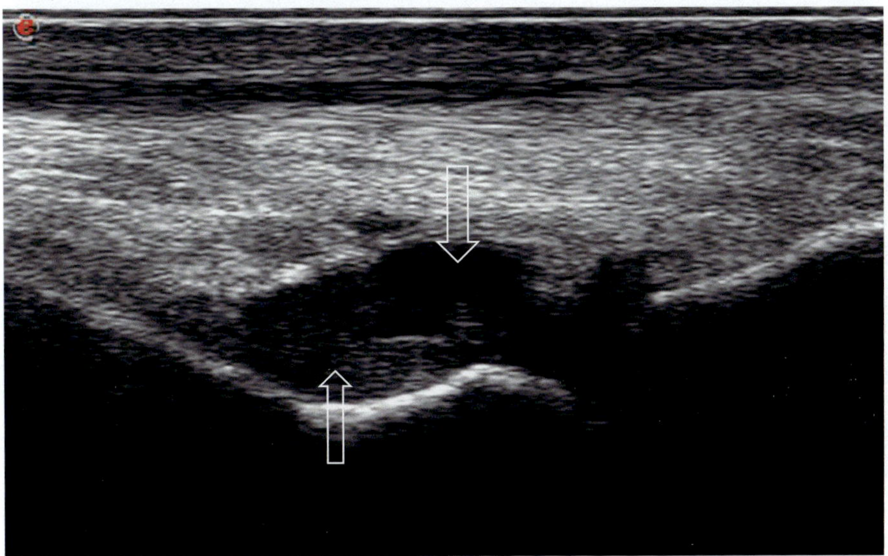

Fig. 12.19 Effusion and synovitis of the second MTP joint (dorsal longitudinal view)

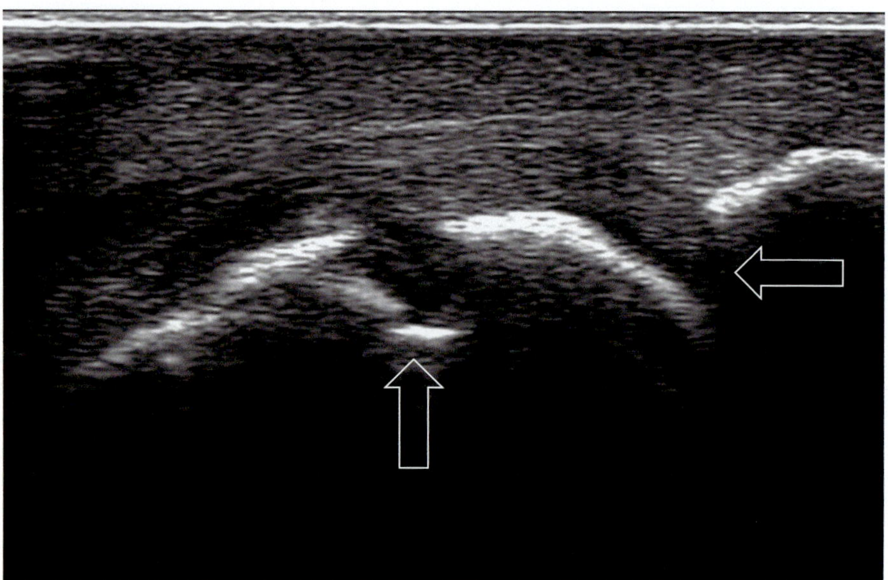

Fig. 12.20 Erosion of the 5th MTP joint in RA (lateral longitudinal view)

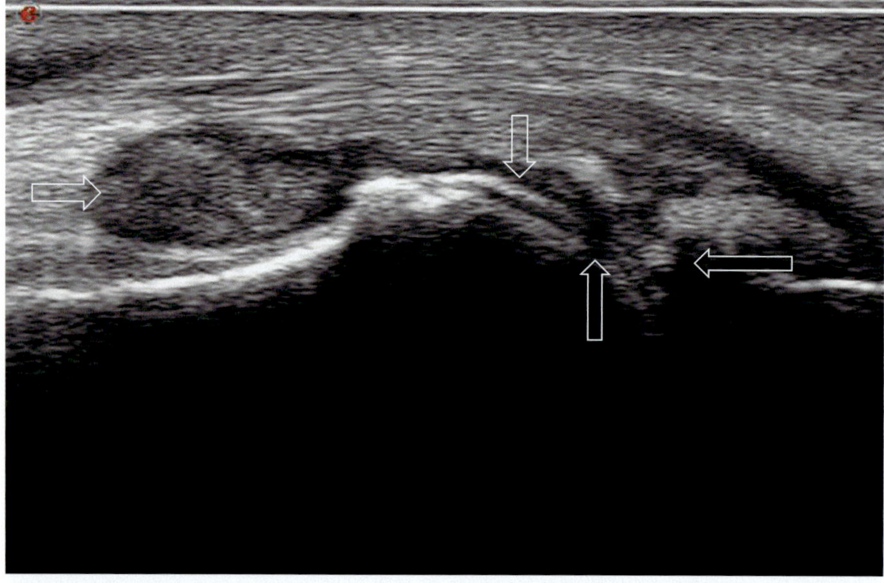

Fig. 12.21 Intraarticular tophi, aggregates and double contour sign of an MTP 1 joint in gout (dorsal longitudinal view)

Chapter 13
Arterial Ultrasound in Rheumatology

13.1 Vasculitis

Primary vasculitides may affect small vessels as in granulomatosis with polyangiitis (GPA), medium-sized arteries as in polyarteritis nodosa, or large arteries as in giant-cell arteritis (GCA) and in Takayasu arteritis (TAK). A clinically suspected diagnosis of large-vessel vasculitis (LVV) needs to be confirmed by imaging or histologically. Ultrasound is the method of choice particularly for cranial GCA provided expertise and adequate equipment are available. Nearly all extracranial arteries can be assessed by ultrasound except the descending thoracic aorta. Many GCA fast-track clinics have been established in specialized rheumatology units. Patients receive an appointment within 24 h. They are examined clinically and with ultrasound with an immediate clearly confirmed diagnosis in most cases. The introduction of such fast-track clinics lead to a significant decrease of permament blindness caused by GCA.

In vasculitis ultrasound shows characteristic concentric, hypoechoic, homogeneous thickening of the arterial wall (halo sign) which remains visible upon compression in superficial arteries like the temporal arteries (compression sign). Stenoses and/or occlusions may simultaneously occur.

13.1.1 Giant Cell Arteritis

Temporal artery ultrasound scans can be obtained by using linear probes with gray scale frequencies of at least 15 MHz. Particularly small probes with >20 MHz provide excellent images.

Several machine adjustments are necessary. For temporal arteries image depth should be 10–15 mm, focus position around 5 mm. The highest B-mode frequency should be applied. The color Doppler frequency should be around 10 MHz. The pulse repetition frequency (PRF) should be set at about 2 to 7 kHz depending on the ultrasound machine. For longitudinal views the color box should be angled for

© The Author(s), under exclusive license to Springer Nature Switzerland AG 2023

G. A. W. Bruyn and W. A. Schmidt, *Musculoskeletal Ultrasound for the Rheumatologist*,

https://doi.org/10.1007/978-3-031-27737-5_13

Fig. 13.1 Anatomy of the
common superficial temporal
artery with its frontal (**a**) and
parietal branches (**b**)

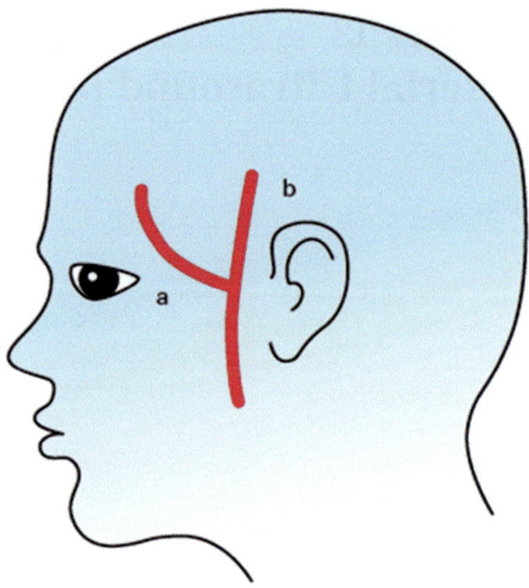

obtaining a good color signal as the temporal artery branches are localized parallel
to the probe. The color signal should completely cover the artery lumen; however, it
should not extend over the artery wall. Color Doppler is preferred to power Doppler
as blood flow velocities are high. With modern very high frequency probes and in
larger arteries normal and abnormal walls can be seen and measured by B-mode
ultrasound without Doppler mode.

The sonographer should examine at least 30 normal subjects to become familiar
with the normal anatomy before using this technology in the diagnosis of GCA.

Figure 13.1 shows the normal anatomy of the common superficial temporal artery
with its frontal and parietal branches.

The sonographer begins with a longitudinal scan anterior to the left ear (Fig. 13.2).
This approach allows the patient to follow the examination on the monitor. The
sonographer then continues distally to the parietal branch and returns scanning the
parietal branch and the common superficial artery in transverse planes (Fig. 13.3).
When doing this the frontal branch can be found. The sonographer follows the frontal
branch in a longitudinal plane (with regard to the course of the artery, Fig. 13.4) and
returns using a transverse plane (Fig. 13.5). Alternatively, the sonographer can scan
the frontal branch first in a transverse scan. Subsequently, the same scans should be
performed on the right side. The temporal arteries should be examined as completely
as possible.

The ultrasound image of a normal temporal artery shows the anechoic lumen and
with high-resolution probes the intima-media complex (IMT; Fig. 13.6). With lower
resolution probes and for finding the artery easier, color Doppler may be applied
(Fig. 13.7). In GCA, ultrasound shows the before mentioned halo sign (Figs. 13.8a
and 13.9) due to edematous wall thickening. The artery lumen is compressible with
the ultrasound probe while the thickened artery wall remains visible with compression. This can be done in longitudinal (Fig. 13.8b) and transverse planes. Compression in a transverse plane is easier as the vessel will still be seen even if the probe

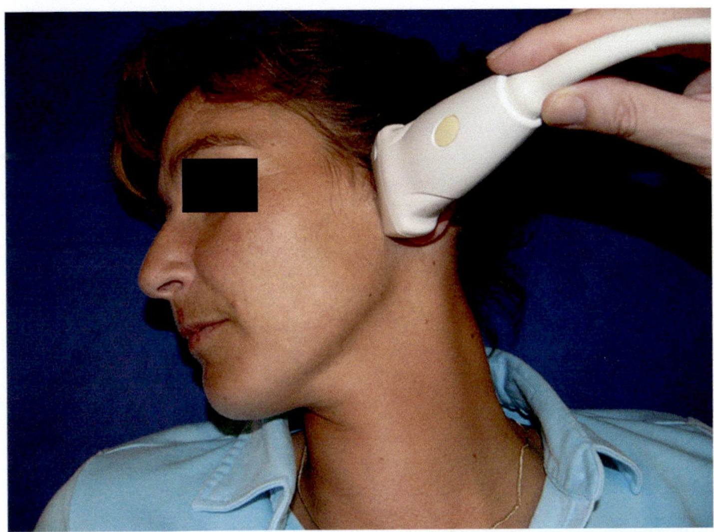

Fig. 13.2 Longitudinal scan of the common superficial temporal artery and the parietal branch

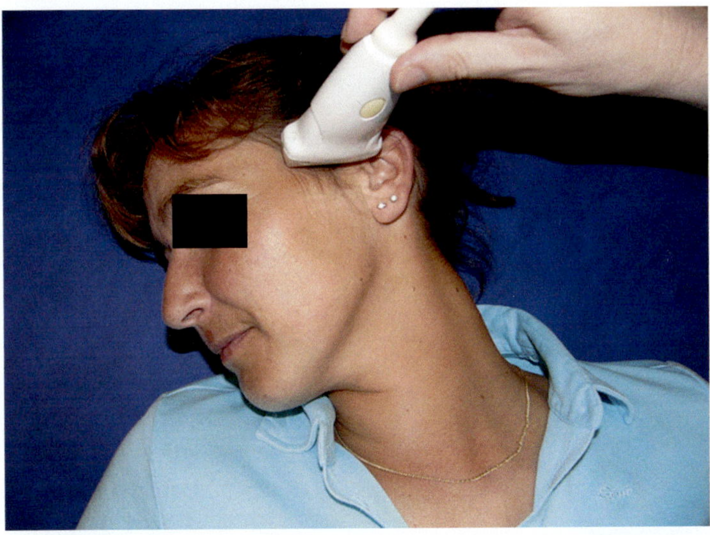

Fig. 13.3 Transverse scan of the parietal branch of the superficial temporal artery

should be shifted away from the original level during the compression which would make the artery invisible in longitudinal scans.

With treatment the halo sign becomes thinner and then disappears after days or weeks. The halo sign is best visible in untreated disease; however, in one third of the patients a small wall swelling is still visible even after 6 months. IMT

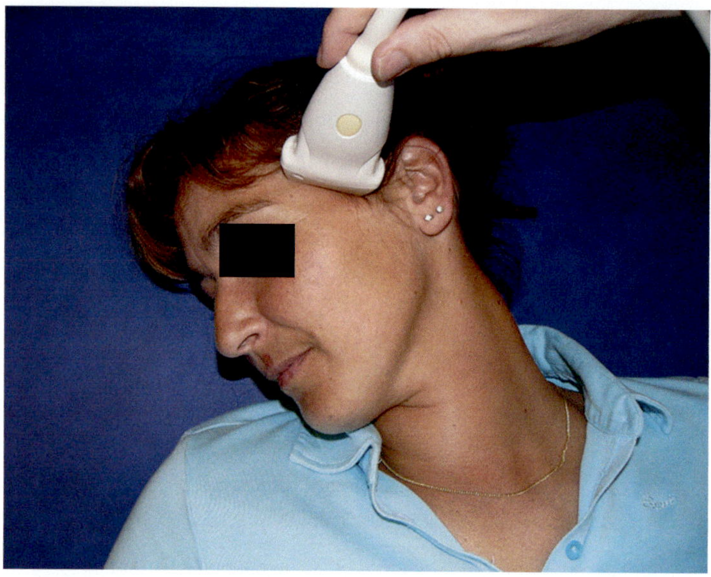

Fig. 13.4 Longitudinal scan in relation to the course of the frontal branch of the superficial temporal artery

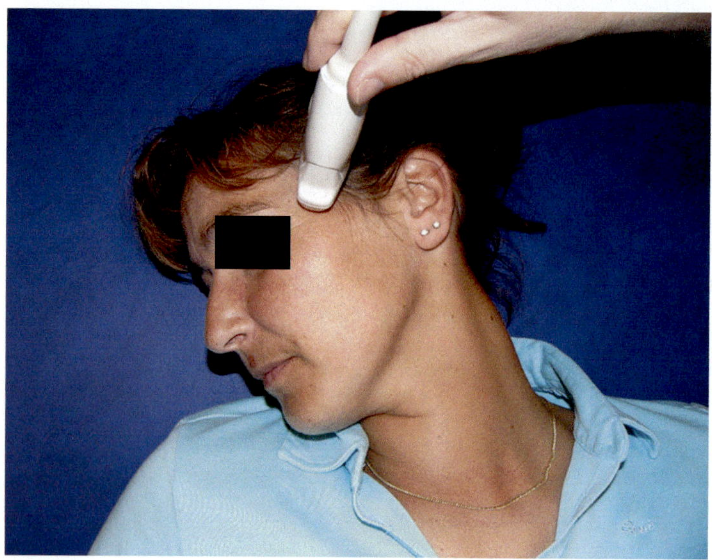

Fig. 13.5 Transverse scan in relation to the course of the frontal branch of the superficial temporal artery

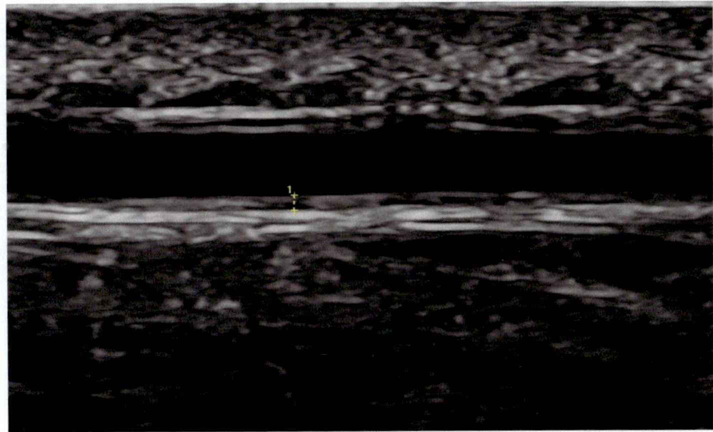

Fig. 13.6 B-mode ultrasound image of a normal frontal branch of the superficial temporal artery in a longitudinal view with measurement of the IMT (0.28 mm); 6–24 MHz hockey stick probe

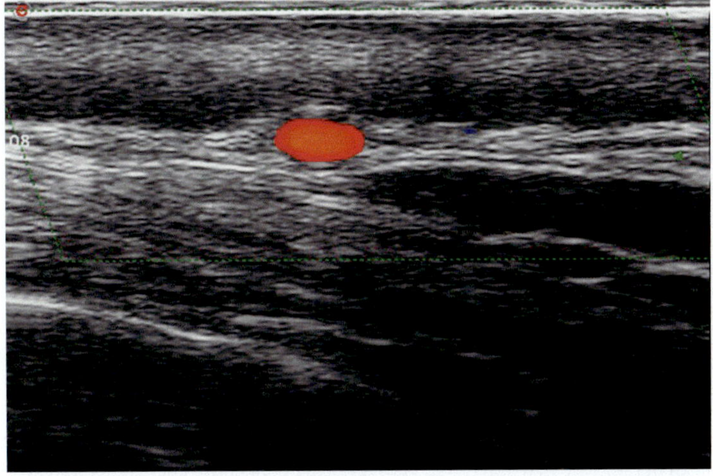

Fig. 13.7 Color Dopper ultrasound image of a normal parietal branch of the superficial temporal artery in a transverse view; 6–18 MHz linear probe

may be measured in order to have a follow-up instrument. IMT decreases with successful treatment and may increase in flares. With high-resolution transducers and in larger arteries measurement of a single wall is possible (Fig. 13.6). Alternatively, the artery may be compressed with measurement of the wall thickness of both walls and following division of the value by 2 (Fig. 13.8b). Table 13.1 lists data on measurements of temporal and axillary arteries.

Cut-off values are 0.7 mm for the vertebral arteries and 1.0 mm for the carotid and subclavian arteries, respectively.

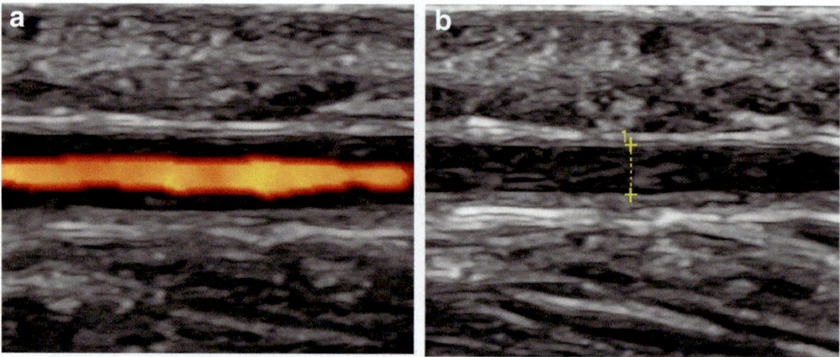

Fig. 13.8 Ultrasound image of the distal common superficial artery in acute GCA in a longitudinal view demonstrating edematous wall swelling (halo sign, left). With compression the hypoechoic material persists (compression sign, right) with a thickness of 0.9 mm for both walls

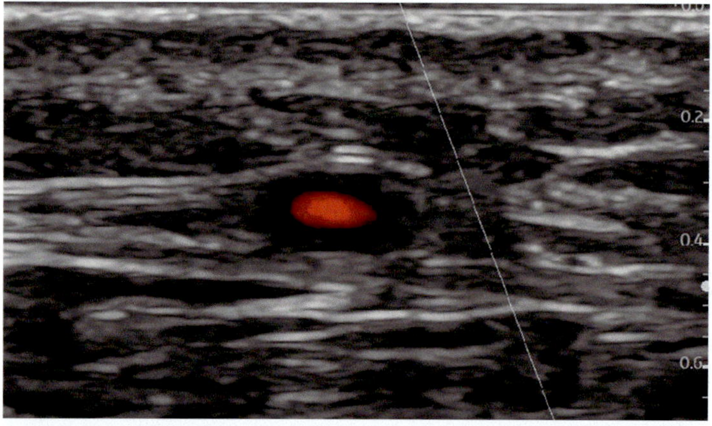

Fig. 13.9 Ultrasound image of the distal superficial common temporal artery in acute GCA in the same patient as in Fig. 13.8 in a transverse view showing concentric edematous wall swelling (halo sign)

Table 13.1 Mean IMT values of arteries commonly involved in GCA in population of persons aged around 70 years (according to Schäfer VS, et al., 2017)

Artery	Normal (mm)	Acute GCA (mm)	Cut-off (mm)
Common superficial temporal artery	0.23	0.65	0.42
Frontal branch	0.19	0.54	0.34
Parietal branch	0.20	0.50	0.29
Facial artery	0.24	0.53	0.37
Axillary artery	0.59	1.72	1.0

If aliasing occurs, i.e., a variety of bright colors due to turbulent flow (Fig. 13.10) together with persistent diastolic flow, the sonographer may use the pulsed wave Doppler mode to determine flow curves for documenting stenosis (Fig. 13.11). In temporal arteries the maximum systolic flow velocity determined within the stenosis by pulsed wave Doppler ultrasound is >2 times higher than the flow velocity proximal or distal to the stenosis. With modern ultrasound equipment a halo sign is usually seen in an area of vasculitis–associated stenosis. In about 15% of newly diagnosed GCA patients acute occlusions occur, which are characterized by the absence of color Doppler signals in a visible artery filled with hypoechoic material, even with low PRF and high color gain (Fig. 13.10).

In addition, facial, occipital and, in part other cranial arteries, can be assessed with ultrasound. Jaw claudication and blindness is more common if ultrasound detects facial artery involvement.

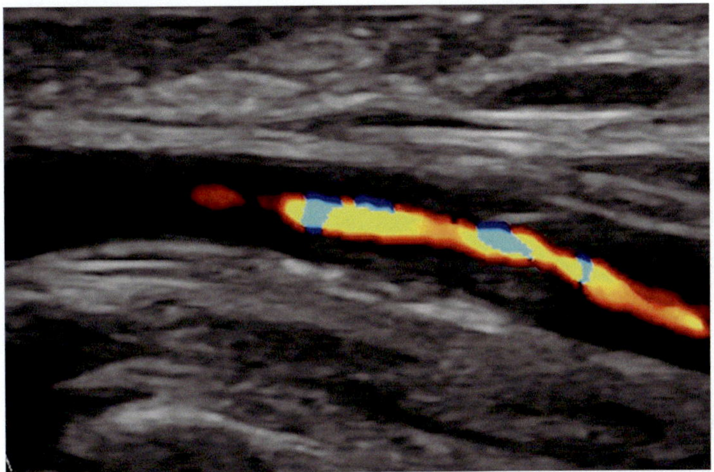

Fig. 13.10 Stenosis with aliasing (right side) and acute occlusion (hypoechoic area without color on left side) of the common superficial temporal artery in active GCA

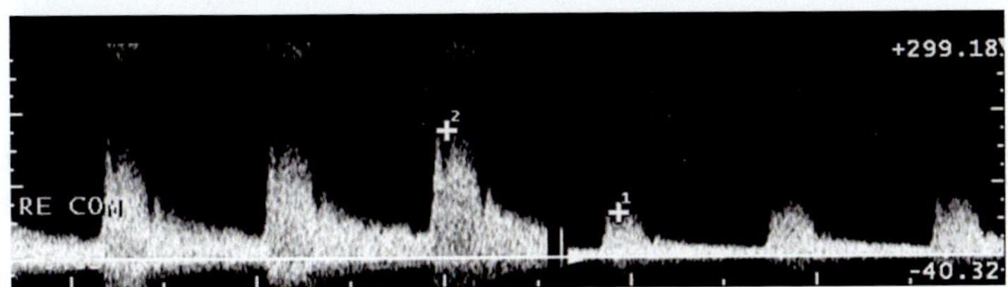

Fig. 13.11 Spectral Doppler ultrasound image of stenotic flow curves of the superficial temporal artery in acute GCA. In the stenosis (left side) maximum systolic flow velocity is 176 cm/s, and diastolic flow velocity is also increased. Outside the stenosis (right side), maximum systolic flow velocity is normal (62 cm/s)

## *13.1.2	Extracranial Giant Cell Arteritis and Takayasu Arteritis*

GCA often affects also extracranial arteries, most commonly the axillary and proximal brachial arteries, but also the subclavian, carotid, vertebral, femoral arteries, the aorta and other arteries. About 20% of our patients have extracranial GCA only, 50% have cranial GCA only, and 30% have mixed GCA with cranial and extracranial involvement. Therefore, at least the axillary region and the temporal arteries should be examined. The axillary arteries can best be seen with the axillary shoulder scan (Standard Scan 5-10). Further arteries like the carotid, subclavian and vertebral arteries are also often examined in fast-track clinics. The arteries of the lower extremities may be examined particularly if the pedal pulses are missing. Figure 13.12 shows a longitudinal view of an axillary artery at the level of the humeral head and neck with halo sign on the left side and an occlusion of the proximal brachial artery on the right side in newly diagnosed GCA.

TAK occurs primarily in young females and most frequently involves the subclavian arteries, the common carotid arteries, and the aorta. The morphology is similar to GCA. The wall swelling may be more hyperechoic in some cases due to an often

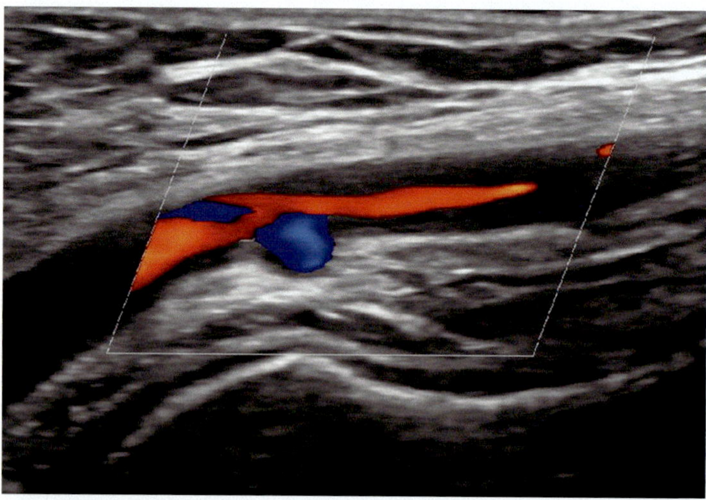

Fig. 13.12 Longitudinal view of an axillary artery at the axillary recess in extracranial GCA with halo sign (left and middle) and occlusion of the proximal brachial artery (right side of the figure)

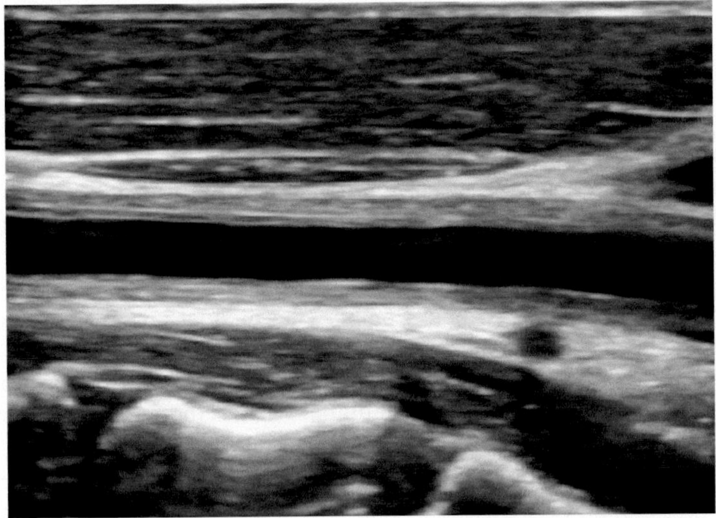

Fig. 13.13 Longitudinal view of a common carotid artery in Takayasu arteritis

more chronic nature of the disease with less vessel wall edema. Figure 13.13 shows a longitudinal view of a common carotid artery in TAK.

13.2 Digital Arteries

Several rheumatic diseases cause damage to digital arteries. Patients with primary Raynaud's phenomenon suffer from vasospasm in cold or wet environments. Secondary Raynaud's phenomenon may occur due to digital artery stenosis or occlusion for instance in systemic sclerosis, in dermatomyositis, in mixed connective tissue disease or due to thrombosis or embolism in anti-phospholipid syndrome, vasculitis, and endocarditis.

The proper palmar digital arteries are larger than the temporal artery branches. The diameter of their lumen is about 1.5 mm. They are located close to finger joints. Figure 13.14 shows the anatomy.

The digital arteries are examined from the palmar side. All ten proper palmar digital arteries, all three common palmar digital arteries, the superficial palmar arch, and the ulnar and radial arteries can be easily visualized by ultrasound. In order to prevent vasospasm, the patient should hold the hands into a water bath at about 37 °C for approximately five minutes directly before the ultrasound examination. Equipment and machine adjustments are comparable with the requirements for temporal artery ultrasound, but the PRF should be lower: about 1.2–2.5 kHz instead of 2–7 kHz as flow velocities in digital arteries are lower.

Figure 13.15 depicts a normal proper palmar digital artery at the level of a PIP joint in a longitudinal scan. The digital arteries are more easily followed on longitudinal scans, but they can be also delineated on transverse scans. Figure 13.16 shows that

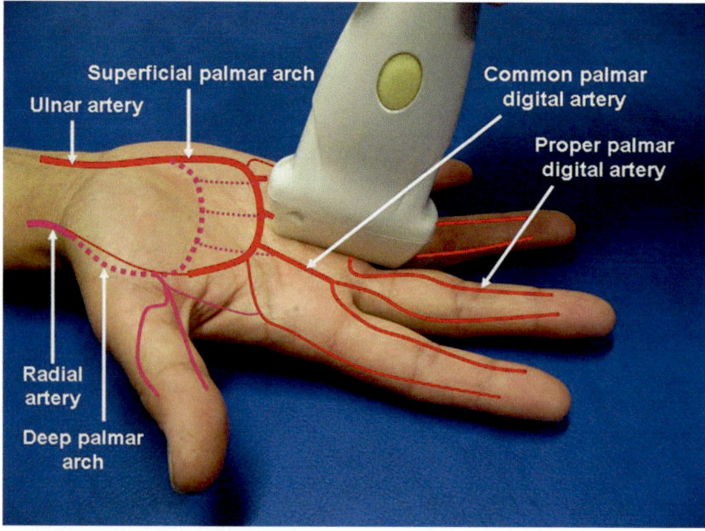

Fig. 13.14 Anatomy of the distal radial, ulnar, palmar and digital arteries. Longitudinal scan of the 3rd/4th common palmar digital arteries

one of the two arteries may be smaller in healthy individuals. In this case the proper palmar digital artery at the ulnar side is smaller than the one on the radial side.

Figure 13.17 depicts a narrowed digital artery with distal occlusion and collateral flow in systemic sclerosis. As pulsation is reduced digital arteries are often not detectable. In advanced stages of systemic sclerosis the ulnar artery and the superficial palmar arch are often occluded. The radial artery is less frequently occluded. The artery walls tend to be slightly thickened when compared with those of normal subjects.

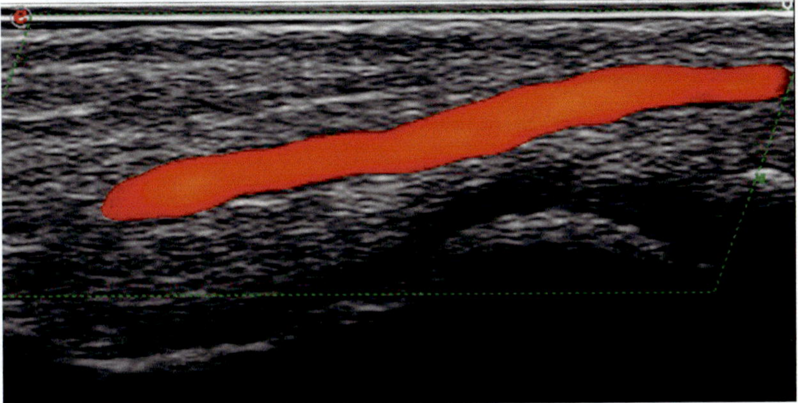

Fig. 13.15 Longitudinal palmar scan of a normal proper palmar digital artery at the level of the PIP joint

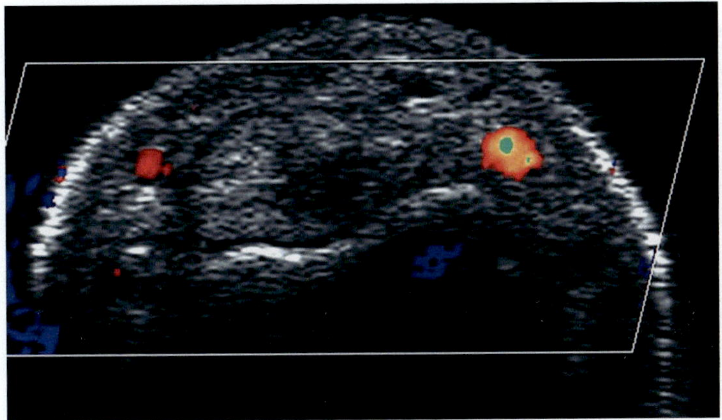

Fig. 13.16 Transverse palmar scan of two normal proper palmar digital arteries close to the PIP joint

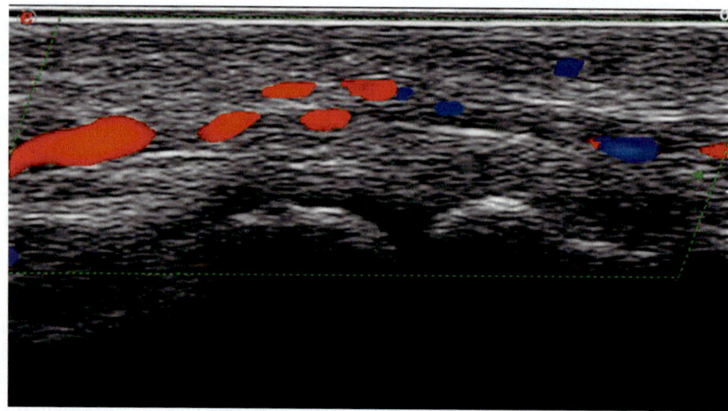

Fig. 13.17 Longitudinal palmar scan of an occluded palmar proper digital artery at the level of the PIP joint in systemic sclerosis

Figure 13.18 depicts an acutely occluded digital artery in a patient with active GPA. Hypoechoic intra-arterial thrombotic material does not display color. The same image occurs for instance in embolism and in anti-phospholipid syndrome.

Turbulent flow and increased diastolic flow velocities are typical of arterial stenoses. Doppler flow curves display increased systolic and diastolic velocities. Normal systolic velocities vary between 10 and 40 cm/s; normal diastolic velocities vary between 0 and 20 cm/s. As velocities differ very much between individuals, the appearance of Doppler curves is only one of several parameters. Increased peripheral resistance causes decreased diastolic flow to appear on inspiration, and, for instance,

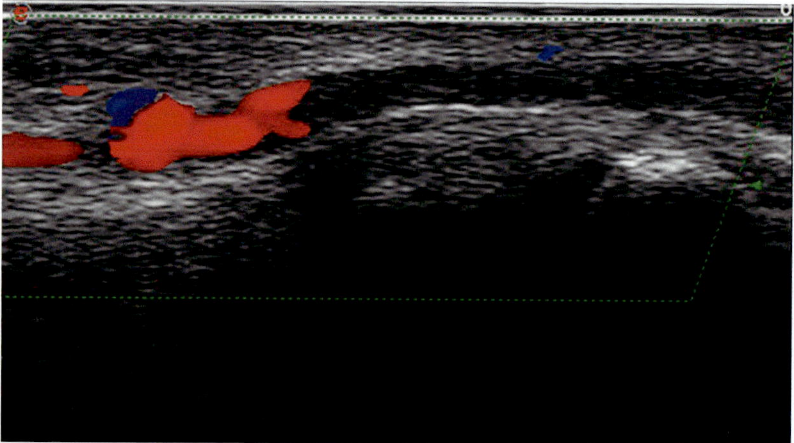

Fig. 13.18 Longitudinal palmar scan of a proper palmar digital artery proximal to the PIP joint with acute digital artery occlusion (right side of the image)

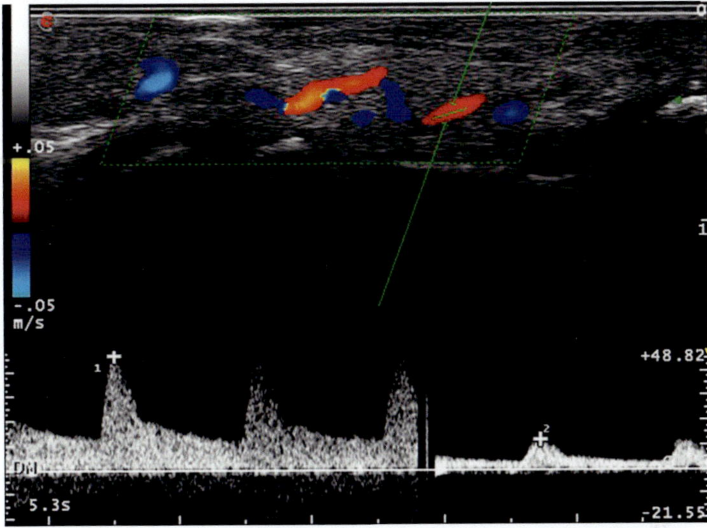

Fig. 13.19 Duplex ultrasound image with Doppler curves of the proper palmar digital artery at the level of the PIP joint. The curves on the left side represent stenotic flow. They correlate with the left bright red portion of the artery. The curves on the right side show poststenotic flow at the portion at the right side which is dark red

if the hands have not been sufficiently warmed up. Figure 13.19 shows the Doppler curves of a digital artery with stenoses in systemic sclerosis.

Digital artery ultrasound correlates well with angiography. It aids in differentiating primary from secondary Raynaud's phenomenon and in assessing patients with acute or chronic ischemia of fingers.

Chapter 14
Ultrasound of the Major Salivary Glands

Sjögren's syndrome is a common rheumatic disease. Diagnosis is based upon history taking (xerostomia, xerophthalmia), measurement of salivary and ocular gland function as well as the detection of antibodies such as anti-Ro- (SSA) and anti-La (SSB) antibodies, and histology of glands. The morphology of the parotid and submandibular glands also changes during the course of the disease. The glands become fibrotic, intraglandular ducts dilate, and lymphatic tissue within the glands increases. The parotid glands are frequently enlarged whereas the submandibular glands may become atrophic.

Ultrasound of the salivary glands is a method that is easy to perform using widely available technology. It is a quick, non-invasive test for assessing the changes in Sjögren's syndrome. The submandibular and parotid glands are easily accessible by ultrasound. All glands should be examined with longitudinal and transverse scans (Figs. 14.1, 14.2, 14.3 and 14.4).

The same linear probes can be used as in musculoskeletal ultrasound with rather low frequencies between 5 and 15 MHz.

The normal ultrasound appearance of parotid and submandibular glands is homogeneous and hyperechoic like thyroid tissue. The glands can be easily distinguished from the surrounding tissue. Figures 14.5 and 14.6 show the echogenicity of normal salivary gland tissue.

In Sjögren's syndrome, glands become hypoechoic and inhomogeneous when compared with the surrounding soft tissue. Thyroid tissue may look similar in chronic thyroiditis. The sagittal diameter of a submandibular gland should be ≥ 0.8 mm, and for a parotid gland this is ≤ 2.0 cm. Mild changes (OMERACT **grade 1**), characterized by mild inhomogeneity without anechoic or hypoechoic areas may be difficult to be distinguished from normal whereas moderate and severe changes are clearly distinguishable from normal. Moderate changes (**grade 2**) are characterized by inhomogeneity with focal anechoic or hypoechoic areas. Severe changes (**grade 3**) are characterized by diffuse inhomogeneity with anechoic or hypoechoic areas occupying the entire gland, which may eventually result in a fibrotic gland.

© The Author(s), under exclusive license to Springer Nature Switzerland AG 2023

G. A. W. Bruyn and W. A. Schmidt, *Musculoskeletal Ultrasound for the Rheumatologist*,
https://doi.org/10.1007/978-3-031-27737-5_14

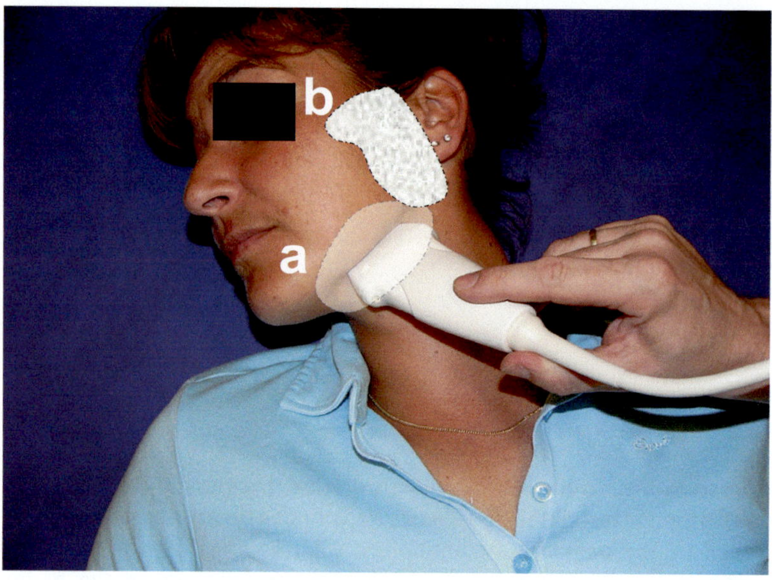

Fig. 14.1 Longitudinal scan of the left submandibular gland (**a**). This figure also shows the localization of the parotid gland (**b**)

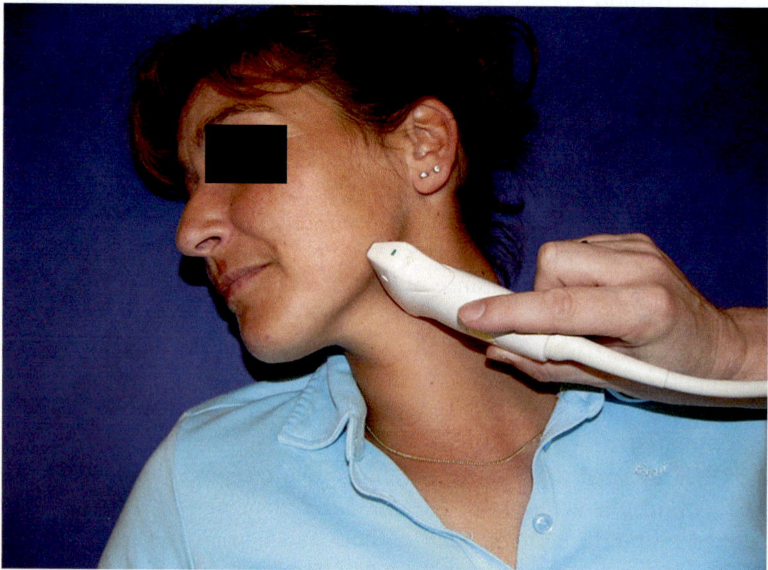

Fig. 14.2 Transverse scan of the left submandibular gland

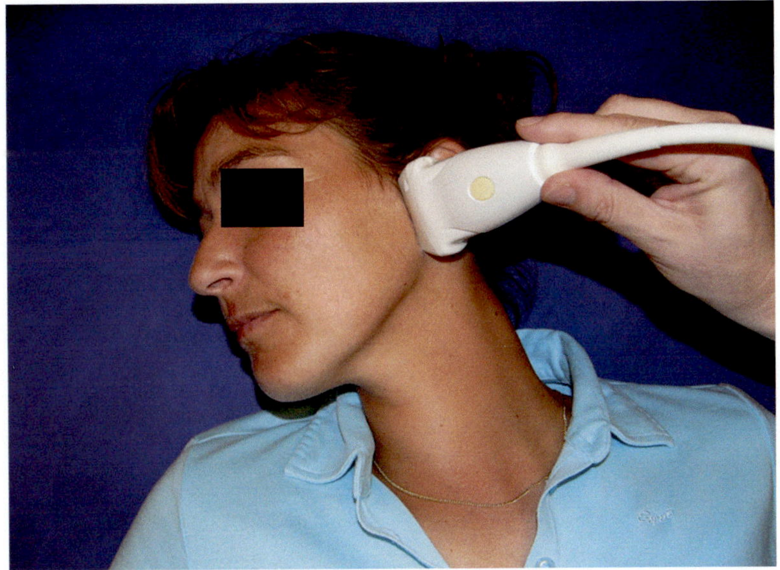

Fig. 14.3 Longitudinal scan of the left parotid gland

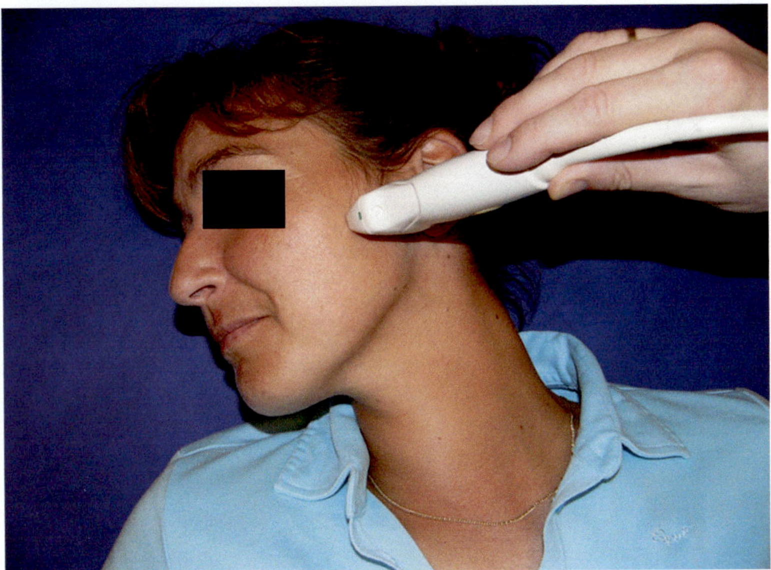

Fig. 14.4 Transverse scan of the left parotid gland

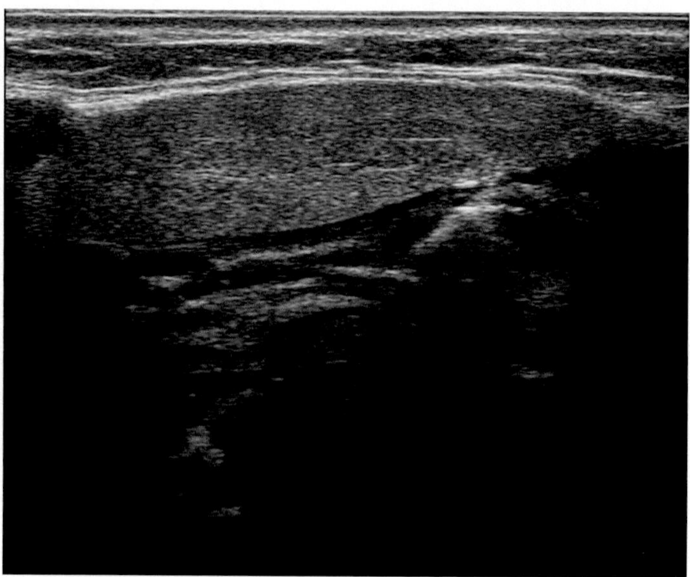

Fig. 14.5 Longitudinal view of a normal submandibular gland

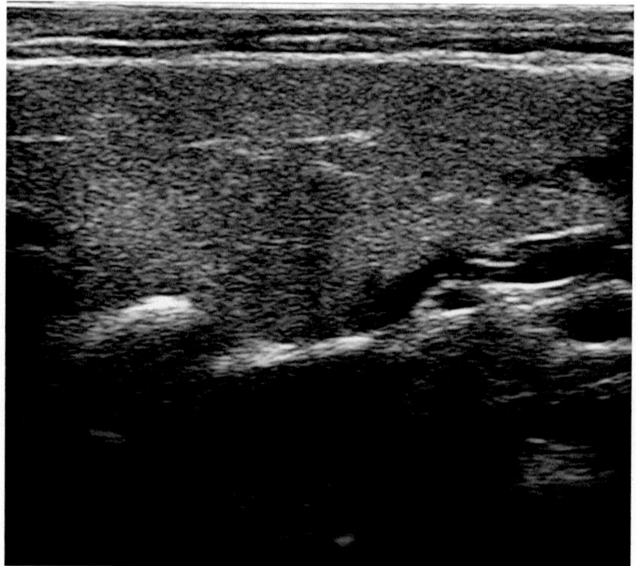

Fig. 14.6 Longitudinal view of a normal parotid gland

It is so far unclear how much the vascularity of the salivary glands correlates with disease activity.

Figures 14.7 and 14.8 show typical ultrasound images of abnormal submandibular and parotid glands in Sjögren's syndrome representing severe pathology. In some patients, changes become more fibrotic showing several horizontal hyperechoic lines within the gland (Fig. 14.9). As a complication of Sjögren's syndrome, malignant lymphoma may develop. Figure 14.10 shows a malignant lymph node characterized by a hypoechoic mass within the parotid gland that shows increased perfusion.

Ultrasound of salivary glands reveals changes that occur due to chronic sialadenitis. Chronic sialadenitis caused by diseases other than Sjögren's syndrome has a similar ultrasound appearance. However, in other conditions all four large salivary glands are very rarely involved. Therefore, abnormal ultrasound images of at least two salivary glands are highly specific for Sjögren's syndrome in rheumatological practice. Sensitivity is about 70%. On ultrasound examination, patients with early or less active disease or without anti-Ro (SSA) antibodies may have normal salivary glands.

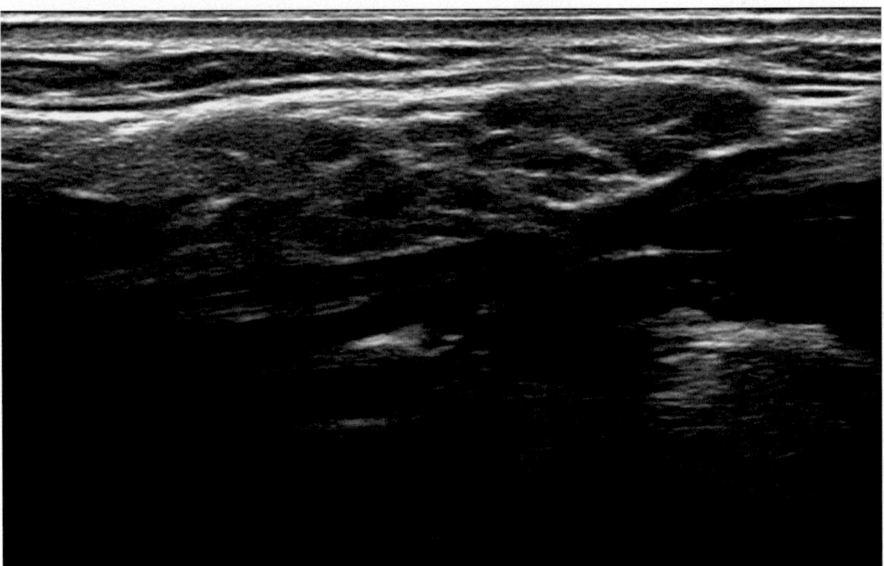

Fig. 14.7 Transverse view of an atrophic, hypoechoic, and inhomogeneous submandibular gland in Sjögren's syndrome

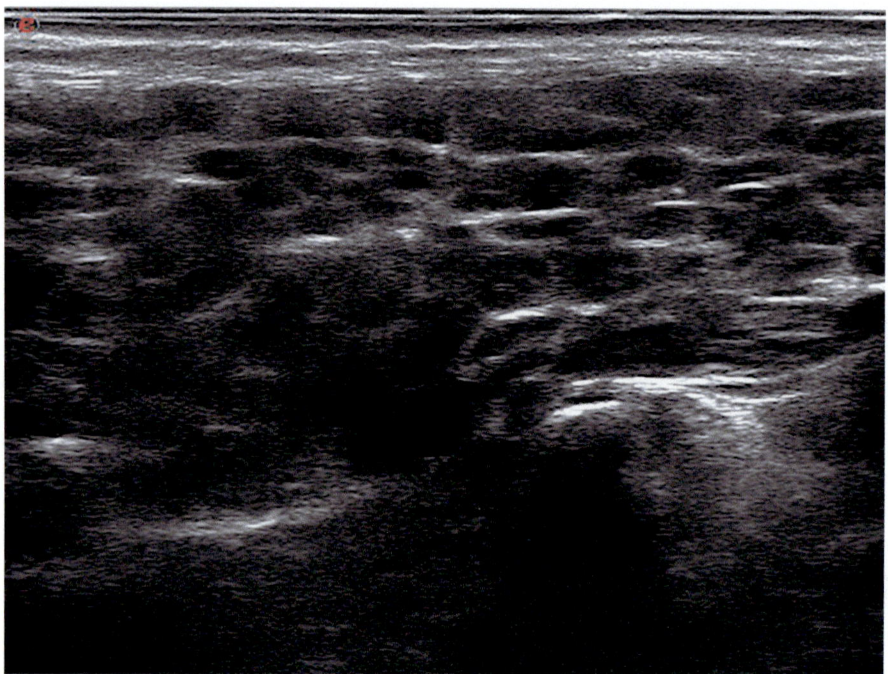

Fig. 14.8 Longitudinal view showing an inhomogeneous parotid gland with many oval hypoechoic areas in Sjögren's syndrome

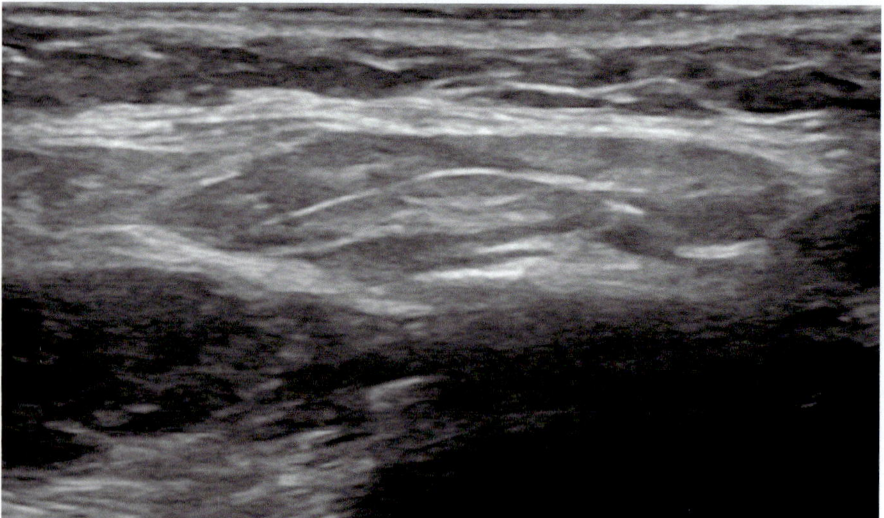

Fig. 14.9 Fibrotic gland in Sjögen's syndrome (transverse view of the submandibular gland)

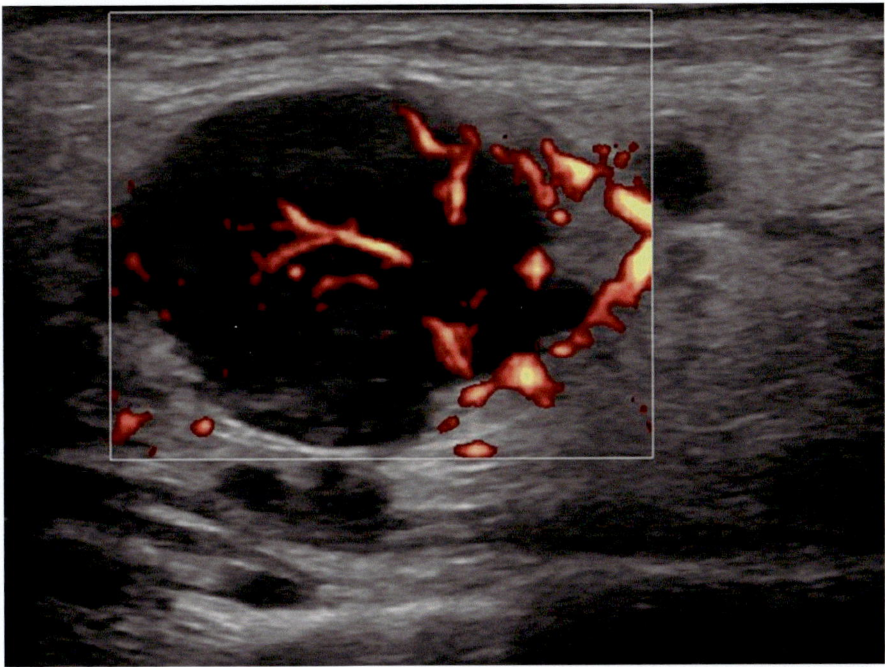

Fig. 14.10 Malignant lymphoma node within the parotid gland (longitudinal view of the parotid gland)

Chapter 15
Lung Ultrasound

As ultrasound plays an increasing role in a variety of disorders, it seems timely to provide a short introduction to lung ultrasound for the rheumatologist. While high resolution CT remains the gold standard for diagnosing interstitial thickening in connective tissue disease, ultrasound may be considered an add-on imaging modality to chest X-ray and chest CT. In addition to detecting signs of interstitial thickening, ultrasound is indicated to pick up pleural effusions or guiding needle aspiration.

The technique is based on imaging the pleura between the ribs. Figure 15.1 shows a normal pleura visualized between two ribs. On dynamic examination, the pleural line is seen sliding with each respiration. Beneath the pleural line, reverberation artifact echoes of the pleura can be observed as hyperechoic lines at regular intervals, called A-lines.

In systemic sclerosis, irregular thickening of the pleura may occur. The foremost typical ultrasound feature in systemic sclerosis is a hyperechoic and fragmented pleura (Fig. 15.4). Secondly, although ultrasound cannot visualize the underlying lung parenchyma, artifacts may demonstrate indirect markers of thickened septa. When the ultrasound beam hits thickened septa underneath the pleura, the beam will be bounced hence and forth between these two linings, i.e., the pleura and the underlying septa. These reverberations will cause the phenomenon of socalled B-lines or comet-tail (Figs. 15.2, 15.3 and 15.4). The B-lines move synchronously with the pleural sliding of each respiration and extend to the bottom of the scan. In addition, the B-lines blur the A-lines.

Various ultrasound scoring systems to assess pulmonary involvement of rheumatic diseases have been introduced, based on counting the number of B-lines in a variable number of lung intercostal spaces. As yet, there is no consensus on the optimal number of intercostal spaces that should be examined to provide a reliable diagnosis.

Patient position:

The patient should be placed in supine/semi recumbent position with arm abducted to facilitate access to the anterior and lateral chest wall. Lateral decubitus position with upper limb moved upwards or laterally is required to expose the lateral chest

© The Author(s), under exclusive license to Springer Nature Switzerland AG 2023 241
G. A. W. Bruyn and W. A. Schmidt, *Musculoskeletal Ultrasound for the Rheumatologist*,
https://doi.org/10.1007/978-3-031-27737-5_15

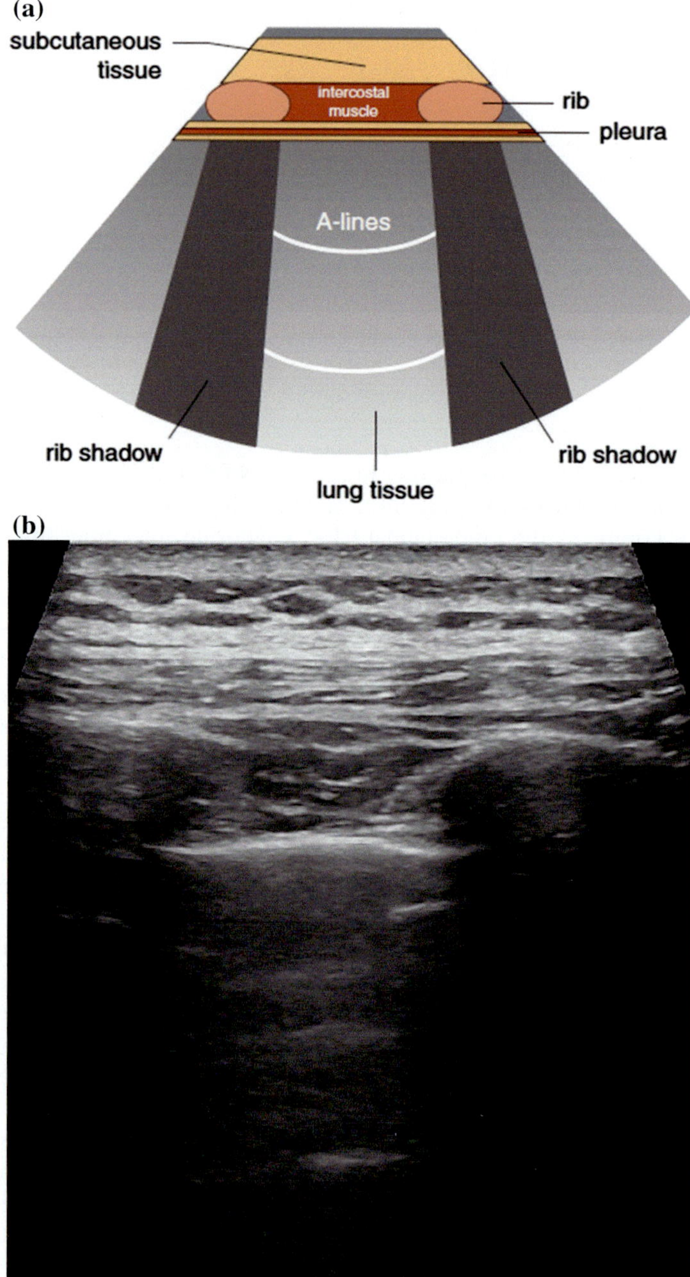

Fig. 15.1 Anatomy (**a**) and normal ultrasound image (**b**) of the pleura

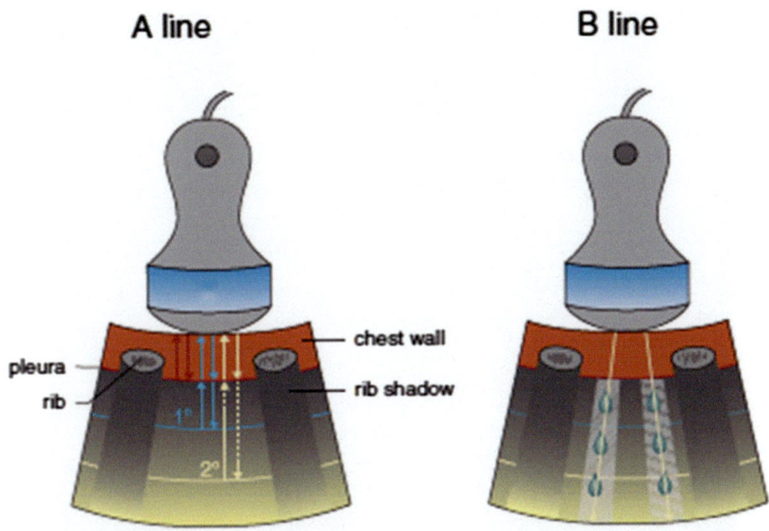

Fig. 15.2 Explanation of A- and B-lines

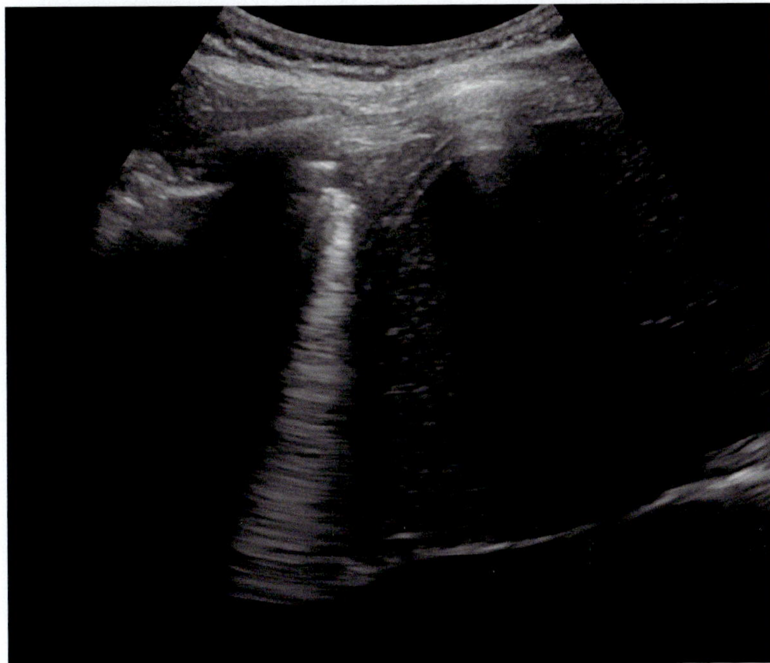

Fig. 15.3 Typical comet-tail B-line

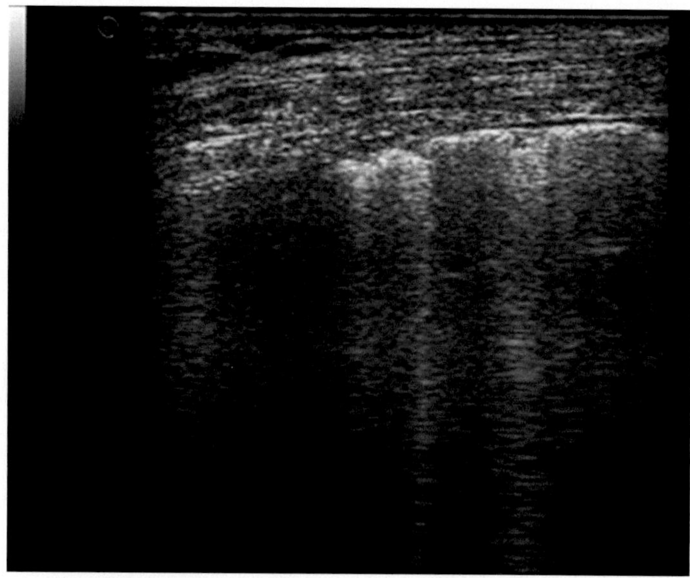

Fig. 15.4 Multiple B-lines and a fragmented pleura in a patient with systemic sclerosis

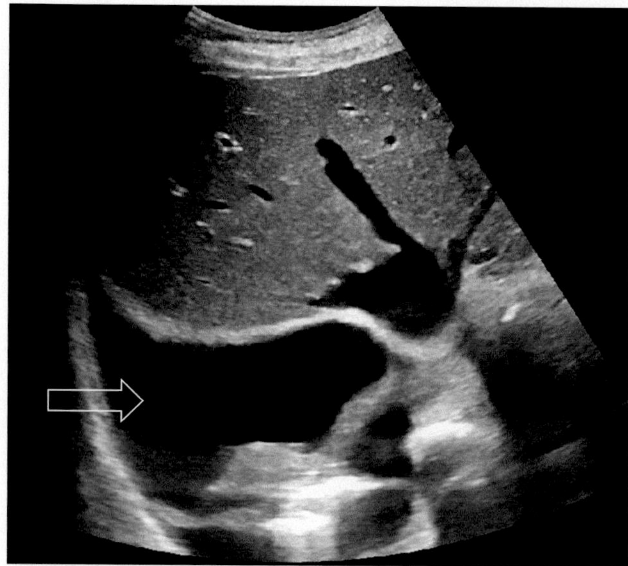

Fig. 15.5 Large pleural effusion ($\rightarrow$) seen with a transverse liver scan with the probe tilted cranially

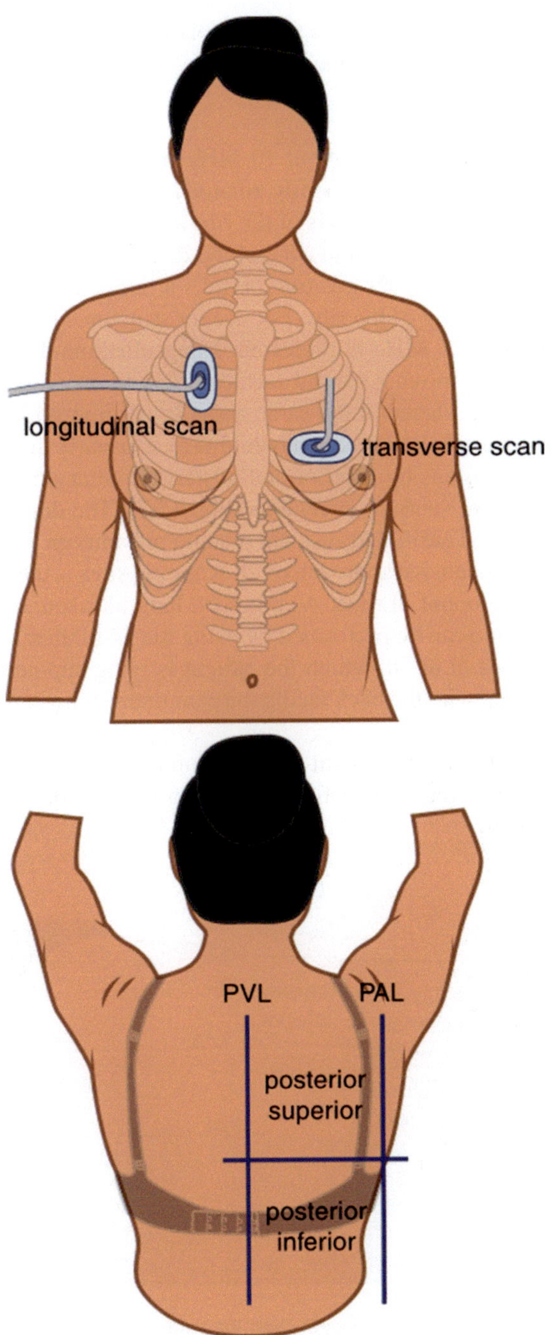

Fig. 15.6 Patient positioning for anterior and posterior chest lung ultrasound. PVL, paravertebral line, PAL posterior axillary line

wall for examination. Pleural effusions and the dorsal region of lower lobes are better appreciated in a sitting position (Figs. 15.5, 15.6).

Probe positioning:

A curved or linear array probe of about 10 MHz should be placed in a sagittal or longitudinal orientation, and subsequently, rotated by 90 degrees into a transverse or slightly oblique position along the axis of the ribs and intercostal spaces (Fig. 15.6). The former view shows the proximal rib and the distal rib shadows and an impression of the pleural line, the latter position permits a larger view of the pleural line, uninterrupted by shadowing of the ribs. For deeper structures like pleural effusions, a curved array of about 5 MHz is preferred. Lung ultrasound is always dynamic because assessment of a moving pleural surface is key to many diagnoses.

The probe should be placed at the same areas in the intercostal spaces where a stethoscope is put for auscultation. Each hemithorax is usually divided into anterior, lateral and posterior regions by anterior and posterior axillary lines. Each region is further divided into upper and lower regions (Fig. 15.7). The dorsal region of upper lobes cannot be assessed easily because the scapula prevents an acoustic window. A systematic and comprehensive approach of 28 scanning sites is the gold standard but takes a considerable amount of time. A shortened lung ultrasound examination in a feasible amount of time can be performed by using the 14 bilateral lung positions as described by Gutierrez et al., in which the patient is lying supine for anterior lung positions and sitting up with the back facing the examiner for posterior lung positions (Table 15.1).

The amount of time for assessment of 14 lung intercostal spaces, i.e., 7 on each side, takes about 8 min, versus an estimated 23 min for the comprehensive 28 lung ultrasound assessment.

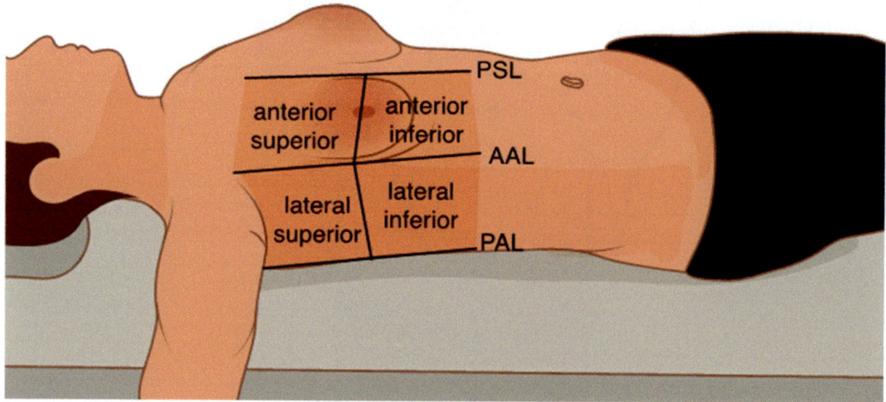

Fig. 15.7 Patient in supine position for lateral chest lung ultrasound. PSL, parasternal line, AAL, anterior axillary line, PAL, posterior axillary line

Table 15.1 Shortened lung ultrasound examination. Anatomical probe position related to intercostal space

Intercostal Space	Position	Anterior/Posterior
2nd	Parasternal	Anterior
4th	Midclavicular	Anterior
4th	Anterior axillary	Anterior
4th	Midaxillary	Anterior
8th	Paravertebral	Posterior
8th	Subscapular	Posterior
8th	Posterior axillary	Posterior

Larger pleural effusions can be seen from the lateral aspects or with a transverse scan of the liver pointing cranially (Fig. 15.5). For detecting smaller effusions, the patient should sit, and the sonographer performs longitudinal scans shifting the probe

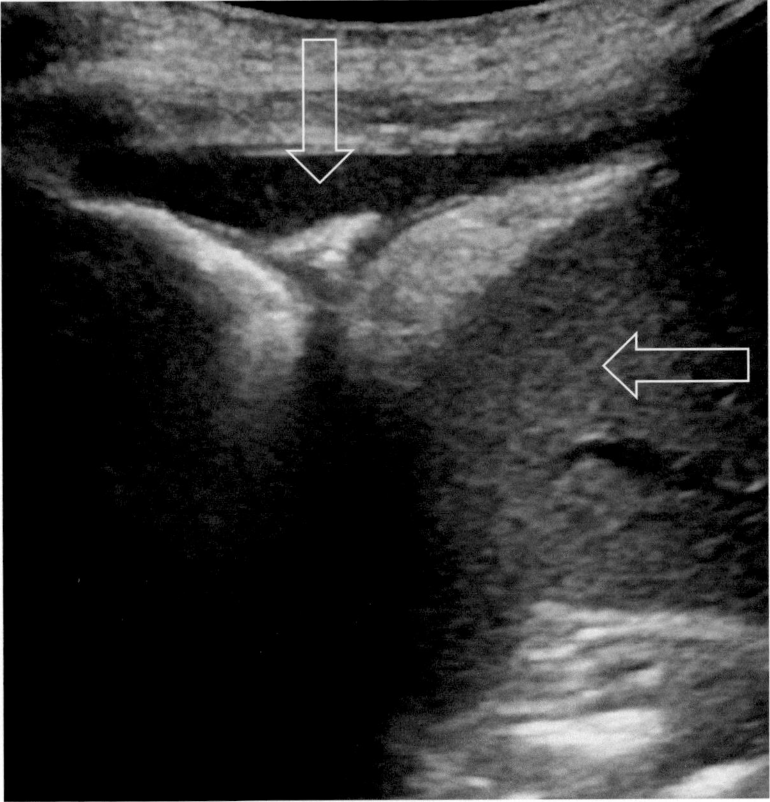

Fig. 15.8 Small left pleural effusion (↑) with dense material cranial to spleen (←) Longitudinal postero-lateral scan with patient sitting

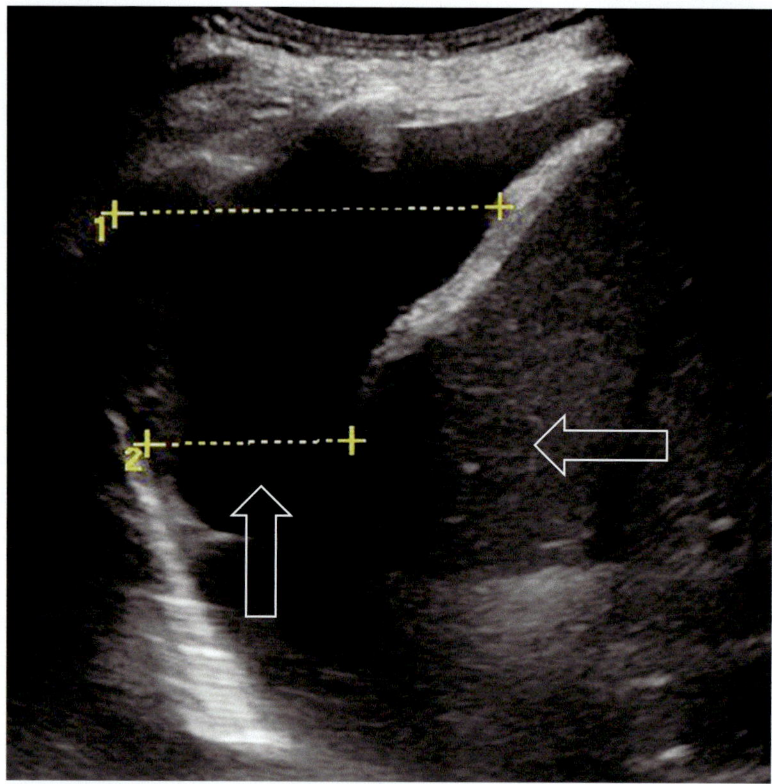

Fig. 15.9 Right pleural effusion (↑) cranial to liver (←). Distance: 1. 6.5 cm, 2. 3.5 cm. Estimation of amount of pleural effusion (6.5 + 3.5) × 70 = 700 ml. Longitudinal postero-lateral scan with patient sitting

from dorsal to lateral (Figs. 15.8 and 15.9). Many ways have been proposed for estimating the pleural effusion volume. One suggestion is shown in Fig. 15.9. The length of the effusion at the dorsolateral chest is added to the distance between lung base to mid-diaphragm. The result is multiplied by 70 for obtaining the estimated pleural effusion volume in ml.

References

Chapter 1. Introduction

Bom, N. (1972). *New concepts in echocardiography*. Ph.D. thesis, Erasmus University Rotterdam.

Bruyn, G. A., Iagnocco, A., Naredo, E., et al. (2019a). OMERACT definitions for ultrasonographic pathologies and elementary lesions 15 years on. *Journal of Rheumatology, 46*, 1388–1393.

Dale, J., Stirling, A., Zhang, R., et al. (2016). Targeting ultrasound remission in early rheumatoid arthritis: The results of the TaSER study, a randomised clinical trial. *Annals of the Rheumatic Diseases, 75*, 1043–1050.

Donald, I., MacVicar, J., Brown, & T. G. (1958). Investigation of abdominal masses by pulsed ultrasound. *Lancet, i*, 1188–95.

Dussik, K. T. (1942). Über die Möglichkeit, hochfrequente mechanische Schwingungen als diagnostisches Hilfsmittel zu verwerten. *Z Neurol Psychiat, 174*, 153–168.

Graf, R. (2017). Hip sonography: Background; technique and common mistakes; results; debate and politics; challenges. *Hip International, 27*, 215–219.

Haavardsholm, E. A., Aga, A. B., Olsen, I. C., et al. (2016). Ultrasound in management of rheumatoid arthritis: ARCTIC randomised controlled strategy trial. *BMJ, 354*, i4205.

Horton, S. C., Tan, A. L., Wakefield, R. J., et al. (2017). Ultrasound-detectable greyscale synovitis predicts future fulfilment of the 2010 ACR/EULAR RA classification criteria in patients with new-onset undifferentiated arthritis. *RMD Open, 3*, E000394.

Kane, D., Balint, P. V., & Sturrock, R. D. (2003). Ultrasonography is superior to clinical examination in the detection and localization of knee joint effusion in rheumatoid arthritis. *Journal of Rheumatology, 30*, 966–971.

Kaproth-Joslin, K., Nicola, R., & Dogra, V. S. (2015). The history of US: From bats and boats to the bedside and beyond. *Radiographics, 35*, 960–970.

Naredo, E., D'Agostino, M. A., Wakefield, R., et al. (2013). Reliability of a consensus-based ultrasound score for tenosynovitis in rheumatoid arthritis. *Annals of the Rheumatic Diseases, 72*, 1328–1334.

Seltzer, S. E., Finberg, H. J., Weissman, B. N., et al. (1979). Arthrosonography: Gray-scale ultrasound evaluation of the shoulder. *Radiology, 132*, 467–468.

Smerilli, G., Cipolletta, E., & Di Carlo, M., et al. (2020). Power Doppler ultrasound assessment of A1 pulley. A new target of inflammation in psoriatic arthritis? *Frontiers Medicine, 7*, 204.

Wakefield, R. J., Gibbon, W. W., Conaghan, P. G., et al. (2000). The value of sonography in the detection of bone erosions in patients with rheumatoid arthritis: A comparison with conventional radiography. *Arthritis and Rheumatism, 43*, 2762–2770.

© The Editor(s) (if applicable) and The Author(s), under exclusive license to Springer Nature Switzerland AG 2023

G. A. W. Bruyn and W. A. Schmidt, *Musculoskeletal Ultrasound for the Rheumatologist*, https://doi.org/10.1007/978-3-031-27737-5

Ziegelasch, M., Eloff, E., Hammer, H. B., et al. (2021). Bone erosions detected by ultrasound are prognostic for clinical arthritis development in patients with ACPA and musculoskeletal pain. *Frontiers in Medicine, 23*(8), 653994.

Chapter 2. Fundamentals of musculoskeletal ultrasound

Schmidt, W. A., & Backhaus, M. (2008). What the practicing rheumatologist needs to know about the technical fundamentals of ultrasonography. *Best Practice & Research Clinical Rheumatology, 22*, 981–999.

Schmidt, W. A. (2007). Technology insight: The role of color and power Doppler ultrasonography in rheumatology. *Nature Clinical Practice Rheumatology, 34*, 839–847.

Taljanovic, M. S., Melville, D. M., Scalcione, L. R., et al. (2014). Artifacts in musculoskeletal ultrasonography. *Semin Musculoskelet Radiol, 18*, 3–11.

Taljanovic, M. S., Gimber, L. H., Becker, G. W., et al. (2017). Shear-wave elastography: Basic physics and musculoskeletal applications. *Radiographics, 37*, 855–870.

Chapter 3. Choosing an ultrasound system

Dejaco, C., Ramiro, S., Duftner, C., et al. (2018). EULAR recommendations for the use of imaging in large vessel vasculitis in clinical practice. *Annals of the Rheumatic Diseases, 77*, 636–643.

European Society of Radiology (ESR). (2019). ESR statement on portable ultrasound devices. *Insights Imaging, 10*, 89.

Joshua, F., Lassere, M., Bruyn, G. A., et al. (2007). Summary findings of a systematic review of the ultrasound assessment of synovitis. *Journal of Rheumatology, 34*, 839–847.

Möller, I., Janta, I., Backhaus, M., et al. (2017). The 2017 EULAR standardised procedures for ultrasound imaging in rheumatology. *Annals of the Rheumatic Diseases, 76*, 1974–1979.

Chapter 4. General Sonoanatomy

Bruyn, G. A. W., & Schmidt, W. A. (2009). How to perform ultrasound-guided injections. *Best Practice & Research Clinical Rheumatology, 23*, 269–279.

Schmidt, W. A., Schmidt, H., & Schicke, B. et al. (2004). Standard reference values for musculoskeletal ultrasonography. *Annals Rheumatic Diseases, 63*, 988–94.

Schmidt, W. A. (2001). Value of sonography in diagnosis of rheumatoid arthritis. *Lancet, 357*, 1056–1057.

Scheel, A. K., Schmidt, W. A., Hermann, K. G., et al. (2005). Interobserver reliability of rheumatologists performing musculoskeletal ultrasonography: Results from a EULAR "Train the Trainers" course. *Annals of the Rheumatic Diseases, 64*, 1043–1049.

Wakefield, R. J., Balint, P. V., Szkudlarek, M. et al. (2005). OMERACT 7 Special Interest Group. Musculoskeletal ultrasound including definitions for ultrasonographic pathology. *Journal of Rheumatology, 32*, 2485–7.

Chapter 5. The Shoulder

Bruyn, G. A. W., Naredo, E., Moller, I., et al. (2009). Reliability of ultrasonography in detecting shoulder disease in patients with rheumatoid arthritis. *Annals of the Rheumatic Diseases, 68,* 357–361.

Bruyn, G. A. W., Pineda, C., Hernandez-Diaz, C., et al. (2010). Validity and measures of adult shoulder function and reliability of ultrasonography in detecting synovitis in patients with rheumatoid arthritis and shoulder using magnetic resonance imaging as gold standard. *Arthritis Care and Research, 62,* 1079–1086.

Dasgupta, B., Cimmino, M. A., Maradit-Kremers, H., et al. (2012). 2012 provisional classification criteria for polymyalgia rheumatica: A European League Against Rheumatism/American College of Rheumatology collaborative initiative. *Annals of the Rheumatic Diseases, 71,* 484–492.

Schmidt, W. A., Schicke, B., & Krause, A. (2008a). Which ultrasound scan is the best to detect glenohumeral joint effusions? *Ultraschall in Der Medizin, 29*(Suppl5), 250–255.

Tamborrini, G., Möller, I., Bong, D., et al. (2017). The rotator interval—a link between anatomy and ultrasound. *Ultrasound International Open, 03,* E107–E116.

Uson, J., Rodriguez-García, S. C., Castellanos-Moreira, R., et al. (2021). EULAR recommendations for intra-articular therapies. *Annals of the Rheumatic Diseases, 80,* 1299–1305.

Chapter 6. The Elbow

Boers, N., Martin, E., Mazur, M., et al. (2022). Sonographic normal values for the cross-sectional area of the ulnar nerve: A systematic review and meta-analysis. *Journal of Ultrasound.* https://doi.org/10.1007/s40477-022-00661-8

De Maeseneer, M., Brigido, M. K., Antic, M., et al. (2015). Ultrasound of the elbow with emphasis on detailed assessment of ligaments, tendons, and nerves. *European Journal of Radiology, 84,* 671–681.

Konin, G. P., Nazarian, L. N., & Walz, D. M. (2013). US of the elbow: Indications, technique, normal anatomy, and pathologic conditions. *Radiographics, 33,* E125–E147.

Chapter 7. The Wrist

Becciolini, A., Ariani, A., & Becciolini, M. (2022). Pisotriquetral arthritis: 'forgotten' joint in ultrasound imaging of the wrist. *Annals of the Rheumatic Diseases, 81,* e97.

Menge, T. J., Rinker, E. B., Fan, K.-H., et al. (2016). Carpal tunnel injections: A novel approach based on wrist width. *Journal of Hand and Microsurgery, 8,* 21–26.

Moritomo, H. (2013). Anatomy and clinical relevance of the ulnotriquetral ligament. *J Wrist Surg, 2,* 186–189.

Yang, F. Y., Shih, Y. C., Hong, J. P., et al. (2021). Ultrasound-guided corticosteroid injection for patients with carpal tunnel syndrome: A systematic literature review and meta-analysis of randomized controlled trials. *Science and Reports, 11,* 10417.

Chapter 8. The Fingers

Boutry, N., Larde, A., Demondion, X., et al. (2004). Metacarpophalangeal joints t US in asymptomatic vounteers and cadaveric specimens. *Radiology, 232*, 716–724.

Bruyn, G. A., Iagnocco, A., Naredo, E., et al. (2019b). OMERACT definitions for ultrasonographic pathologies and elementary lesions of rheumatic disorders 15 years on. *Journal of Rheumatology, 46*, 1388–1393.

Colebatch, A. N., Edwards, C. J., Østergaard, M., et al. (2013). EULAR recommendations for the use of imaging of the joints in the clinical management of rheumatoid arthritis. *Annals of the Rheumatic Diseases, 72*, 804–814.

D'Agostino, M. A., Terslev, L., Aegerter, P., et al. (2017). Scoring ultrasound synovitis in rheumatoid arthritis: A EULAR-OMERACT ultrasound taskforce-Part 1: Definition and development of a standardised, consensus-based scoring system. *RMD Open, 3*, e000428.

Furlan, A., & Stramare, R. (2018). The thickening of flexor tendons pulleys: A useful ultrasonographical sign in the diagnosis of psoriatic arthritis. *Journal of Ultrasound, 21*, 309–314.

Hunter-Smith, D. J., Slattery, P. G., Rizzitelli, A., et al. (2015). The dorsal fibrocartilage of the metacarpophalangeal joint: A cadaveric study. *Journal of Hand Surgery American, 40*, 1410–1415.

Terslev, L., Naredo, E., Aegerter, P., et al. (2017). Scoring ultrasound synovitis in rheumatoid arthritis: A EULAR-OMERACT ultrasound taskforce-Part 2: Reliability and application to multiple joints of a standardised consensus-based scoring system. *RMD Open, 3*, e000427.

Chapter 10. The Hip

Dasgupta, B., Cimmino, M. A., Maradit-Kremers, H., et al. (2012). 2012 provisional classification criteria for polymyalgia rheumatica: A European League Against Rheumatism/American College of Rheumatology collaborative initiative. *Annals of the Rheumatic Diseases, 71*, 484–492.

Iagnocco, A., Filippucci, E., & Meenagh, G., et al. (2006). Ultrasound imaging for the rheumatologist III. Ultrasonography of the hip. *Clinical Experimental Rheumatology, 24*, 229–32.

Schäfer, V. S., Fleck, M., Kellner, H., et al. (2013). Evaluation of the novel ultrasound score for large joints in psoriatic arthritis and ankylosing spondylitis: Six month experience in daily clinical practice. *BMC Musculoskeletal Disorders, 14*, 358.

Wink, F., Arends, S., Maas, F., et al. (2019). High prevalence of hip involvement and decrease in inflammatory ultrasound lesions during tumour necrosis factor-α blocking therapy in ankylosing spondylitis. *Rheumatology (Oxford), 58*, 1040–1046.

Chapter 11. The Knee

Berthaume, M. A., & Bull, A. M. (2020). Human biological variation in sesamoid bone prevalence: The curious case of the fabella. *Journal of Anatomy, 236*, 228–242.

Cipolletta, E., Filippou, G., Scirè, C. A., et al. (2021). The diagnostic value of conventional radiography and musculoskeletal ultrasonography in calcium pyrophosphate deposition disease: A systematic literature review and meta-analysis. *Osteoarthritis Cartilage, 29*, 619–632.

Filippou, G., Scirè, C. A., Adinolfi, A., et al. (2018). Identification of calcium pyrophosphate deposition disease (CPPD) by ultrasound: Reliability of the OMERACT definitions in an extended set of joints-an international multiobserver study by the OMERACT Calcium Pyrophosphate Deposition Disease Ultrasound Subtask Force. *Annals of the Rheumatic Diseases, 77,* 1194–1199.

Karim, Z., Wakefield, R. J., Quinn, M., et al. (2004). Validation and reproducibility of ultrasonography in the detection of synovitis in the knee: A comparison with arthroscopy and clinical examination. *Arthritis and Rheumatism, 50,* 387–394.

Koski, J. M., Kamel, A., Waris, P., et al. (2016). Atlas-based knee osteophyte assessment with ultrasonography and radiography: Relationship to arthroscopic degeneration of articular cartilage. *Scandinavian Journal of Rheumatology, 45,* 158–164.

Mandl, P., Brossard, M., Aegerter, P., et al. (2012). Ultrasound evaluation of fluid in knee recesses at varying degrees of flexion. *Arthritis Care Res (Hoboken), 64,* 773–779.

Meenagh, G., Iagnocco, A., & Filippuci, E., et al. (2006). Ultrasound imaging for the rheumatologist IV. Ultrasonography of the knee. *Clinical Experimental Rheumatology, 24,* 357–60.

Najm, A., Orr, C., Gallagher, L., et al. (2018). Knee joint synovitis: Study of correlations and diagnostic performances of ultrasonography compared with histopathology. *RMD Open, 4,* e000616.

Schmidt, W. A., Völker, L., Zacher, J., et al. (2000). Colour Doppler ultrasonography to detect pannus in knee-joint synovitis. *Clinical and Experimental Rheumatology, 18,* 439–444.

Terslev, L., D'Agostino, M. A., Brossard, M., et al. (2012). Which knee and probe position determines the final diagnosis of knee inflammation by ultrasound? Results from a European multicenter study. *Ultraschall in Der Medizin, 33,* E173–E178.

Chapter 12. The Ankle, Foot and Toes

Bruyn, G. A. W., Siddle, H. J., Hanova, P., et al. (2019c). Ultrasound of subtalar joint synovitis in patients with rheumatoid arthritis: Results of an OMERACT reliability exercise using consensual definitions. *Journal of Rheumatology, 46,* 351–359.

Khosla, S., Thiele, R. G., & Baumhauer, J. F. (2009). Intra-articular injection of the foot and ankle. *Foot and Ankle International, 30,* 886–890.

De Miguel, E., Munoz-Fernandez, S., Castillo, C., et al. (2011). Diagnostic accuracy of enthesis ultrasound in the diagnosis of early spondyloarthritis. *Annals of the Rheumatic Diseases, 70,* 434–439.

Mandl, P., Bong, D., Balint, P. V., et al. (2018). Sonographic and anatomic description of the subtalar joint. *Ultrasound in Medicine and Biology, 44,* 119–123.

Terslev, L., Naredo, E., Iagnocco, A., et al. (2014). Defining enthesitis in spondyloarthritis by ultrasound: Results of a Delphi process and of a reliability reading exercise. *Arthritis Care Res (Hoboken), 66,* 741–748.

Midfoot and Toes

Bowen, C. J., Hooper, L., Cullifor, D., et al. (2010). Assessment of the natural history of forefoot bursae using ultrasonography in patients with rheumatoid arthritis: A twelve-month investigation. *Arthritis Care and Research, 62,* 1756–1762.

Christiansen, S. N., Filippou, G., Scirè, C. A., et al. (2021). Consensus-based semi-quantitative ultrasound scoring system for gout lesions: Results of an OMERACT Delphi process and web-reliability exercise. *Seminars in Arthritis and Rheumatism, 51,* 644–649.

Gutierrez, M., Schmidt, W. A., Thiele, R. G., et al. (2015). International Consensus for ultrasound lesions in gout: Results of Delphi process and web-reliability exercise. *Rheumatology (Oxford), 54*, 1797–1805.

Thiele, R. G., & Schlesinger, N. (2007). *Diagnosis of gout by ultrasound. Rheumatology (Oxford), 46*, 1116–1121.

Chapter 13. Arterial Ultrasound in Rheumatology

Chrysidis, S., Duftner, C., Dejaco, C., et al. (2018). Definitions and reliability assessment of elementary ultrasound lesions in giant cell arteritis: A study from the OMERACT Large Vessel Vasculitis Ultrasound Working Group. *RMD Open, 4*, e000598.

Dejaco, C., Ponte, C., Monti, S., et al. (2022). The provisional OMERACT ultrasonography score for giant cell arteritis. *Annals of the Rheumatic Diseases.* https://doi.org/10.1136/ard-2022-223367

Friedrich, S., Lüders, S., Glimm, A. M., et al. (2019). Association between baseline clinical and imaging findings and the development of digital ulcers in patients with systemic sclerosis. *Arthritis Research & Therapy, 21*, 96.

Jcše, R., Rotar, Ž, Tomšič, M., et al. (2021). The cut-off values for the intima-media complex thickness assessed by colour Doppler sonography in seven cranial and aortic arch arteries. *Rheumatology (Oxford), 60*, 1346–1352.

Langholz, J., Landleif, M., Blank, B., et al. (1997). Colour coded duplex sonography in ischemic finger artery disease–a comparison with hand arteriography. *Vasa, 26*, 85–90.

Ponte, C., Monti, S., Scirè, C. A., et al. (2021). Ultrasound halo sign as a potential monitoring tool for patients with giant cell arteritis: A prospective analysis. *Annals of the Rheumatic Diseases, 80*, 1475–1482.

Schäfer, V. S., Juche, A., Ramiro, S., et al. (2017). Ultrasound cut-off values for intima-media thickness of temporal, facial and axillary arteries in giant cell arteritis. *Rheumatology (Oxford), 56*, 1479–1483.

Schmidt, W. A., Kraft, H. E., Vorpahl, K., et al. (1997). Color duplex ultrasonography in the diagnosis of temporal arteritis. *New England Journal of Medicine, 337*, 1336–1342.

Schmidt, W. A. (2018). Ultrasound in the diagnosis and management of giant cell arteritis. *Rheumatology (Oxford), 57*(suppl_2), ii22–ii31.

Schmidt, W. A., & Nielsen, B. D. (2020). Imaging in large-vessel vasculitis. *Best Practice & Research Clinical Rheumatology, 34*, 101589.

Schmidt, W. A., Nerenheim, A., Seipelt, E., et al. (2002). Diagnosis of early Takayasu arteritis with sonography. *Rheumatology (oxford), 41*, 496–502.

Schmidt, W. A., Wernicke, D., Kiefer, E., et al. (2006). Colour duplex sonography of finger arteries in vasculitis and in systemic sclerosis. *Annals of the Rheumatic Diseases, 65*, 265–267.

Schmidt, W. A., Krause, A., Schicke, B., et al. (2008b). Color Doppler ultrasonography of hand and finger arteries to differentiate primary from secondary forms of Raynaud's phenomenon. *Journal of Rheumatology, 35*, 1591–1598.

Chapter 14. Ultrasound of the Major Salivary Glands

Finzel, S., Jousse-Joulin, S., Costantino, F., et al. (2021). Patient-based reliability of the Outcome Measures in Rheumatology (OMERACT) ultrasound scoring system for salivary gland assessment in patients with primary Sjögren's syndrome. *Rheumatology (Oxford), 60*, 2169–2176.

Hočevar, A., Bruyn, G. A., Terslev, L., et al. (2022). Development of a new ultrasound scoring system to evaluate glandular inflammation in Sjögren's syndrome: An OMERACT reliability exercise. *Rheumatology (Oxford), 61*, 3341–3350.

Inanc, N., Bruyn, G. A. W. (2022). Imaging of Sjögren's syndrome, with special reference to ultrasound. In: G. A. W. Bruyn (ed.), *Sjögren's Syndrome and the Salivary Glands.* Springer Nature Switzerland AG.

Jousse-Joulin, S., D'Agostino, M. A., Nicolas, C., et al. (2019). Video clip assessment of a salivary gland ultrasound scoring system in Sjögren's syndrome using consensual definitions: An OMERACT ultrasound working group reliability exercise. *Annals of the Rheumatic Diseases, 78*, 967–973.

Makula, E., Pokorny, G., Kiss, M., et al. (2000). The place of magnetic resonance and ultrasonographic examinations of the parotid gland in the diagnosis and follow-up of primary Sjögren's syndrome. *Rheumatology (Oxford), 39*, 97–104.

Wernicke, D., Hess, H., Gromnica-Ihle, E., et al. (2008). Ultrasonography of salivary glands—a highly specific imaging procedure for diagnosis of Sjogren's syndrome. *Journal of Rheumatology, 35*, 285–293.

Chapter 15. Lung Ultrasound

Buda, N., Piskunowicz, M., Porzeninska, M., et al. (2017). Lung ultrasound in the evaluation of interstitial lung diseases in the course of connective tissue diseases. *Eur Resp J, 50*, PA1520. https://doi.org/10.1183/1393003

Gargani, L., & Volpicelli, G. (2014). How I do it: Lung ultrasound. *Cardiovascular Ultrasound, 12*, 25.

Gutierrez, M., Salaffi, F., Carotti, M., et al. (2011). Utility of a simplified ultrasound assessment to assess interstitial pulmonary fibrosis in connective tissue disorders: Preliminary results. *Arthritis Research & Therapy, 13*, R134.

Ibitoye, B. O., Idowu, B. M., Ogunrombi, A. B., et al. (2018). *Ultrasonography, 37*, 254–260.

Mathis, G. (2011). Pleura. In: Mathis, G. (ed.), *Chest Sonography.* 3rd ed. Heidelberg: Springer, 30–2.

© The Editor(s) (if applicable) and The Author(s), under exclusive license
to Springer Nature Switzerland AG 2023
G. A. W. Bruyn and W. A. Schmidt, *Musculoskeletal Ultrasound for the Rheumatologist*,
https://doi.org/10.1007/978-3-031-27737-5

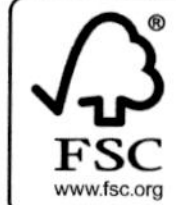

MIX
Papier aus verantwortungsvollen Quellen
Paper from responsible sources
FSC® C105338

If you have any concerns about our products,
you can contact us on
ProductSafety@springernature.com

In case Publisher is established outside the EU,
the EU authorized representative is:
Springer Nature Customer Service Center GmbH
Europaplatz 3, 69115 Heidelberg, Germany

Printed by Libri Plureos GmbH
in Hamburg, Germany